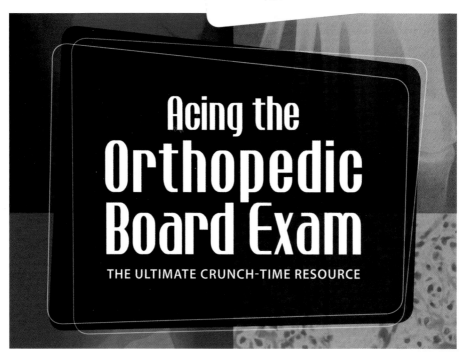

Acing the
Orthopedic
Board Exam

THE ULTIMATE CRUNCH-TIME RESOURCE

Brett R. Levine, MD, MS

Associate Professor
Rush University Medical Center
Chicago, Illinois

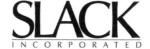

www.Healio.com/books

ISBN: 978-1-55642-993-4

Published by: SLACK Incorporated
                  6900 Grove Road
                  Thorofare, NJ 08086 USA
                  Telephone: 856-848-1000
                  Fax: 856-848-6091
                  www.Healio.com/books

Contact SLACK Incorporated for more information about other books in this field or about the availability of our books from distributors outside the United States.

Library of Congress Cataloging-in-Publication Data
Levine, Brett R., author.
  Acing the orthopedic board exam : the ultimate crunch-time resource / Brett R. Levine.
      p. ; cm.
  Includes bibliographical references and index.
  ISBN 978-1-55642-993-4 (alk. paper)
  I. Title.
  [DNLM: 1. Musculoskeletal Diseases--Examination Questions. 2. Orthopedics--methods--Examination Questions. WE 18.2]
  RC925.7
  616.70076--dc23
                      2015022664

Printed in the United States of America.

Last digit is print number: 10   9   8   7   6   5   4   3   2   1

DEDICATION

To my loving wife, Kari, and my children, AJ and Kylie, for their devotion and support. Without the support and understanding of my family, this book would not be possible.

CONTENTS

ACKNOWLEDGMENTS

The content of this book has been inspired by the many colleagues I have worked with during my career. I am especially grateful to all of my mentors who have taught me to be an orthopedist and a physician along the way. Without the guidance of Drs. Jack Delahay, William Jaffe, Joseph Zuckerman, Wayne Paprosky, Aaron Rosenberg, Craig Della Valle, Richard Berger, and Joshua Jacobs, I would not be in the position to write and edit this book. I would like to thank the contributing authors for their thoughtful insights and exceptional writing skills (and for being on time). Special thanks to Carrie Kotlar for supporting this book and Dr. Brennan Spiegel for starting this series of Acing the Boards books.

ABOUT THE AUTHOR

Brett R. Levine, MD, MS is an Associate Professor of Orthopaedics in the Adult Reconstruction Division at Rush University Medical Center in Chicago, Illinois. He is the former Residency Program Director and participates in one of the largest adult reconstruction fellowships in the country. He also served as the Chairman of the American Academy of Orthopaedic Surgeons Knee Instructional Course Lectures Subcommittee, serves on the Communication and Patient Education Committees for AAHKS, is a participant in the AAOS Leadership Fellowship Program, and is a member of the Council of Orthopaedic Residency Directors Education Committee.

Dr. Levine received his undergraduate degree in chemistry from American University in Washington, DC. He later earned his master's degree in physiology and biophysics and his medical degree from Georgetown University, also in Washington, DC. After completing a general surgery internship at New York University, Bellevue Hospital (New York, New York), he received his orthopedic training at New York University, Hospital for Joint Diseases (New York, New York). This was followed by a Fellowship in Adult Reconstructive Surgery at Rush University Medical Center. He is Board certified in Orthopedic Surgery. Dr. Levine's research interests have focused on porous biomaterials in hip and knee arthroplasty, corrosion and metal ion release in total hip arthroplasty, and operative techniques in revision hip and knee surgery. He is a peer reviewer for numerous orthopedic and basic science journals. He has contributed more than 80 peer-reviewed papers, as well as numerous book chapters, posters, and podium presentations at national and international meetings.

Contributing Authors

Amir M. Abtahi, MD
Department of Orthopaedic Surgery
University of Utah
Salt Lake City, Utah

Frank R. Avilucea, MD
Assistant Professor of Orthopaedic Surgery
Division of Trauma
University of Cincinnati
Cincinnati, Ohio

James T. Beckmann, MD, MS
Department of Orthopaedic Surgery
University of Utah
Salt Lake City, Utah

Michael J. Beebe, MD
Orthopaedic Resident
University of Utah
Salt Lake City, Utah

Sanjeev Bhatia, MD
Director
Hip Arthroscopy and Joint Preservation Center
Cincinnati Sports Medicine and Orthopaedic Center
Cincinnati, Ohio

Andrew A. Brief, MD
Orthopaedic Foot and Ankle Surgeon
Ridgewood Orthopedic Group
Ridgewood, New Jersey

Nicholas M. Brown, MD
Orthopaedic Surgery Resident
Rush University Medical Center
Chicago, Illinois

Peter N. Chalmers, MD
Orthopaedic Surgery Resident
Rush University Medical Center
Chicago, Illinois

Dan J. Del Gaizo, MD
Assistant Professor of Orthopaedic Surgery
University of North Carolina Chapel Hill
Chapel Hill, North Carolina

Michael B. Ellman, MD
Orthopedic Surgery
Panorama Orthopedics and Spine Center
Golden, Colorado

Brandon J. Erickson, MD
Orthopaedic Surgery Resident
Rush University
Chicago, Illinois

Jonathan M Frank, MD
Fellow Orthopaedic Sports Medicine
Steadman Philippon Research Institute
Vail, Colorado

Rachel Frank, MD
Orthopaedic Surgery Resident
Rush University Medical Center
Chicago, Illinois

James M. Gregory, MD
Assistant Professor
Department of Orthopaedic Surgery
University of Texas Medical School at Houston
Houston, Texas

Christopher E. Gross, MD
Assistant Professor
Medical University South Carolina
Charleston, South Carolina

Wyatt Lee Hadley, MD
Musculoskeletal Radiologist
Alliance Radiology
Kansas City, Kansas

Justin M. Haller, MD
Department of Orthopaedic Surgery
University of Utah
Salt Lake City, Utah

Marc Haro, MD
Assistant Professor
Department of Orthopedics
Division of Sports Medicine
Medical University of South Carolina
Charleston, South Carolina

Bryan D. Haughom, MD
Orthopaedic Surgery Resident
Rush University Medical Center
Chicago, Illinois

Andrew R. Hsu, MD
Assistant Clinical Professor of Orthopaedic Surgery
University of California–Irvine
Orange, California

Benjamin R. Koch, MD
Staff Pathologist
Essentia Health
Duluth, Minnesota

Monica Kogan, MD
Assistant Professor
Residency Program Director
Department of Orthopaedics
Rush University Medical Center
Chicago, Illinois

Erik N. Kubiak, MD
Associate Professor
University of Utah
Salt Lake City, Utah

Simon Lee, MD
Assistant Professor
Department of Orthopaedics
Rush University Medical Center
Chicago, Illinois

Brett Lenart, MD
Department of Orthopaedic Surgery
Metropolitan Hospital
New York, New York

David Levy, MD
Orthopaedic Surgery Resident
Rush University Medical Center
Chicago, Illinois

Randy Mascarenhas, MD, FRCSC
Assistant Professor of Orthopaedic Surgery and Sports
    Medicine
University of Texas Health Sciences Center at Houston
Houston, Texas

Benjamin J. Miller, MD, MS
Assistant Professor
Department of Orthopedics and Rehabilitation
University of Iowa
Iowa City, Iowa

Shane J. Nho, MD, MS
Assistant Professor
Section Head, Young Adult Hip Surgery
Division of Sports Medicine
Department of Orthopaedic Surgery
Rush University Medical Center
Chicago, Illinois

Dan K. Park, MD
Assistant Professor
Department of Orthopaedic Surgery
Oakland University–Beaumont School of Medicine
Royal Oak, Michigan

David L. Rothberg, MD
Clinical Instructor
Department of Orthopaedics
University of Utah
Salt Lake City, Utah

Zachary M. Working, MD
Department of Orthopaedic Surgery
University of Utah
Salt Lake City, Utah

Thomas Wuerz, MD, MSc
Clinical Instructor
Tufts Medical School
New England Baptist Hospital
Boston, Massachusetts

Robert Wysocki, MD
Assistant Professor
Division of Hand, Upper Extremity and Microvascular
    Surgery
Rush University Medical Center
Chicago, Illinois

Adam B. Yanke, MD
Assistant Professor
Assistant Director, Cartilage Restoration Center
Department of Orthopedics, Sports Medicine Division
Rush University Medical Center
Chicago, Illinois

Joseph D. Zuckerman, MD
Professor and Chairman
Department of Orthopaedic Surgery
NYU Hospital for Joint Diseases
NYU Langone Medical Center
New York, New York

PREFACE

If you are preparing to read this book, you are likely studying for part I of the Boards, taking the recertification exam, or reviewing for the upcoming Orthopaedics In-Training Exam (OITE). Either way, you are likely very busy with limited time to prepare. You have spent years studying textbooks, sitting through lectures, scrubbing in on cases, and working with patients. With the basics already ingrained, the goal is to learn the information you don't know and not review the stuff you already know.

Yet, we often take an inefficient approach to studying for such examinations. This typically consists of comprehensively reviewing topics in their entirety without focusing on facts that will likely appear on the test or areas of orthopedics in which our knowledge is more suspect. Knowing the basics of orthopedics and clinical practice will only get you so far on standardized tests. During crunch time, we need to focus on what it will take to overcome the upcoming hurdle and pass—or better yet, ace—the Boards!

There is no time for an inefficient approach to studying, which is often fostered in traditional Board review books and chapter-laden textbooks. Looking back at my notations within my old review books, it is impossible to decipher the hieroglyphics that I created. Most often, simple facts were outlined across the page with a variety of stars, circles, and other annotations. Most of this information is well known, yet we find something self-gratifying about rereading the facts we already know. Don't get me wrong: I have no problems highlighting and scribbling throughout a Board review textbook. However, during crunch time, the goal should be to gain high-yield facts and knowledge that you don't already possess.

The goal of this book is to cut to the chase and eliminate information not likely to be on the test, of personal interest only, or too immature to include on current Board exams. We have attempted to dispense with novel speculations, new epidemiological oddities, and cutting-edge hypotheses and focus on time-tested pearls and prime-time material. This book is set up to be different and aims to fill in the holes between what you already know and what you do not know or have forgotten. You may find that you know some of the data in this book; if so, that means you are well prepared for the test. However, you will also find many facts that you don't know or have forgotten, which should bolster your chances of passing your upcoming exam.

The information in this book has been pooled from my experiences in teaching and taking these exams, as well as those of the contributing authors. The contributing authors have all recently taken the Board review or recertification exam and are well versed on its content and what it takes to conquer the test. We train many residents and fellows at Rush University who go on to successful careers and are generally considered to be top of their class during training. However, we typically do not "teach for the Boards" during everyday training; instead, we teach the skills and knowledge that support rational and evidence-based decision making in clinical practice. Unfortunately, Board exams don't always pull directly from these skill sets, and some great clinicians do poorly on Board exams. Conversely, great test takers can be suboptimal clinicians. In the end, I believe we all recognize that it is of utmost importance to be a great clinician and of secondary importance to be a great test taker.

This book consists of a series of high-yield vignettes, relevant factoids, pearls, and basic questions targeted toward the tough stuff that you don't know. They are based on perennial favorite topics that may be found on the Boards, recertification exam, or OITE. These are all original questions and vignettes, but they generally reflect typical information you will be presented with in these exams. It goes without saying that I do not have a crystal ball and have no idea what topics will be emphasized on your particular exam. The contributing authors and I feel that the information included in this book will be in the ballpark of things you should know to be prepared for your test.

Here are some highlights of this book:

- Focus on clinical vignettes. Board questions are typically associated with a scenario that you might see in the clinical setting. Such vignettes are the foundation of this book and replace the fact-laden blocks of text found in a typical review book.

- Relatively short. Most Board review books are dense, thick, and weigh as much as a typical dumbbell found in the gym. This is not conducive for rapid and effective learning during crunch time. Unlike traditional didactic volumes, this book is meant for more casual reading in more casual settings (some would classify it as bathroom reading material). The hope is that you can read through the text and take in high-yield information in an entertaining and interactive format in short order. This book can be used in accord with longer-volume review texts for more extensive topic coverage.

- Focus on the stuff you don't know. The goal of this book is to take things one step beyond the average knowledge base and touch on high-yield, less well-known facts. Although some of the data will rehash what you already know, it is meant to be dense with material you might have forgotten or do not know yet. That's the point: learn stuff you don't know yet, and don't keep reading and rereading that which you have known forever.

- Emphasis on pearl after pearl after pearl. Students, residents, fellows, and even attendings like to skip to the conclusion when reading articles or the plan when reading clinical notes. It is human nature to want to see what the bottom line is. After every vignette in this book, there is a pearl called "Here's the Point!"

- Random order of vignettes. Standardized examinations are not topically presented in nice, neat chapters; they are presented in a random order. This book is meant to emulate the Board experience by providing vignettes in a random order in the anticipated percentage of topics suggested by the American Board of Orthopaedic Surgery (ABOS). It is a way to introduce cognitive dissonance into your learning experience by constantly switching directions. Considering patients present to us in random order, why not review for the Boards in a similar manner? If you find the need to focus on a specific topic, you may use the index to find relevant pages for specific topics.

- No multiple-choice questions. Although standardized tests are laden with multiple-choice questions, these can be boring to study. They also often test the process of elimination reasoning more than knowledge and aptitude. During our typical conferences, I use the Socratic method in prying information and answers from unyielding residents. This is a more realistic approach to patient care, as patients in the office do not present with a multiple-choice grid floating over their heads. Open-ended questions are more entertaining, thought provoking, and memorable. If you can answer these questions correctly without the multiple-choice options present, then you will most definitely get them right on the test. Self-assessment and old OITE exams provide the ability to test your multiple-choice test-taking skills.

- Content reflective of ABOS proportions. The ABOS writes the Board and recertification examinations. In the instructions for Part I, there is an explicit percentage breakdown of content, as shown in Table P-1. I tried to maintain this proportion of vignettes presented in this book. For complete instructions, please reference the printed instructions published by the ABOS at http://www.abos.org.

- Emphasis on clinical thresholds/relevant values. This concept is borrowed from the original book in this series, *Acing the GI Boards*, by Dr. Brennan Spiegel. The idea is that there are many Board-type questions that require the test taker to memorize some numerical threshold values. For example, "If an XX-year-old patient presents with an XX degree of scoliosis, the treatment is surgical correction." Or, "XX is the common translocation associated with Ewing's sarcoma." There are a minimum of 10 clinical threshold/relevant values for each subspecialty in orthopedics that are commonly seen on OITE and Board exams. These are emphasized throughout the vignettes and are separately cataloged toward the end of the book. The catalog is a one-stop shop for all the little numerical and relevant facts that everyone forgets but needs to know.

- Comprehensive yet parsimonious explanations. This book tries to provide a comprehensive answer to a non–multiple-choice question while keeping it succinct and emphasizing the key clinical pearls. The relatively informal discussions should give enough information to understand the question in its entirety without overwhelming the reader with superfluous details. Board review is not about ruminating forever about personal areas of interest; it is about cutting to the chase and staying on target with the information presented.

- Avoidance of mind-numbing prose. Too many textbooks are difficult to read in the setting of review for the Boards. Those studying for these tests are often tired and trying to cram Board review into an already packed schedule. We have all had the experience of resting our eyes while hoping to learn from osmosis as we use our latest text as a pillow. This book is written in a more entertaining way to remove some of the pain associated with studying for the Boards. We have tried to include interesting

Table P-1.	
TOPICS AND ESTIMATED PERCENTAGE OF **QUESTIONS ASKED ON PART I OF THE BOARDS**	
Topic	*Percentage of ~300 Questions*
Adult reconstruction	33%
Basic orthopedic knowledge (includes tumors)	30%
Pediatrics (includes disease, trauma, and sports medicine)	17%
Rehabilitation	4%
Trauma and musculoskeletal system	16%

vignettes, provide answers that are based on real clinical encounters, and avoid unnecessary jargon or verbose academic descriptions.

- Emphasis on images. Orthopedic review is difficult without the presence of appropriate images. Many of the vignettes are accompanied by a carefully selected image designed to bring the content to life and aid in understanding the key points of the case.

FOREWORD

As physicians and orthopedic surgeons, lifelong learning is an essential component of our professionalism in order to provide proper care for our patients. For us, learning is not complete at the end of our residency or fellowship; rather, it continues throughout our careers. There are some who would consider lifelong learning to be an aspirational goal. This is certainly not true; instead, it is a mandatory responsibility for each one of us.

There are some practical components in the continuity of learning that begin with the completion of the 5-year orthopedic residency with Part I of the certification examination of the American Board of Orthopaedic Surgery (ABOS). After successful completion of the Part II exam, which follows 2 to 3 years later, we become Board certified—but we are not finished. From that point forward, we are required to recertify every 10 years by either written or practice-based oral examination. Dr. Levine and his contributing authors have given us an innovative, creative, and even enjoyable approach to learning that will greatly facilitate achieving the requirements of certification and recertification.

For more than 30 years, I have had conversations with residents about preparing for the Part I ABOS exam. I have my own formula for successful completion of this important requirement. However, through the years I have noted that more and more residents seem to focus on multiple-choice questions or brief review outlines as a basis for study and learning. This is often chosen to avoid the perceived overwhelming effort of reading textbooks and journal articles to acquire the information. Fortunately, Dr. Levine has provided us with an approach that will overcome the natural aversion to reading textbooks by using a comprehensive vignette-based approach that is clinically driven while at the same time providing the basic science component. In addition, a Facts and Figures section provides information that is often needed to answer direct recall (memorization) questions. This approach–clinical vignettes and facts and figures–provides an efficient, effective, and engaging way to study.

By titling this textbook *Acing the Orthopedic Board Exam*, Dr. Levine has emphasized its use by fifth-year orthopedic surgery residents preparing for the Part I ABOS exam. I have no doubt it will be used extensively for this purpose. However, I would highlight its value for practicing orthopedic surgeons preparing for the written recertification exam. Having just completed my third written recertification exam, I only wish *Acing the Orthopedic Board Exam* had been available sooner. It would have made my own preparations so much more efficient and less painful. Rest assured, when I prepare for my next recertification exam, *Acing the Orthopedic Board Exam* will be by my side.

I am particularly proud of Dr. Levine because he is a graduate of the NYU Hospital for Joint Diseases Orthopaedic Surgery Residency Program. His career has flourished as a clinician and as an educator. *Acing the Orthopedic Board Exam* is another of his many important scholarly contributions to the field of orthopedic surgery.

Joseph D. Zuckerman, MD
Walter A.L. Thompson Professor of Orthopaedic Surgery
New York University School of Medicine
Chair, Department of Orthopaedic Surgery
NYU Hospital for Joint Diseases
New York, New York

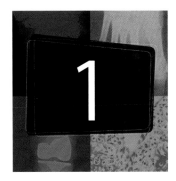

IMPORTANT FACTS ABOUT THE ORTHOPEDIC BOARDS

The orthopedic Boards are harder than the Orthopaedic In-Training Exam (OITE). The OITE often consists of repeating questions with similar themes, whereas Part I of the Boards tends to go one step further. It is important to have a wide breadth of knowledge because this will allow you to make good choices on the exam. It is impossible to predict which subspecialty will receive a greater number of questions each year, so the best thing to do is cover the topics in which you tend to underperform on the OITE. Although it is easier to get a greater number correct on the OITE, your percentile score on the OITE is predictive of your success in passing Part I of the Boards. As a rule of thumb, those typically scoring greater than 50th percentile on the OITE are safe on the Boards (but please study and do not get cocky if you fall into this category). Those between the 30th and 50th percentiles are likely safe, those between the 20th to 30th percentiles are a bad day away from failing, and those below the 20th percentile are in the high-risk category.

- Details regarding Part I. The examination is offered one day a year to 750 to 800 candidates at various test sites across the country. You are allotted 9 hours for the test, which breaks down into 40 minutes of break time, a 20-minute tutorial, and 8 hours for answering the questions. If you pass Part I, you then become eligible for 5 years, not including your fellowship year. If you do not pass Part II during these 5 years, you have to reapply and pass Part I again. Typical pass/fail rates for Part I are listed in Table 1-1.

- Playing the odds. In reviewing the content of Part I, it is imperative to look at what areas of weakness you had on your OITE. Then, correlate this with the rough percentage of questions anticipated to be on the Boards regarding this topic. For example, if your strong suit is not in the rehabilitation world and this only represents 4% of the test, I am not sure dedicating extended time to this topic is wise. Essentially, this comes down to picking and choosing your battles; if you want to win the war, pick the battles that help you win. In this case, adult reconstruction and basic orthopedic knowledge are the biggest players on the test; thus, it is probably a good idea to be secure on those fronts. Trauma and pediatrics are the next 2 well-represented topics typically found in Part I. Try to cover the kinks in your armor without spending too much time on topics not well represented historically on the exam. Also, remember that each question requires at least 2 references to support the answer, so they will be based on peer-reviewed literature.

Levine BR. *Acing the Orthopedic Board Exam: The Ultimate Crunch-Time Resource* (pp 1-2).
© 2016 SLACK Incorporated.

Table 1-1.

PASS/FAIL RATES FOR PART I OF THE ORTHOPEDIC BOARDS: 2007-2013

	2007	2008	2009	2010	2011	2012	2013
Examinees	728	715	719	779	832	865	832
Passed	641 (88%)	610 (85%)	643 (89%)	628 (81%)	660 (79%)	736 (85%)	701 (84%)
Failed	87 (12%)	105 (15%)	76 (11%)	151 (19%)	172 (21%)	129 (15%)	130 (15%)

Adapted from the American Board of Orthopaedic Surgery website: www.abos.org.

- The 18 content domains include the following:
  - Adult trauma
  - Adult disease
  - Ankle, foot
  - Basic science
  - Clavicle, scapula, shoulder
  - Diagnosis
  - Humerus, elbow, forearm
  - Knee, tibia, fibula
  - Neoplasms
  - Nonoperative management
  - Operative management
  - Pediatric disease
  - Pediatric trauma
  - Pelvis, hip, femur
  - Rehabilitation
  - Spine
  - Sports
  - Wrist, hand

- The proof is in the pudding. Read the questions and vignettes carefully in this book and on your examination. There are often key phrases and adjectives that should instantly trigger specific thoughts as to where the question writers were headed. For example, historically, upon viewing an x-ray showing osteolysis distal to the femoral stem, several thoughts should immediately enter your mind, such as patch coating of the implant and effective joint space. Simple things in the history will often eliminate answers; a history of inflammatory arthropathy immediately rules out the possibility of unicompartmental knee arthroplasty or high tibial osteotomy as answers on a joint question. I use examples from my personal specialty because this hits home, but for each subspecialty, there are phrases that should evoke immediate responses in your mind. Even if you do not ultimately know the correct answer, the description, images, or both will guide you to eliminating 2 to 3 answers right off the bat, and then you can make an educated guess (50/50).

- Maintenance of certification. Make sure you know your 10-year cycle and where you stand for recertification. I will refer you to the American Board of Orthopaedic Surgery website (www.abos.org). Essentially, there are 2 three-year cycles for Continuing Medical Education credits following case collection and enrollment to take the oral or written Boards.

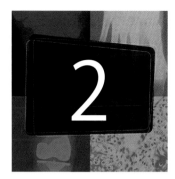

"TOUGH STUFF" VIGNETTES

The following are "tough stuff" vignettes that are set to take you through all of orthopedics. These vignettes have been prepared by Board-certified orthopedic surgeons as well as orthopedic surgery residents. The final products were reviewed for content and worded to be easy to read. The topics reviewed are high-yield and cover what is likely to be encountered in some form on the Boards and/or Orthopaedic In-Training Examination (OITE) tests.

The vignettes are meant to be tough and cover some of the more difficult concepts and forgotten facts. Although you may know some of the information, this means you are aptly prepared to take the test. The vignettes should build on the knowledge you already have while skipping over the "gimmie" questions that everybody gets right.

Just like the standardized examinations, the vignettes are in random order. There is no rhyme or reason to the order in which they are presented, and, overall, they represent the correct percentage of topics as per the American Board of Orthopaedic Surgery.

The vignettes are listed on the first page with questions following each one. The following page has the answer, but you should postulate your own observations and answers prior to flipping the page. It is important to think about the answer and critically read the vignettes for the key words. Actively devising your own answers is a useful way of learning and is better than just flipping to the answer page and reading through the discussion.

At the end of each answer, there is a short section titled "Why Might This Be Tested?" The purpose of this short section is to explain why you might see something similar to this vignette on your test. It puts you in the mind of the Board examiners for a second to better understand their potential reasoning. Furthermore, it may allow you to better remember each vignette.

At the bottom of each answer page there is a box titled, "Here's the Point!" This is meant to summarize the key issues that appear in the vignette. During crunch time, this may be the most important part to review, although it is not suggested to skip reading the whole discussion. The "Crunch-Time" Self-Test in Chapter 4 helps complement the facts in this section.

There are also clinical thresholds and important facts listed in Chapter 3. These factoids help support the vignettes so your study time is maximized. Again, "gimmies" are not necessarily included so that the tough stuff can be covered.

Levine BR. *Acing the Orthopedic Board Exam:*
The Ultimate Crunch-Time Resource (pp 3-406).
© 2016 SLACK Incorporated.

Vignette 1: Why Are My Legs So Bowed?

A 55-year-old male status post open meniscectomy at the age of 20 presents with worsening right knee pain and deformity. He has gradually developed a bowlegged deformity and decreasing ability to perform his activities of daily living. His range of motion (ROM) is 20 to 90 degrees. He reports occasional lower back pain and has had a prior anterior cervical diskectomy and fusion (ACDF) at C6-C7. Laboratory values sent over by his primary care physician reveal the following: white blood cell (WBC) count, 7 cells/uL; erythrocyte sedimentation rate (ESR), 35 mm/hr; C-reactive protein (CRP), <0.8 mg/L. Nonsteroidal anti-inflammatory drugs (NSAIDs), corticosteroid injections, and activity modification have proven unsuccessful. A bilateral x-ray is shown in Figure 1-1.

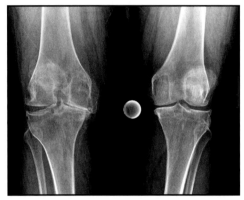

Figure 1-1. Anteroposterior x-ray of bilateral knees.

► *What is the diagnosis?*

► *What is the pathogenesis of the disorder?*

► *What are the current treatment options?*

Vignette 1: Answer

Don't read too much into this vignette because there are several distractors meant to confuse you. The history of open meniscectomy, a progressive varus deformity, and knee pain all point to osteoarthritis (OA) or degenerative joint disease (DJD). The elevated ESR is nonspecific in this case because there are no other findings consistent with a knee infection or inflammatory arthropathy. The neck problems are more indicative of a generalized OA picture rather than a contributing cause to his knee pain. The hallmark symptoms of OA include activity-related pain, stiffness, mechanical symptoms (locking and buckling), and joint effusions. This typically occurs as a primary process or a secondary disease that ultimately leads to the common endpoint of articular cartilage breakdown and progressive deformity of the knee. OA afflicts more than 27 million Americans, with the treatment of this condition representing a large burden to the health care system.[1] The x-rays show classic findings of severe endstage degenerative changes, with joint space narrowing, osteophyte formation, and subchondral sclerosis/cysts.

The pathogenesis of OA is multifactorial, with no definitive mechanism leading to endstage disease that requires treatment. In this case, the 2 biggest factors are his history of an open meniscectomy and aging. As we get older, the water content of articular cartilage decreases as a result of a reduced proteoglycan (PG) presence. The cartilage becomes less resilient to trauma, starting a progressive degradation pathway leading to joint space narrowing and deformity. OA displays a greater prevalence between siblings in a family, with up to 60% of cases having some genetic predisposition to this condition.[2] In this vignette, the open meniscectomy is likely responsible for the onset of DJD and progressive varus deformity. Classically open procedures involved a complete meniscectomy of the affected side of the knee. Studies have shown that complete meniscectomy (6-fold greater chance than unoperated knees) can lead to future OA, with better results being reported for arthroscopic partial meniscectomies.[2,3] The main concept behind this process is that removal of the meniscus makes the knee more susceptible to cartilage breakdown because there is less shock absorption by the meniscus. This leads to greater forces on the affected compartment of the knee with a subsequent deformity (knock-knee if lateral compartment or bow-leg if medial compartment). As the deformity progresses, there is greater force being applied to that compartment of the knee, leading to a vicious cycle.

On a molecular biology level, which is where many of the tests are heading, there is an increase in cytokines (interleukin [IL]-1 and tumor necrosis factor alpha [TNF-α]) that upregulate the gene expression of matrix metalloproteinases (MMPs). Other markers that have been hypothesized (and you should file in your memory banks) to play a role in the development of OA are receptor activator of NF-κB ligand (RANKL), IL-6, and MMP13.[4] Pharmaceutical agents are being developed to target these molecules, as are other modalities (physiologic loading of joints has been shown to modify MMP expression) in the hopes of being able to slow or reverse the progression of OA. Cartilage oligomeric matrix protein (COMP) is another marker of OA in synovial fluid. COMP is degraded by ADAMTS-7 and ADAMTS-12, and recent studies show that antibodies to these molecules inhibit the breakdown of COMP induced by IL-1 and TNF-α and may provide treatment options in the future. Other pathways include neurogenic and vascular growth factors that may stimulate pain and angiogenesis leading to aspects of the pathophysiology associated with OA. Vascular endothelial growth factor (VEGF) may play a role in the increase of MMPs and tissue inhibitory metalloproteinases as well as angiogenesis and chondrocyte death during the development of OA. These factors are of greater interest because platelet-rich plasma (contains a wide constituent of host growth factors) and mesenchymal stem cell (MSC) injections have become new options in managing knee OA. Understanding the molecular pathways and interactions at the microscopic level will likely be where test questions head in the future, as will OA treatments.

Current treatment options have been reviewed in 22 specific recommendations in the Amercan Academy of Orthopaedic Surgeons (AAOS) guidelines.[5] This includes nonoperative and operative management (Table 1-1).

Guideline recommendations are as follows:

1. Education: Attend programs to educate oneself on OA and modify activities accordingly.

2. Promote self-care through regular contact.

3. Patients who are overweight, with a body mass index (BMI) greater than 25 kg/m^2, should be encouraged to lose weight via dietary modification and exercise.

4. Low-impact aerobic fitness should be encouraged.

Table 1-1.

MANAGEMENT OPTIONS OF OSTEOARTHRITIS OF THE KNEE

Nonoperative Management	Operative Management
Nutraceuticals	Arthroscopy
Nonsteroidal anti-inflammatory drugs, acetaminophen, pain medications	High tibial osteotomy
Unloader braces	Unicompartmental knee arthroplasty
Corticosteroid injections	Total knee arthroplasty
Viscosupplementation	
Weight loss	
Assistive devices	

5. Enhance and maintain ROM.

6. Quadriceps strengthening.

7. Patellar taping.

8. Limited data exist to support the use of lateral heel wedges to treat symptomatic medial compartment DJD.

9. Inconclusive data exist to support or refute the use of unloader braces for medial compartment DJD.

10. Inconclusive data exist to support or refute the use of unloader braces for lateral compartment DJD.

11. Inconclusive data exist to support or refute the use of acupuncture to treat DJD.

12. Glucosamine and/or chondroitin sulfate or hydrochloride are not recommended to treat symptomatic DJD.

13. Tylenol or NSAIDs should be used to manage DJD pain.

14. In those with gastrointestinal (GI) risk, acetaminophen, topical NSAIDs, NSAIDs with a GI protectant, or COX-2 inhibitors can be used successfully.

15. Intra-articular corticosteroid injections are useful in the short term.

16. With mild to moderate DJD, there is inconclusive evidence to support or refute the use of viscosupplementation injections.

17. Isolated aspiration is not suggested to treat knee DJD.

18. Arthroscopic debridement for DJD is not recommended.

19. Arthroscopic management is feasible in those with primary signs and symptoms of a torn meniscus or a loose body.

20. Tubercle osteotomy is not supported or refuted in the literature regarding tibial tubercle osteotomy for patellofemoral OA.

21. High tibial osteotomy (HTO)/realignment is a good option in active patients with unicompartmental DJD and a knee malalignment.

22. Free-floating interpositional devices are not recommended.

In this case with severe tricompartmental degenerative changes, a greater than 10-degree varus deformity, and a 20-degree flexion contracture, thus eliminating arthroscopy, HTO or unicompartmental knee arthroplasty (UKA) as viable options. The description states nonoperative management has been unsuccessful and that the best management option at this time would be total knee arthroplasty (TKA).

Why Might This Be Tested? OA is such a common diagnosis and represents a large cost to society. Molecular pathways and modes of cartilage breakdown are now testable items. In addition, AAOS clinical practice guidelines must be known because these recommendations will be tested in upcoming years.

Here's the Point!

OA is a common diagnosis. Recognize and understand/memorize the common molecular elements involved. Know the clinical practice guidelines. Reasonable nonoperative options include NSAIDs, weight loss, activity modification, and corticosteroid injections. Surgical options include TKA, HTO, and UKA when indicated.

Vignette 2: Doc, How Does My Broken Arm Heal?

A 14-year-old right-hand-dominant male presents with pain, swelling, and deformity of the left forearm after falling off a skateboard. On exam, he is neurovascularly intact with soft left forearm compartments. An x-ray of the forearm is shown (Figure 2-1).

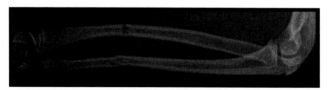

Figure 2-1. AP x-ray of the left forearm showing a middle distal third radius and ulna fracture.

▶ *What is the patient's underlying diagnosis?*

▶ *What is the structure of bone?*

▶ *What are the potential bone healing pathways?*

▶ *What are the treatment options?*

Vignette 2: Answer

The patient has a displaced left middle third radius and ulna fracture.

Normal bone is lamellar (highly organized) and comprises 2 different types of bone: cortical and cancellous. In contrast, pathologic bone is woven (haphazard arrangement). Cortical bone, also known as compact bone, composes 80% of the skeleton and is made up of tightly packed bone units called osteons. Haversian canals containing arterioles, capillaries, venules, and nerves connect osteons. Cement lines define the outer border of an osteon, and canaliculi are small tubules that connect lacunae of ossified bone. In comparison with cortical bone, cancellous bone is spongier and more elastic, has a lower Young's modulus, and has a higher turnover rate.[6]

Osteoblasts lay down new bone, while osteoclasts resorb it. Bone is constantly formed and broken down by these cells in response to environmental and mechanical stressors. Wolff's law explains that bone will increase in density to cope with increasing mechanical stress; conversely, bone loss will ensue with removal of stress. The Hueter-Volkmann law dictates that longitudinal bone growth is stimulated by tension and inhibited by compression.[6]

There are 3 sources of vascular supply to long bones, including the nutrient artery, metaphyseal-epiphyseal system, and periosteal system. Nutrient arteries branch from larger systemic vessels and enter long bones in the diaphysis through the nutrient foramen. Upon entrance, the vessel divides into arterioles, with the nutrient artery supplying the inner two-thirds of the diaphyseal cortex (high-pressure system). A vascular plexus that derives from periarticular blood vessels supplies the metaphyseal-diaphyseal area of bone, and the periosteum contains capillaries that supply the outer one-third of the diaphyseal cortex (low-pressure system). The inner portion of the periosteum, the cambium, also contains osteoblast progenitor cells.[7]

Bone healing occurs through 2 pathways (direct and indirect). Direct healing occurs with absolute rigid fixation, whereas indirect healing occurs with more dynamic types of fixation and with casting. Regardless of the type of healing, adequate bone blood flow is paramount to healing (remember the pneumonic for nonunion: motion, avascular, gap, and infection [MAGI]). Initially, there is a decrease in blood flow to the area of injury, primarily as a result of the traumatic vascular disruption. However, blood flow then resumes with an increased rate, with a peak at about 2 weeks, and returns to normal around 5 to 6 months.[8]

There are 3 stages to fracture healing: inflammation, repair, and remodeling. During the inflammation stage, a hematoma forms, providing the hematopoietic cells capable of releasing growth factors.[8] Fibroblasts and mesenchymal cells infiltrate the fracture site and form granulation tissue around the fracture fragments. Osteoblasts and fibroblasts proliferate as well.

During the repair stage, a soft callus forms within 2 weeks postinjury of surgical fixation. The extent of this callus is inversely proportional to the degree of fracture stability; absolute stability with a direct compression plate, for example, will have very little, if any, callus, whereas cast immobilization will develop a robust callus. The soft callus is converted to a hard callus via enchondral ossification, supplemented by medullary callus. For more rigid fixation, the repair stage involves primary cortical healing (ie, cutting cones and Haversian remodeling), rather than callus formation and maturation.

Remodeling begins to occur during the repair stage and continues even after clinical healing has occurred. Lamellar bone replaces woven bone, with Wolff's law and piezoelectric remodeling helping to shape this stage. Piezoelectric remodeling refers to the tension side of bone having a positive charge, which stimulates osteoclasts, whereas the compression side has a negative charge, which stimulates an osteoblast reaction.

Treatment choice depends on several factors, including patient age, time from original injury, fracture site, degree of comminution and displacement, and patient comorbidities (tobacco and NSAID use can adversely contribute to these concerns), among others. Options range from cast immobilization (Figure 2-2) and flexible rodding (intramedullary [IM] fixation) to absolute stability constructs such as compression plating (Figure 2-3).

At the same time, patient comorbidities must be optimized because these may adversely affect fracture healing and overall outcomes. Nicotine use may decrease the rate of fracture healing and strength of the callus, thereby leading to an increased risk of nonunion. Malnourishment has been shown to impede healing in a rat model.[9] Diabetics are known to have higher complication rates for most surgeries, but they are also reported to have a higher risk of nonunion.[10] Furthermore, attempts should be made to limit use of NSAIDs or COX-2 inhibitors as COX-2 has been shown to promote fracture healing by causing MSCs to differentiate into osteoblasts.[11]

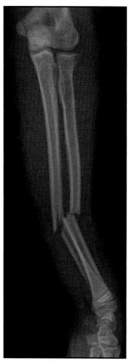 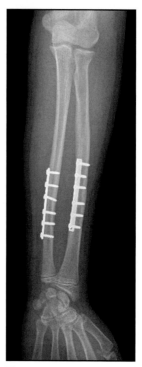

Figure 2-2. Lateral x-ray of the left forearm showing a middle distal third fracture of the radius and ulna with 90 degrees of rotational displacement.

Figure 2-3. AP x-ray of the left forearm showing compression plating of the forearm fracture and complete healing of both fracture sites.

Why Might This Be Tested? Bone remodeling and structure are the basic fundamentals in orthopedics. Many disorders stem from abnormalities in these processes, which makes this ripe testing ground. In addition, this topic is chock full of basic science, so just know it!

Here's the Point!

The 2 types of bone include lamellar and woven. Bone remodels according to Wolff's law and the Hueter-Volkmann law. There are 3 stages to fracture repair: inflammation, repair, and remodeling. Bone heals by direct apposition with cutting cones and Haversian remodeling or via bridging callus and interfragmentary enchondral ossification. The most important factor in fracture healing is blood supply.

Vignette 3: Can't Even Lift My Morning Cup of Coffee With These Hands

A 71-year-old male presents to your hand clinic with a 2-year history of bilateral hand pain. He says the pain started 2 years prior and has been getting worse ever since. He wakes up with significant stiffness in both of his hands every morning, which lasts longer than 1 hour. The patient denies any trauma to the hands and says they feel as if grip strength is declining in both hands. The pain is mostly in his proximal interphalangeal (PIP) and metacarpophalangeal (MCP) joints of both hands. He says he has general aches and pains all over, but the hands are the worst. He denies any other symptoms. Vital signs are normal. On physical exam, you notice swollen, tender PIP and MCP joints bilaterally with some ulnar deviation of both hands. There is no erythema seen around the joints. Notably, the distal interphalangeal (DIP) joints seem to be normal. He also has a small, nontender, rubbery nodule near his elbow. Neurovascular exam in both upper extremities is normal.

▶ *What is the presumed diagnosis?*

▶ *What tests are required to confirm the diagnosis?*

▶ *What are the treatment options?*

Vignette 3: Answer

The presumed diagnosis in this case is rheumatoid arthritis (RA). The clues that point to this are the history of bilateral (symmetrical) hand swelling that has been getting progressively worse, involvement of the MCP and PIP joints with sparing of the DIP joints, ulnar deviation of the hand, and rheumatoid nodule in his elbow. The history of morning pain lasting 1 hour or so is classic of RA. The gradual onset with no history of trauma and a normal neurovascular exam should point you away from more acute things, and the fact that it is symmetrical should lead you away from a tumor. One thing that makes the diagnosis a little more difficult is the lack of systemic manifestations (pleuritis, pericarditis, vasculitis, etc), although these are infrequently present and seen more in patients with very active disease. RA is an inflammatory arthritis that leads to destruction of cartilage via thickened synovium and an abundance of IL-1 and TNF-α. It is a bone-wasting disease (as opposed to bone-forming OA).[12] There are several other types of inflammatory arthritis (Table 3-1).

Juvenile idiopathic arthritis (JIA) has several subsets, with each subset affecting a different age group or a different number of joints. This is the only inflammatory arthropathy that could require surgery in the early period. If a child has a limb-length discrepancy secondary to JIA, an epiphysiodesis may be performed to ensure proper limb biomechanics. Reactive arthritis (Reiter's syndrome) is seen in conjunction with a systemic infection. Treating the infection will treat the arthritis. Likewise, in systemic lupus erythematosus (SLE), controlling the lupus will help control the arthritis, as will the addition of disease-modifying antirheumatic drugs (DMARDs).

The diagnosis of RA is made with several tests. First, plain x-rays of the affected joints should be ordered. Like OA, there will be joint space narrowing. However, a difference from OA is that in RA, as well as in the other inflammatory arthropathies, you will see bone erosion. This can also be seen in gout, so the presence of bony erosion in and of itself is not pathognomonic for inflammatory arthritis but should lead you away from a diagnosis of OA. Protrusio is often seen in the hip. Periarticular osteopenia and soft tissue swelling can also be seen in RA. Joint aspiration can be performed to diagnose RA or other inflammatory arthropathies, but many times the plain x-rays and laboratory tests will give the diagnosis. However, in very active RA, patients may present with a blurred clinical picture, and a joint aspiration can be performed to rule out septic arthritis. The white blood cell count will be between 1500 and 50,000, with a predominance of polymorphonuclear leukocytes (PMNs). Although a cell count greater than 50,000 is possible in RA, this should alert the clinician to possible septic arthritis.[13] Gram stain and crystal analysis of the synovial fluid will be negative in RA. If these are positive, a diagnosis of septic arthritis, gout, or pseudogout should be considered.

Laboratory tests are also key to diagnosing RA. Rheumatoid factor (RF), which is an autoantibody (immunoglobulin [IgM]) to the Fc portion of IgM G, is present in 75% to 80% of patients with RA. The sensitivity and specificity of this test have been reported at 60% to 70% and 80% to 90%, respectively.[12] RF can also be present in Sjögren's syndrome, lupus, and inflammatory conditions, so its presence does not definitively diagnose RA. Anticitrullinated peptide antibodies can also be seen in RA. This test carries a similar sensitivity to RF but has a specificity approaching 98%, meaning that if this test is positive, the patient has a high likelihood of having RA.[12] Furthermore, ESR and CRP may be elevated in patients with RA, which signals more active disease.[12]

Treatment for inflammatory arthritis is largely medical with DMARDs, such as methotrexate, TNF-α antagonists, and immunosuppressant agents, which should be monitored by a rheumatologist. The surgical options for inflammatory arthritis include synovectomy of the involved joints and, ultimately, a total joint arthroplasty (TJA). Patients should understand that synovectomy will not restore function to the joint and is simply used to relieve pain.

Why Might This Be Tested? It is important to differentiate between inflammatory and noninflammatory arthropathies early on when caring for a patient as the treatments for these conditions are markedly different. Also, the sooner the diagnosis and appropriate referrals are made, the sooner the patient can begin treatment.

Here's the Point!

RA usually involves the MCP and PIP joints and spares the DIP joints. It is almost always symmetrical. Diagnose with x-rays showing bony erosions and blood tests for RF and anticitrullinated peptide antibodies. Refer the patient to the rheumatologist for appropriate DMARD therapy; reserve synovectomy and joint replacement for refractory cases.

Table 3-1.

INFLAMMATORY ARTHROPATHIES

Type	Pathophysiology	Physical Findings	Diagnosis
RA	Hypertrophic synovium with auto-immune cartilage destruction (IL-1 and TNF-α cascade)	MCP and PIP swelling/tenderness, morning stiffness, rheumatoid nodules, systemic manifestations, symmetric polyarthropathy	• X-rays: Periarticular osteopenia and erosions, protrusio acetabuli • Labs: +RF/ACPA, increased ESR and CRP • Proper history, usually ≥3 joints
Psoriatic	Associated with psoriasis; HLA B27 associated; seronegative spondyloarthropathy	Preceded by skin rash with plaques (silvery), asymmetric swelling of joints, nail pitting, dactylitis (sausage digit)	• X-rays: DIP arthritis, pencil-in-cup deformity, bone erosions (small joints) • Labs: HLA B27 in 50%, RA/ANA negative • Only 5% to 20% with psoriasis develop psoriatic arthritis
AS	HLA B27 positive (90%); autoimmune; likely due to reaction to environmental pathogen	Bilateral sacroiliitis, progressive spinal kyphosis, cervical spine fractures and large joint DJD noted	• X-rays: Marginal syndesmophytes, bamboo spine, bilateral sacroiliac erosion, sometimes protrusio acetabuli • Limitation of chest wall expansion can be pathognomonic for AS
Reiter	Associated pathogens: mycoplasma, salmonella, shigella, chlamydia, campylobacter	Urinary symptoms (discomfort), inflammation or dry eyes (conjunctivitis/uveitis) and joint pain common	• X-ray: DJD of joints • Labs: HLA B27 in 75%, ESR and CRP elevated • Usually in men aged <40 years; "can't cry, pee, or climb a tree"
JIA	Autoimmune destruction of cartilage lasts >6 weeks in patients aged <16 years	• Still's disease: rash, fever, splenomegaly • Iridocyclitis (anterior uveitis) • Polyarticular (30%): >5 joints • Pauciarticular (50%): ≤4 (large) joints • Systemic: Poor prognosis, systemic symptoms present	• X-ray: Often negative early on; may see periarticular osteopenia; check c-spine films for atlantoaxial instability • Labs: RF+ in <15%, serology often negative • HLA markers: o DR4→polyarticular o DR8, DR5, DR2.1→pauciarticular
SLE	Autoimmune disorder; leads to accumulation of complexes in joints, skin, kidneys, lungs, and nervous system	• >75% of patients have joint involvement; seen in PIP, MCP, knee • Pancytopenia, pericarditis, kidney disease, Raynaud's • Fever, butterfly malar rash, synovitis, hand and wrist swelling (90%)	• X-ray: Often negative early on; osteonecrosis common • Labs: ANA (95%), anti-DNA antibodies • HLA markers: o HLA-DR3 o HLA Class II o HLA Class III o HLA-DQ • Common in Black women aged 15 to 25 years

AS = ankylosing spondylitis.

Vignette 4: Doctor, My Feet Are Flat

A 52-year-old obese female presents with a 3-year history of intermittent medial ankle pain and swelling. The pain radiates into the arch of her foot. Her pain is exacerbated by prolonged periods of walking, standing, or exercise. She has worn over-the-counter and custom orthotics for many years. The patient has been told by her family that she has flat feet. On physical examination, she is noted to have a pes planus deformity that is passively correctable. In the weight-bearing position, her heel is in slight valgus. She is unable to perform a single heel/toe raise and has a positive "too many toes" sign. She has limited dorsiflexion of the ankle compared with the opposite side.

▶ *What is the patient's underlying disease?*

▶ *What is the pathophysiology of this disease process?*

The patient was ultimately scheduled for reconstructive surgery to address her pathology.

▶ *How does the patient's disease stage affect the surgical algorithm?*

Vignette 4: Answer

The underlying pathology in this case is posterior tibial tendon insufficiency (PTTI).[14] This is overwhelmingly the most common cause of an adult-acquired flatfoot deformity. Other causes of the painful pes planovalgus foot include inflammatory arthropathy, DJD of the midfoot and hindfoot, and Charcot neuroarthropathy. Many patients describe a history of flat feet or an inciting overuse episode (eg, "I felt a pop on the inside of my ankle while playing tennis on my Wii!").

The posterior tibial tendon acts to adduct and supinate the forefoot and to stabilize the hindfoot against valgus forces. Through chronic, repetitive microtrauma, the posterior tibial tendon lengthens, substantially diminishing the inversion force of the tendon. This insult leads to longitudinal arch collapse, and a flatfoot deformity results. Unopposed pull of the peroneus brevis tendon creates a valgus deformity of the hindfoot, altering the mechanical pull of the tendo-Achilles complex lateral to the axis of the subtalar joint. This renders the Achilles tendon an evertor of the hindfoot, which accelerates the valgus deformity and exerts a downward force on the talonavicular joint, weakening the calcaneonavicular (spring) ligament.

Although PTTI can be congenital or acutely traumatic in origin, the most common presentation is seen with chronic pain in overweight, middle-aged women. This condition is often misdiagnosed as a sprained ankle or foot. Clinical manifestations include pain and boggy swelling along the course of the tendon, from posterior to the medial malleolus to the instep of the foot. Arch collapse is a common complaint, as is painful lateral impingement of the talus and calcaneus as medial stability deteriorates. (Patients look like they are walking on the talus.)

Physical examination, initiated with the patient in standing position, often reveals a prominent medial malleolus with an abducted forefoot and a "too many toes" sign. (This is where you see too many toes when looking at the patient's foot from behind due to the aforementioned deformity.) Inability of the patient to initiate a single heel/toe raise, or absence of heel inversion with single heel/toe raise, indicates an insufficient posterior tibial tendon. Typically, the tendo-Achilles complex is tight, and one tests for an isolated gastrocnemius contracture or a fulminant equinus contracture. In the seated position, ROM is assessed to determine if the deformity is passively correctable. Fixed varus of the forefoot is common in longstanding disease and has implications in the management of this problem.

Clinical staging of PTTI is critical to guiding treatment. Stage I patients present with pain and swelling along the medial ankle in the absence of clinical deformity. Tenosynovitis is the cause of pain, and the patient can perform a single heel/toe raise. Stage II patients have undergone tendon elongation and exhibit obvious deformity. Although hindfoot valgus and forefoot abductus are evident, the deformity remains passively correctable. Medial symptoms with ability to perform single heel/toe raise may be present in early stage II disease (stage II, subclass "a"), whereas lateral symptoms develop later in the presence of subfibular impingement (subclass "b"). The hallmark of stage III disease is the development of a rigid deformity. Heel valgus and forefoot varus are fixed, and the gastrocsoleus complex is tight. Pain at rest is common as hindfoot arthritis sets in. In stage IV, chronic eccentric loading of the ankle creates lateral ankle compartment wear patterns and failure of the deltoid ligament. Insufficiency fracture of the distal fibula is a common development at this stage.

Imaging studies consist of standard weight-bearing x-rays of the foot and ankle. As PTTI progresses, the anteroposterior (AP) foot view will demonstrate increasing talonavicular uncoverage (yes, this is a word; it describes the lack of coverage of the talonavicular joint). On the lateral view, plantarflexion of the talus is often noted, plantar gapping is often noted at the medial column (talonavicular and/or naviculocuneiform joints), and calcaneal pitch also diminishes. It had been noted that calcaneal pitch is the most reliable radiographic measurement with the least interobserver variability.[14] Plain x-rays are useful in determining the presence or absence of degenerative changes in the midfoot, hindfoot, and ankle joints. Magnetic resonance imaging (MRI) is helpful in diagnosing PTT pathology and quantifying DJD.

Treatment for stage I and early stage II PTTI consists of immobilization, NSAIDs, activity, and shoewear modifications. Physical therapy is used when the acute swelling has subsided. Custom orthotics can be useful in this phase in an attempt to ease the strain across the tendon by eliminating pronation and elevating the medial arch. As the deformity becomes more pronounced, a flexible, total-contact, rigid orthotic (ie, University of California Biomechanics Laboratory) brace may become necessary. The biomechanical principle of this device is to stabilize the heel in neutral position to prevent forefoot abduction.

With advancing PTTI, surgical options are recommended. Isolated soft tissue procedures are seldom indicated. The algorithm for bony reconstruction typically begins with medial displacement calcaneal osteotomy in order to restore the mechanical axis by eliminating hindfoot valgus. Flexor digitorum longus tendon transfer to the navicular is recommended as the most appropriate substitute for the nonviable posterior tibial tendon. The spring ligament, rendered incompetent by chronic pressure from the uncovered talar head, is often primarily repaired. Lateral column lengthening (Evans osteotomy), is a viable option in stage IIb disease as lateral symptoms develop. The Evans procedure has been shown to provide additional bony support to the soft tissue reconstruction and is often considered in more youthful, active patients, as well as in obese individuals. In the setting of medial column instability (plantar gapping on weight-bearing lateral x-rays), plantarflexion opening wedge osteotomy of the medial cuneiform (Cotton procedure) or isolated naviculocuneiform fusion are performed. The equinus contracture is corrected by means of a gastroc recession or tendo Achilles lengthening. For stage III disease, arthrodesis (talonavicular, double, or triple) is required to salvage the rigid deformity. In stage IV disease, in addition to hindfoot arthrodesis, deltoid ligament reconstruction is performed, often with the use of allograft.

Why Might This Be Tested? PTTI is the most common cause of medial ankle and foot pain and the most common etiology of pes planovalgus.

Here's the Point!

If the patient is middle-aged, overweight, flatfooted, and has medial ankle and foot pain, think PTTI! If the deformity is flexible and passively correctable, think reconstruction. If it is rigid and arthritis is present, think fusion.

Vignette 5: Fall Onto an Outstretched Hand While Skiing

A 28-year-old female sustained a fall onto an outstretched dominant right hand while skiing. She was found to have a distal radius and ulnar styloid fracture. There is dorsal comminution and a 50-degree apex volar angulation deformity but no intra-articular displacement. She was closed reduced and treated in a cast for 6 weeks at another facility. She is now 3 months out from her injury and presents to you for a second opinion, primarily reporting a lack of wrist flexion and forearm supination and a visible wrist deformity. Her physical exam shows a mild clinical deformity, no tenderness radially or ulnarly, mild pain with forced ulnar deviation, a stable distal radioulnar joint (DRUJ), and full digital motion with no trophic signs. Her x-rays show a healed primarily extra-articular distal radius fracture with 50 degrees of apex volar angulation as well as loss of radial height and inclination but no arthritic changes of the wrist (Figure 5-1).

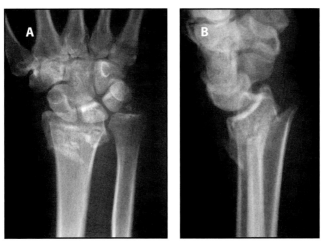

Figure 5-1. (A) AP and (B) lateral x-rays of the wrist.

▶ *What are the effects of a distal radius fracture healing in this malunited position?*

▶ *What operative treatment options are available, and what are the advantages of each?*

Vignette 5: Answer

The patient has developed a distal radius malunion. The presence of dorsal comminution at the time of injury and an ulnar styloid fracture served as risk factors for this as an unstable injury. If the first closed reduction achieved acceptable alignment, the patient should have been observed weekly for 3 to 4 weeks to assure the reduction was maintained. In this case, at some point the fracture fell back into the dorsal comminution and displaced. Oops!

Apex volar angulation is the most common pattern for distal radius malunion and most typically presents clinically with loss of supination, wrist flexion, and grip strength. Shortening, whether from true axial loss of length or from relative shortening from malangulation, results in functionally increased ulnar variance, which places the patient at risk of ulnocarpal abutment and DRUJ dysfunction.[15] Although there is variability, the average wrist typically has 10 degrees of apex volar angulation, 20 degrees of radial inclination, and neutral ulnar variance. It is well known that in the normal setting, approximately 80% of the load across the wrist occurs through the radiocarpal articulation, with the remainder across the ulnocarpal joint. Either 2.5 mm of radial shortening or 20 degrees of dorsal angulation past neutral has been shown to increase the load borne by the ulna to between 40% and 50%, increasing the risk of ulnar-sided wrist dysfunction, especially in young patients.[16,17]

The surgical consideration in this case is corrective osteotomy. Although osteotomy may be contraindicated in a low-demand patient, in the presence of established arthritic change or severe intra-articular comminution or when signs of complex regional pain syndrome are present, this young, active patient would likely benefit from restoration of more normal wrist kinematics. The goal of treatment is to re-establish more normal radiographic parameters of the distal radius itself (tilt, height, inclination) as well as to restore a more normal relationship with the distal ulna (variance). A closing-wedge osteotomy has the benefit of more reliable union because no defect is created and bone graft is usually not required; however, it makes multiplanar correction more difficult and invariably leads to shortening. Thus, when used alone, it is unable to restore appropriate ulnar variance.[15,18] Restoration of ulnar variance would require an ulnar shortening osteotomy or, in severe cases, salvage procedures; a distal ulna resection or the Sauve-Kapandji procedure may be required to prevent ulnar-sided dysfunction.

An opening-wedge osteotomy has the advantage of allowing multiplanar correction and restoration of ulnar variance as a single procedure, but it results in a dorsal defect that is subject to collapse in the setting of poor bone stock and is also at greater risk of nonunion than closing-wedge procedures.[15,18] In the past, it would be performed from a dorsal (Thompson) approach with corticocancellous structural grafting, but the advent of volar fixed-angle constructs has allowed for the procedure to be performed through a volar Henry approach (proximally between the brachioradialis and pronator teres and distally between the brachioradialis and flexor carpi radialis), and most authors agree that cancellous autograft or allograft dorsally can be used rather than structural graft. This is primarily the preferred technique for most malunion corrections. Correction of primarily extra-articular defects is technically less demanding than intra-articular fractures with reproducible outcomes. There is increasing research that intra-articular osteotomy can be beneficial, but this is primarily in the setting of simple articular patterns, such as die punch or displaced volar lunate facet fragments. The procedure requires meticulous fluoroscopic evaluation or a dorsal arthrotomy for confirmation of the quality of the reduction and is mainly indicated in trying to achieve 2 mm or less articular displacement in young patients.[19]

Why Might This Be Tested? Given how common distal radius fractures are, malunion is frequently seen. Cadaveric studies have demonstrated the effects of malunion (especially extra-articular) on wrist kinematics and function. Its treatment tests basic principles of osteotomy.

Here's the Point!

The most common malunion undergoing surgical correction is an apex volar deformity with resultant shortening and loss of radial length and inclination. Left untreated, this increases load on the ulnar wrist and frequently limits wrist and forearm ROM. The most popular osteotomy technique is a dorsal opening-wedge from a volar approach with a fixed-angle device.

Vignette 6: My Child Fell Down the Stairs!

A 3-year-old male presents with pain and swelling in his right knee after a fall down a couple of stairs at home. The child refuses to bear weight on his right lower extremity and holds the knee in a slightly flexed position. An AP x-ray was obtained of the right knee (Figure 6-1).

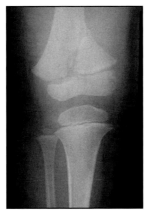

Figure 6-1. AP x-ray of the right knee.

▶ *What should the initial management be?*

▶ *This fracture pattern has a high chance of what long-term problem?*

The patient presents 1 year later with a progressive deformity of his right lower extremity. X-rays and a clinical photograph were obtained (Figure 6-2).

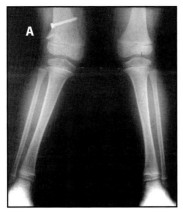
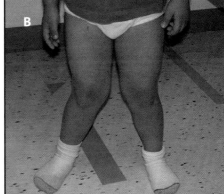

Figure 6-2. (A) Plain x-ray of both lower extremities showing overall limb alignment. (B) Clinical picture of the patient's lower extremities showing the progressive deformity.

▶ *What is the diagnosis?*

▶ *What is the treatment of this secondary deformity?*

Vignette 6: Answer

Making the diagnosis is the first step in this case because not all distal femoral fractures are the same in children. To nail down the diagnosis and corresponding recommended treatment options, one must first classify this fracture. The most common system for distal femoral epiphyseal fractures is the classic Salter-Harris scheme. In a type I fracture, there is a separation through the growth plate; in type II (most common), the fracture crosses the physis and exits obliquely across one of the corners of the metaphysis; in type III, the fracture line extends through the growth plate and exits through the epiphysis into the joint; in type IV, a vertical fracture crosses the epiphysis, physis, and metaphysis; and type V are crush fractures of the growth plate.[20] Based on the x-ray, the patient sustained a displaced Salter-Harris II fracture of his distal femur. Because this fracture is displaced, the likelihood of growth arrest and formation of a physeal bar are quite high, thus necessitating anatomic alignment of the fracture. This is typically accomplished via an open reduction (if adequate closed reduction cannot be achieved) and pinning of the fracture.

Often, type II fractures reduce with longitudinal traction, and smooth transphyseal pins can be placed when the metaphyseal piece is small. In cases with a large metaphyseal fragment, K-wires or cannulated screws can be used to fix the fracture without violating the growth plate. Unlike Salter-Harris II fractures elsewhere in the body, in the distal femur, even with anatomic alignment, there is a high chance of growth arrest. This physis maintains an undulating shape and is more susceptible to shearing and compressive forces.[20]

Surveillance follow-up is recommended, with an evaluation around 6 months after the injury for early detection of a potential growth disturbance. It is even suggested that follow-up should continue until skeletal maturity because both growth acceleration and arrest have been seen with distal femur physeal fractures. If a bony bar is identified, indications for excision are when less than 50% of the bar is affecting the physis and more than 2 years of growth remain (as in our case).[20] An MRI is the best modality to determine the extent of a physeal bar formation. In older children, it is commonly viewed that girls stop growing at 13 years of age and boys stop at 16 years of age. Typically, projected leg-length discrepancies of less than 2 cm can be managed nonsurgically, between 2 and 5 cm can be treated with a contralateral epiphysiodesis, and greater than 5 cm may need a limb-lengthening procedure.

If the bar is excised, it is usually filled with a substance that will prevent the bar from reoccurring (fat is commonly used). If Harris growth arrest lines are present, you will see them starting at the bar and extending outward. (A Harris growth arrest line is a linear increased density seen above the growth plate on x-rays. It represents temporary slowing or cessation of growth due to insult from the fracture.) Once the bar is excised and the growth resumes, the Harris growth arrest lines will become more horizontal, indicating that the bar is no longer acting as a tether. An osteotomy may be performed depending on the child's age and extent of deformity. Some believe that by merely removing the physeal bar, the limb will continue to grow and the deformity will improve. Others believe that if the deformity is clinically unacceptable, then an osteotomy should be performed. In patients approaching skeletal maturity, an osteotomy and/or a hemiepiphysiodesis may be the better treatment option.

Why Might This Be Tested? Question writers typically focus on pediatric fractures that may lead to secondary deformities and complications. It is important to be aware of which distal femur fractures have a higher likelihood of future issues (growth arrest and deformity) and to know which ones need to be followed closely and what to do if the issues arise.

Here's the Point!

If you inherit a patient with a distal femoral physeal fracture, you have bought that patient until skeletal maturity because growth acceleration or deceleration are common. Anatomic reduction and secure fixation is a must. Physeal bars should be resected when less than 50% of the growth plate and more than 2 more years of growth are left.

Vignette 7: Increased Pain and Swelling After a Primary Total Knee Arthroplasty

A 72-year-old male who underwent a left TKA 3 days prior started to complain of some increased pain and swelling in his left lower extremity overnight. The patient's postoperative course to this point has been uncomplicated, although his physical therapy has been progressing slowly. He has been receiving aspirin twice daily for anticoagulation. The patient denies any chest pain or shortness of breath and states the pain started about 4 hours ago. It has been getting slightly better. His heart rate is elevated to 115 bpm, with an oxygen saturation of 93% on room air. His other vital signs are within normal limits. On physical examination, the patient is obese and has normal postoperative swelling of the knee with some mild swelling and tenderness in the posterior aspect of the left calf. Homans' sign is negative.

▶ *What is the presumed diagnosis?*

▶ *What tests are required to confirm the diagnosis?*

▶ *What are the treatment options?*

Vignette 7: Answer

The presumed diagnosis in this case is a deep venous thrombosis (DVT) with question of a pulmonary embolism (PE). The clues in the vignette that point toward this are the history of a TKA 3 days ago, increased pain and swelling in left lower extremity, tachycardia, lack of movement with physical therapy, and decreased oxygen saturation. The fact that the patient was doing fine and then complained of increased pain and swelling in his calf is a clue toward DVT. The negative Homans' sign (pain on forced dorsiflexion of the foot) and current use of anticoagulation are used as distractors in this case. Given the slight elevation in heart rate with a mild decrease in oxygen saturation, a PE is a definite possibility in this patient who likely has a DVT.

DVT and PE are well documented complications following THA and TKA, occurring in approximately 50% of patients not receiving thromboprophylaxis and roughly 1% of those receiving some form of chemical prophylaxis.[21] There are many options for chemical prophylaxis after surgery (Table 7-1).

Table 7-1.

CHEMICAL PROPHYLAXIS OPTIONS AFTER SURGERY

Anticoagulant	Effect	Monitoring
Aspirin	Inhibits platelet aggregation	None
Warfarin	Inhibits factors II, VII, IX, X	INR
LMWH	Inhibits factor Xa and thrombin via antithrombin	None
Fondaparinux	Indirect factor Xa inhibitor	None
Rivaroxaban	Direct factor Xa inhibitor	None
Heparin	Binds antithrombin III, inhibits factors IIa, Xa	PTT
INR = international normalized ratio; LMWH = low-molecular-weight heparin; PTT = partial thromboplastin time.		

DVT and PE are also commonly seen in patients who sustain a hip fracture. This relatively high rate of DVT/PE can be attributed to several predisposing factors. The 3 most important factors that increase a person's risk for DVT are known as Virchow's triad. These include stasis, hypercoagulable state (surgery, pregnancy, malignancy, oral contraceptive use, smoking, obesity, hypercoagulable disorder, etc), and endothelial/vessel wall injury. Our patient has at least 2 of the 3 predisposing factors (stasis from his lack of movement and hypercoagulable state secondary to his obesity and recent surgery) and could potentially have the third in vessel wall injury if his vessels were damaged at the time of surgery.

One cannot rely solely on physical exam for diagnosis of DVT or PE. Homans' sign is neither sensitive nor specific for a DVT, and somewhere between 50% and 80% of DVTs are clinically silent. Although tachycardia, tachypnea, and fevers are often seen with PE, their presence or absence from the clinical picture cannot confirm or refute this diagnosis. Chest pain, shortness of breath, dyspnea, anxiety, and other signs and symptoms are variably present/absent with PE as well. In order to confirm the diagnosis of a DVT, a venous ultrasound of the lower extremity in question should be performed. Some people advocate starting with a D-dimer; and if this is negative; it can rule out a DVT. In the acute postoperative setting, this is frequently positive, so it has little value in the evaluation of our patient. Although the gold standard for diagnosis of DVT is contrast venography, this is an invasive and time-consuming test. Therefore, a venous ultrasound is the first-line test for a suspected DVT.[22]

In order to diagnose a PE, one must rule out other disease processes first. Start with a chest x-ray to rule out any other causes of hypoxia and obtain an electrocardiogram (EKG) to rule out cardiac pathology. An arterial blood gas (ABG) on room air should be drawn, and the alveolar-arterial gradient should be calculated $(150-1.25[PaCO_2]) - PaO_2$. The ABG in a patient with a PE will show a hypoxic, hypocapnic patient secondary to hyperventilation with an increased alveolar-arterial gradient (> 20 mm Hg). Once these tests have been performed and there is no better explanation for the patient's vague symptoms of shortness of breath, tachycardia, etc, computed tomography (CT) pulmonary angiography is the diagnostic test of choice for its speed and reliability. Although a ventilation perfusion scan is an option, this test is not performed at all institutions, often gives indeterminate results, and is not as quick to perform as a CT scan. However, CT requires contrast and exposes the patient to radiation, so it is not without its pitfalls.

Once the diagnosis of a DVT or PE is confirmed with a venous ultrasound or CT, respectively, the patient should be started on either a heparin drip or treatment dose; low-molecular-weight heparin (LMWH) should be given for 5 days along with oral warfarin to achieve a goal of international normalized ratio (INR) of 2 to 3.[22] This should be maintained for a minimum of 3 months because the patient had a provoked DVT/PE (provoked by surgery). If the patient had sustained a DVT/PE without provocation (no surgery or some other inciting event that placed him in a hypercoagulable state), then he would need to be on warfarin for significantly longer and be referred to a hematologist for workup of his potential hypercoagulable disorder.

Why Might This Be Tested? DVT/PE are relatively common occurrences after TKA and THA (seen in approximately 1% of patients receiving therapeutic anticoagulation), so most physicians will have to deal with this on a regular basis. Rapid diagnosis and management is important to minimize complications and maximize patient outcomes.

Here's the Point!

Physical exam is unreliable to detect both DVT (Homans' sign only seen in 50% of patients with DVT) and PE (tachycardia and tachypnea can be present but do not have to be). If suspicion for DVT is high, diagnose with lower extremity venous ultrasound, and if positive, therapeutically anticoagulate the patient. If suspicion for PE is high, order a chest CT with PE protocol, and if positive, start the patient on a heparin drip and bridge to warfarin.

Vignette 8: Where's My Kneecap Going?

A 59-year-old female is now 1 year post TKA for advanced DJD with a valgus deformity. She reports persistent pain and poor motion "ever since surgery." She denies any history of draining wounds or infections postoperatively. Her pain is worse with activities, such as walking, arising from a seated position, and going up and down stairs. She has had extensive physical therapy and a course of NSAIDs without much improvement. Physical examination demonstrates a well-healed incision, mild effusion, and ROM of 15 to 85 degrees of flexion with pain at the extremes of motion. She has no varus/valgus or AP laxity. Periprosthetic infection has been ruled out with the appropriate laboratory studies and/or negative aspiration results. Follow-up x-rays demonstrate a neutral mechanical axis, no component loosening, and mild lateral patella tilt on the Merchant's view.

▶ *What are other possible etiologies of this patient's pain and poor motion?*

▶ *What clues from the history may lead one to be concerned about component malrotation?*

▶ *What is the optimal rotation of the femoral and tibial components?*

▶ *What is the diagnostic study of choice to determine component rotation?*

▶ *What is the treatment of choice for component malrotation?*

Vignette 8: Answer

After infection has been ruled out, other etiologies for painful and stiff TKA should be explored, including loosening, arthrofibrosis, failure to complete physical therapy, mechanical failure, and malrotation. Given that the patient has never done well after surgery, a technical error at the time of surgery must be considered. Technical errors during TKA are often related to poorly balanced soft tissues (midflexion instability) and/or component malposition (most often internal rotation of one or both of the implants). In this patient, the knee appears to be well balanced, and the x-rays demonstrate no major coronal or sagittal malposition of the components. Unless gross maltracking is seen on physical examination or the Merchant's x-ray, rotational malposition can be difficult to detect. More subtle forms of malrotation are often undetectable on plain x-rays.

The patient's history of a valgus deformity preoperatively increases the index of suspicion that the femoral component may have been placed in internal rotation.[23,24] The femoral component should have rotation matching that of the transepicondylar axis, and the tibial component should have rotation aligning the center of the baseplate with roughly the medial third of the tibial tubercle. A valgus deformity of the knee is often accompanied by hypoplasia of the lateral femoral condyle. If the surgeon uses the common technique referencing 3 degrees off of the posterior condylar axis, the femoral component would be placed in internal rotation (which medializes the trochlea groove leading to poor tracking and increased retinacular strain). In the setting of valgus deformity, surgeons should use additional checks when setting femoral component rotation, such as Whiteside's line, the transepicondylar axis, and/or making sure the anterior distal femoral resection represents a grand piano sign.[25,26] In this case, anterior knee pain and a preoperative valgus deformity screams component malrotation.

CT is the diagnostic study of choice to determine component rotation.[27] The goal is to measure femoral and tibial rotation combined with the grading as follows: mild (1 to 4 degrees, lateral patella tilt), moderate (3 to 8 degrees with patellar subluxation), and severe (7 to 17 degrees, patellar dislocation or early failure). Additional hints on rotation include the foot progression angle. If the patient walks with an externally rotated foot, this can be due to internally rotated components and vice versa for an internally rotated foot. All malrotated components should be revised. Optimal placement includes lateralizing the femoral component, appropriate implant external rotation (femur and tibia), medializing the patella component, and a neutral mechanical axis.

Why Might This Be Tested? Despite having a lower incidence, the valgus knee is commonly tested, particularly in relation to component rotation, maltracking, and peroneal nerve palsy. The diagnosis can be difficult to pin down with limited options for studies to make a diagnosis.

Here's the Point!

The valgus knee is associated with femoral condylar hypoplasia, which can lead to significant internal rotation of the femoral and/or tibial components during TKA. Follow Whiteside's line, check the epicondylar axis, and make sure there is a grand piano sign on the femur to assure good component positioning is maintained.

Vignette 9: Pedestrian Struck With A Knee Injury

A 22-year-old intoxicated female is brought to the trauma unit by the police after sustaining injuries from a hit-and-run by a car while walking home from a party. The patient does not recall specifics of the accident. On physical examination, the patient has severe swelling about the left knee but no open wounds. A posterior sag sign is evident. Tenderness is noted throughout the knee with palpation but is particularly evident on the medial side. Ligamentous testing is limited by guarding, but severe laxity is noted with varus stress testing, anterior/posterior drawer testing, Lachman's test, and dial test in 30 and 90 degrees of flexion. Good 2+ dorsalis pedis and posterior tibialis pulses are palpable in the left foot and ankle-brachial index (ABI) is 0.98. She is neurologically intact to motor and sensory function on exam. Additional workup and secondary survey is negative for any other orthopedic injuries or head trauma. Initial x-rays and advanced imaging are shown in Figures 9-1 and 9-2.

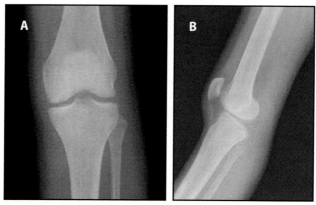

Figure 9-1. (A) AP and (B) lateral x-rays of the left knee.

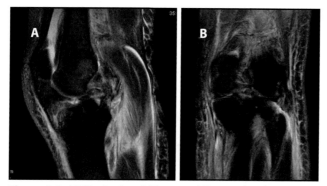

Figure 9-2. (A) Sagittal and (B) coronal T2-weighted images of the affected knee.

▶ *What is the diagnosis?*

▶ *What other aspects of the physical exam are important to note?*

▶ *What other tests should be ordered?*

▶ *What is the classification of these injuries?*

▶ *What are the treatment options? What are the advantages and disadvantages of each?*

Vignette 9: Answer

The diagnosis is a multiligament knee injury stemming from a femorotibial knee dislocation. History and exam are suspicious for injury to both cruciate ligaments, the medial collateral ligament (MCL), and the posterolateral corner. X-ray demonstrates that the knee is currently relocated, suggesting that spontaneous reduction occurred prior to evaluation. MRI exam of the knee is most notable for complete tearing of the anterior and posterior cruciate ligaments (ACL and PCL), lateral collateral ligamentous complex (LCL), and popliteus tendon (grade IIIL).

Most knee dislocations result from high-energy events, such as motor vehicle or industrial trauma. However, lower-energy mechanisms, such as those seen in contact sports, have also been capable of producing knee dislocations. Spontaneous reduction of knee dislocation occurs in approximately 20% to 50% of cases. In order for a knee to dislocate, significant soft tissue injury must be incurred; typically, injury to at least 3 of 4 major ligamentous structures of the knee must be damaged. Most cases result in rupture of the ACL and PCL but often have associated injuries to the collateral ligaments, capsular elements, and menisci. In addition, fractures of the tibial eminence, tibial tubercle, and fibular head or neck have been reported.

Given the popliteal vascular bundle's narrow course through a fibrous tunnel at the level of the adductor hiatus, thorough vascular examination and workup is paramount in any patient with suspected knee dislocation. The popliteal artery is made vulnerable by its numerous, tethering branches at the level of the popliteal fossa, particularly at the moment of dislocation. All patients with suspected knee dislocations should have a thorough vascular examination documented at initial presentation. If a pulse is present, ABIs should be measured. Those with an ABI greater than 0.9 can be observed, whereas patients with an ABI less than 0.9 should undergo angiogram or exploration in the operating room. If no pulse is palpable and the knee is dislocated, immediately perform closed reduction on the knee and reassess; if the pulse returns, the patient may then undergo an angiogram. If no pulse is palpable and the knee is reduced, then the patient should proceed to the operating room for exploration and vascular consultation. When performing the workup, it is imperative to be prompt and thorough because the maximum warm ischemic time is only 8 hours.

Classification of multiligament knee injuries is most commonly based on the anatomic classification (class I to V) put forth by Schenck.[28] Class I injuries are defined as pathology involving a single cruciate and a collateral ligament. Class II is termed as injury to both cruciates but no collateral ligaments. Class III is divided into 2 categories: IIIM and IIIL. Class IIIM is defined by injury to the ACL, PCL, and MCL, whereas class IIIL is notable for injury to the ACL, PCL, LCL, and posterolateral corner. Class IV involves injury to all 4 major ligamentous complexes about the knee: ACL, PCL, MCL, LCL, and posterolateral corner. Finally, class V includes any fracture-dislocation. In addition to these classifications, further descriptions are provided by subcategories: arterial injuries are denoted as "C" and nerve injuries are denoted as "N."

Acute management of a multiligament knee injury stemming from a knee dislocation first involves achieving reduction as soon as possible if not already present. Most knee dislocations can be closed reduced, but certain variants (posterolateral dislocations) may require open reduction. Knees should then be placed in a splint or an external fixator to maintain reduction and guard against further neurovascular injury.

Definitive treatment of multiligament knee injuries is complex and depends on the number and type of ligaments torn.[29] Prior to any soft tissue reconstruction procedure, all vascular injuries should be assessed and addressed. Most authors recommend surgical reconstruction or repair of torn knee ligaments because nonoperative treatment has been shown to have poor outcomes. Treatment recommendations for specific patterns of injury have been proposed. Class I injuries (ACL + MCL) are generally treated with delayed ACL reconstruction because the MCL has fairly predictable healing potential. Class I injuries (ACL + LCL/PLC) are treated with cruciate ligament reconstruction and open PLC repair at 2 weeks to allow for capsular healing. Class II injuries are managed initially with a hinged knee brace. After 6 weeks, the PCL is reconstructed; in high-demand patients, concomitant ACL reconstruction is also performed. Class IIIM, IIIL, and IV multiligament knee injuries are also treated with surgical reconstruction and repair after a brief immobilization period. A shorter period of immobilization allows improved ROM, but residual laxity often results. A longer period of immobilization, in contrast, frequently yields better stability in exchange for limited ROM.

Why Might This Be Tested? Multiligament knee injuries frequently result from knee dislocation injuries and are commonly seen in orthopedic trauma centers. Many questions can arise from this topic, particularly as it relates to associated anatomy, classification, vascular injury, general treatment principles, and outcomes.

Here's the Point!

Be very suspicious of a prior knee dislocation in any patient who presents with a multiligament knee injury. Assessment of concomitant vascular injury is paramount and should take precedence over ligament injury evaluation. For testing purposes, early reconstruction can lead to less stiffness but more laxity; the converse is true of late reconstructions.

Vignette 10: Anterior Knee Pain in a Collegiate Basketball Player

A healthy 21-year-old male collegiate basketball player complains of anterior right knee pain. He has a history of prior knee pain with recurrent effusions. He has not experienced locking, catching, or feelings of instability. On physical exam, he was ligamentously intact and had a positive patellar grind test. AP and lateral knee x-rays failed to show any lesions or fracture. His MRI showed a lesion, and he underwent arthroscopic microfracture and debridement of this unipolar trochlear lesion without bone loss (Figures 10-1 to 10-3). At that time, a prophylactic cartilage biopsy was taken in case of future procedures. The patient is 1 year posttreatment with continued pain and effusions that are recalcitrant to nonoperative management.

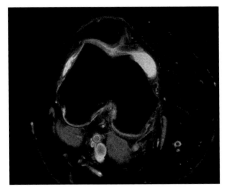

Figure 10-1. MRI of patient with a 3-cm irregular trochlear lesion, unipolar with no bone loss, and lateral maltracking of the patella.

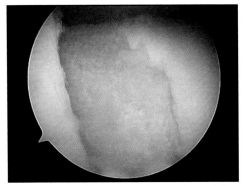

Figure 10-2. Arthroscopic picture of a trochlear defect after a thorough debridement.

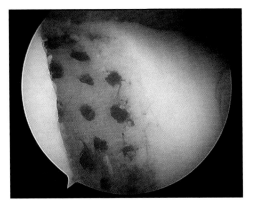

Figure 10-3. Arthroscopic picture of microfracture of the trochlear groove defect.

▶ *What other studies would you order?*

▶ *What are the available treatment options given this patient's age and lesion location?*

▶ *If the same injury was in other locations in the knee, how would this change your treatment?*

Vignette 10: Answer

The patient presents with symptoms of a unipolar chondral defect of the trochlea without bone loss. Imaging should begin with plain x-rays, including AP, flexion lateral, Rosenberg (45-degree flexed postero-anterior [PA]), mechanical axis, and axial patellar views. The usefulness of a CT scan is 2-fold because it can evaluate associated bone loss along with an abnormal tibial tubercle to trochlear groove distance (TT-TG). The presence of bone loss is a game changer and eliminates certain modalities as treatment options. In the setting of a patellofemoral lesion with a TT-TG distance greater than 20 mm,[30] one should consider a concurrent realignment procedure, such as anteromedialization. It has been shown that the TT-TG distance is more accurate than using the Q-angle described in the past. MRI is most commonly used because it allows evaluation of lesion size along with ligament and meniscus integrity. Although these studies are important, it is key to remember that arthroscopy is the gold standard for diagnosis and evaluation, which this patient has already undergone.

Ideal treatment should take into account patient age, occupation, activity level, joint alignment, ligamentous stability, meniscus status, and lesion characteristics. The latter include the size, depth, and amount of symptoms from the lesion. Depth of cartilage involvement is classified most commonly by the Outerbridge classification. The more active or high-demand a patient is, the more the practitioner should err on the side of a more durable and faster incorporating options (autologous chondrocyte implantation [ACI], osteochondral [OC] allograft, OC autograft).

In general, ACI is indicated in Outerbridge grade III or IV defects greater than 2 to 3 cm^2 without associated bone loss located on the femoral condyles, trochlea, and patella. The use of ACI on the patella is not currently approved by the Food and Drug Administration. The procedure requires 2 stages, the first involving a cartilage biopsy from the intercondylar notch and the second being reimplantation. Although the literature is varied, the outcomes tend to be good to excellent in 70% to 80% of patients.[31]

OC autograft transplantation is useful for Outerbridge grade III or IV defects less than 2 to 3 cm^2 with or without bone loss. The donor tissue is harvested from nonweight-bearing portions of the knee and is press-fit into the defect site. Larger defects may require implantation of multiple adjacent plugs. This method does not have the risk of disease transmission that accompanies OC allograft transplantation; however, it may result in donor site morbidity. Outcomes have been superior in the condyles, followed by the tibia and trochlea, with relative contraindication to patellar usage.[32]

OC allografts can be used for defects greater than 2 to 3 cm^2 with associated bone loss (typically seen in osteochondritis dissecans [OCD], osteonecrosis [ON], and trauma). Another important indication for OC allograft over ACI is a lesion that is not contained. Allografts allow for more accurate matching of surface topography and avoid the risk of donor site morbidity while adding the concern of disease transmission (< 1/1.6 million).[33] Results are good to excellent in about 85% of patients receiving OC allografts.[34]

Assuming these exams are normal and knowing the patient's meniscus and ligaments are intact via the physical exam and prior arthroscopy, the lesion characteristics should be taken into account. If the lesion is small (< 2 to 3 cm^2) and involves bone loss, then osteochondral autograft transfer is a good option. For larger lesions (> 2 to 3 cm^2) with or without bone loss, one should consider using an osteochondral allograft or ACI, respectively. These options are summarized in Table 10-1 and take into account lesion location, size, and depth. Given our healthy, active (high-demand), young patient with normal alignment, symptomatic cartilage defect that is 3 cm and irregular, and failed microfracture, ACI would be the treatment of choice.

Why Might This Be Tested? While the technology of treating cartilage lesions continues to evolve, taking into account a patient's physiologic age and predisposing factors will always be important. Lesions should be treated based on their location, size, and depth of involvement.

	Table 10-1.			
CARTILAGE DEFECT MANAGEMENT BASED ON DEFECT SIZE, GRADE, AND LOCATION				
Cartilage Procedure	Defect Size	Outerbridge Grade	Location	Other
Osteochondral autograft	<2 to 3 cm^2	III or IV	WB FC, T	Limited tissue available, donor site morbidity
Autologous chondrocyte implantation	>3 cm^2	III or IV	WB FC, T, P	Expensive, 2-stage
Osteochondral allograft	>3 cm^2	IV with bone loss	WB FC, T, P	Disease transmission
FC = femoral condyle; P = patella; T = tibia; WB = weight bearing.				

Here's the Point!

First-line treatment for lesions smaller than 2 to 3 cm^2 should be microfracture; if this fails, it should be ACI. For lesions larger than 2 to 3 cm^2, ACI is preferred for the patellofemoral joint and OC allograft is preferred for high-demand patients.

Vignette 11: Hip Pain After a Motor Vehicle Collision

A 23-year-old male is the restrained driver in a motor vehicle accident and is transferred to the emergency department, where he reports right hip pain. The primary survey reveals that the patient is stable. Your physical exam identifies a neutral-positioned right lower extremity with a palpable dorsalis pedis pulse and normal motor and sensory function in all distributions. Examination of the soft tissue is found to be without injury. An AP x-ray of the patient's pelvis is shown in Figure 11-1.

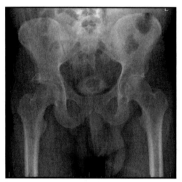

Figure 11-1. AP x-ray of the patient's pelvis.

▶ *What is the patient's underlying diagnosis?*

▶ *What is the mechanism for such an injury?*

▶ *Should any other x-rays be ordered?*

▶ *What associated injuries should clinical and radiographic evaluation address?*

In the emergency room, to further assess the patient's injury, Judet views are obtained (Figure 11-2) to help characterize the patient's injury. The patient is diagnosed with a posterior acetabular wall fracture. Following appropriate resuscitation, he underwent open reduction and internal fixation (ORIF).

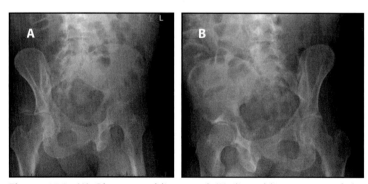

Figure 11-2. (A) Obturator oblique and (B) iliac oblique x-rays of the patient's injury.

▶ *What role does advanced imaging, particularly CT, play in assessing these injuries?*

▶ *What are common complications related to this class of injuries?*

Vignette 11: Answer

The underlying diagnosis in this case is a posterior wall acetabular fracture. The most widely used classification of acetabular fractures is that of Letournel and Judet (Table 11-1).[35] This system divides fractures of the acetabulum into 5 elementary and 5 associated patterns. The elementary patterns are defined as those that separate all or part of a single column of the acetabulum. The anterior and posterior column fractures separate the entire column from the intact innominate bone, whereas the anterior and posterior wall fractures separate only a portion of the column's articular surface. The integrity of the obturator foramen and ischiopubic ramus may aid the surgeon in making this distinction. Also included in the elementary patterns are transverse acetabular fractures that disrupt the anterior and posterior column.

Table 11-1.	
LETOURNEL ACETABULAR CLASSIFICATION	
Simple Type Fractures	*Associated Type Fractures*
Anterior column Anterior wall	T-type
Posterior column Posterior wall	Transverse + posterior wall Posterior column + posterior wall
Transverse	Anterior + posterior hemitransverse Both columns

Radiographic assessment of acetabular fractures includes AP, iliac oblique, obturator oblique, inlet, and outlet images to characterize the fracture pattern and evaluate for joint displacement; the inlet and outlet views allow the surgeon to assess for pelvic injuries that may affect acetabular injury management and are not routinely obtained. CT scans, particularly the axial sections, have a distinct advantage in showing the site and degree of displacement of fractures, their orientation in these dimensions, the relationship of small fragments, the amount of articular surface involvement (beware of the marginal impaction—crushing of the posterior acetabular articular), and whether loose bodies reside within the joint. Three-dimensional (3D) reconstructions may help to better understand the fracture pattern and delineate any rotational deformity.

Upon initial evaluation, a careful and thorough examination documenting complete neurologic assessment of the patient (including rectal exam, reflexes, and full motor and sensation testing) and lower extremity soft tissue integrity (beware the dreaded Morel-Lavallée lesion—a closed degloving injury, with the skin and subcutaneous tissues being stripped off of the underlying fascia, allowing for a blood-filled cavity to form) in the trochanteric and gluteal regions, and resting position of the lower extremity should be completed. The sciatic nerve, which is injured in up to 20% of acetabular fractures affecting the posterior wall or column, should be carefully examined in motor and sensory distributions. Because the peroneal division is at risk for stretch injury, foot dorsiflexion and eversion must be tested.

In general, acetabular fractures occur as a result of a severe force to the femur that is transmitted through the femoral neck, resulting in femoral head impaction against the acetabulum; the magnitude and force vector impacting the acetabulum determines the resultant fracture pattern. Commonly, in the setting of a head-on motor vehicle collision, the knee strikes the dashboard, resulting in a proximally directed force that potentially results in acetabular injury. By virtue of the mechanism, the potential for patella fracture, chondral injuries, knee ligamentous injuries, and femoral neck fracture should also be kept in mind when evaluating any patient with an acetabular fracture resulting from a dashboard-type injury. The pelvic CT used to assess the acetabular injury often extends to the proximal femur; these images should be carefully reviewed to help identify subtle fractures of the femoral neck prior to proceeding to the operating suite.

There are several known complications. The primary complication following acetabular fracture is posttraumatic arthrosis. Long-term studies demonstrate that articular reductions within 1 mm of displacement have a better long-term outcome and a lower incidence of arthritis compared with those with greater than 1 mm of residual displacement.[36]

Injury of the sciatic nerve associated with acetabular fracture occurs most often when the femoral head is dislocated posteriorly. Iatrogenic nerve palsy, however, is caused almost exclusively by prolonged retraction of the sciatic nerve. This most often occurs through a Kocher-Langenbeck approach and primarily affects the peroneal division. To reduce the risk for such injury, tension to the sciatic nerve is minimized by flexing the knee at least 60 degrees and maintaining the hip in an extended position. Traumatic and iatrogenic nerve injuries to the sciatic nerve are most often a form of axonotmesis. If a nerve palsy develops, an ankle-foot orthosis (AFO) is used because some nerve function recovery is expected in the first year.

Heterotopic ossification (HO) is another complication related to the degree of soft tissue disruption from the injury or the surgical approach utilized. Prophylactic treatments for HO include indomethacin for 6 weeks, low-dose external radiotherapy (single dose, 700 to 800 cgy, can be given pre- or postoperatively), or a combination of both. Finally, ON of the femoral head may occur following fracture-dislocation. Immediate reduction of the hip decreases the rate of ON.

Why Might This Be Tested? Numerous aspects of an acetabular fracture may be tested, including fracture pattern identification based on x-rays, an axial CT section of the acetabulum, surgical approach used to complete ORIF, and complications related to injury and surgical intervention.

Here's the Point!

Acetabular fractures are high-energy injuries diagnosed with x-rays. High suspicion should be held for associated injuries, including soft tissue, neurologic, and bony injuries. Correctly characterizing the fracture pattern allows for the correct surgical approach to allow for anatomic reduction. Posttraumatic arthritis is the most common complication.

Vignette 12: Pedestrian Struck and Sustains an Open Leg Fracture

A 27-year-old female pedestrian is struck by a motor vehicle. Comprehensive trauma evaluation reveals an isolated injury to the right lower leg. AP and lateral x-rays show a proximal third metadiaphyseal fracture of the tibia with comminuted fibula fracture at the same level. There is 20-degree apex anterior and 30-degree apex medial angulation with 2 cm of shortening. She is comfortable and neurovascularly intact with palpable pulses and has no pain with passive stretch of her toes. There is a 3-cm open wound over the tibial crest with an exposed tibia.

▶ *What is the first sign of compartment syndrome?*

▶ *What Gustilo-Anderson type is this fracture, and how should the local soft tissues be treated?*

▶ *What radiographic parameters allow for cast treatment of a stable tibial shaft fracture?*

The patient is taken to the operating room for definitive management.

▶ *What are your operative treatment options?*

▶ *What deformity is expected in proximal metadiaphyseal tibia fractures, and what reduction methods may be used in its prevention?*

Irrigation and debridement with definitive closure and IM nailing of the tibia are performed without complication.

▶ *How long until union of this fracture occurs?*

Vignette 12: Answer

The first sign of compartment syndrome is pain out of proportion to the injury. Decreased sensation and pain with passive stretch of muscles in the affected compartment are the best early signs of compartment syndrome. Other common exam findings include paresthesia/hypoesthesia, paralysis, palpable swelling, and absent pulses. Diagnosis is clinical, while a measured ΔP (ΔP = diastolic pressure − intracompartmental pressure) less than 30 mm Hg may serve as a diagnostic adjunct in equivocal cases or in cases in which clinical exam is impossible or unreliable. Treatment is emergent for compartment fasciotomy.[37]

This is a type II Gustilo-Anderson open fracture. See Table 12-1 for complete classification.[38] (Wound size is not really that important in defining the type of open fracture; it's really more about energy, periosteum, and overall soft tissues, not the wound length.) All patients with open fractures should receive tetanus prophylaxis, intravenous (IV) antibiotics, and irrigation and debridement of the open fracture. Historic recommendations for specific antibiotic use and timing of irrigation and debridement have recently been challenged. The previous standard was for a first-generation cephalosporin, adding an aminoglycoside for higher grade and a clostridial species–specific antibiotic for farmyard injuries. The timing of irrigation and debridement for type I injuries may be delayed until the following morning because evidence does not mandate emergent management. Most surgeons feel that type II or III or any grossly contaminated wound should be treated with urgent surgical irrigation and debridement.

Table 12-1.		
GUSTILO-ANDERSON CLASSIFICATION		
Type	Wound	Note
I	<1 cm	
II	1 to 10 cm	
IIIA	>10 cm	Does not need soft tissue coverage
IIIB	>10 cm	Needs soft tissue coverage
IIIC	Any size	Vascular injury requiring repair present

Primary closure of open wounds may be performed at the surgeon's discretion. Minimal to noncontaminated wounds may be closed at the index procedure, whereas grossly contaminated wounds require serial debridement with or without local antibiotic delivery and/or negative pressure wound therapy. When the open wound is unable to be closed primarily, adjunctive procedures, such as skin grafting with or without rotational muscle flap coverage, fasciocutaneous flap, or free tissue transfer, must be considered. The timing of coverage is largely dictated by the wound and fracture stability. Every attempt should be made to provide definitive fracture stability prior to soft tissue coverage to allow for uninterrupted soft tissue healing. Definitive coverage should be performed as soon as possible but ideally within 7 to 10 days because infection rates and flap failures increase with increasing coverage time.

Coronal plane deformity less than 5 degrees, sagittal plane deformity less than 10 degrees, malrotation less than 5 degrees, and shortening less than 1 cm allow for nonoperative treatment of a tibial shaft fracture, whether through cast treatment or functional bracing.

IM nail, plate, and external fixation have all been used successfully for tibia fractures. External fixation may be used in the setting of a narrow canal diameter (<8 mm), excessive contamination, severe open fractures, open physes, and complex periarticular injury. Plate fixation may be preferred in proximal or distal metadiaphyseal fractures, especially with articular extension or when access to the IM canal may be compromised. Nail fixation is preferred in diaphyseal fractures to prevent soft tissue and periosteal stripping, blood supply disruption, and wound breakdown/infection. When external fixation is chosen as initial management, conversion to a definitive IM nail should be performed within 28 days to reduce the chance of secondary infection from contaminated pin tracts.

Proximal metadiaphyseal tibia fractures tend to present in procurvatum, posterior translation, and valgus deformity secondary to the pull of the extensor mechanism and hamstrings insertion on the proximal tibia. A more vertical and lateral start point, coupled with a semiextended knee position, will allow for good control of the tibial deformity. Blocking screws enable control of IM nail placement, particularly at the proximal and distal tibia, where a nail-to-cortical-diameter mismatch exists. In the proximal fragment, typical blocking screw placement is lateral in the coronal plane and posterior in the sagittal plane (this may vary depending on the fracture location and angular deformity). Anterior unicortical plates may be used for provisional fixation prior to reaming and IM nail placement, especially in the setting of an open wound.

Average time to union in a nonoperatively treated tibia fracture is 26 weeks vs 18 weeks in those treated with an IM nail. Some have advocated for bone grafting at 8 to 10 weeks if little to no callus is seen and low-intensity pulsed ultrasound has been used successfully in nonoperatively treated closed tibia fractures to increase healing times. Adjuncts to healing, such as bone morphogenetic protein, have not shown differences in healing rates or time to union in open tibia fractures treated with a reamed nail. Smoking and NSAIDs have been shown to increase healing time.

Why Might This Be Tested? Open fractures frequently occur, and the type is often tested. Appropriate management of tibial shaft fractures and potential sequelae are commonly handled problems by many orthopedists. Recognizing compartment syndrome is important, and the definition and ability to recognize this injury are common test questions.

Here's the Point!

Compartment syndrome requires urgent recognition and emergent fasciotomies. Open fractures are not based on the length of the wound but more the associated soft tissue damage and energy absorbed during the injury. Understand the deforming forces on tibial shaft fractures because this will help with reduction and fixation techniques.

Vignette 13: The Back of My Knee Swelled Up After My Pregnancy

A 34-year-old female reports an area of fullness in the posterior aspect of her knee. She can palpate this area and feels tightness when she moves the knee into deep flexion. It is occasionally painful, but she is still able to perform activities of daily living. She first noticed it 2 years ago and states that it enlarged during her most recent pregnancy. It does not limit her knee ROM. Plain x-rays appear normal. MRI slices and a histology slide are shown in Figures 13-1 to 13-3.

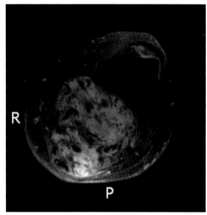

Figure 13-1. Axial T2-weighted knee MRI.

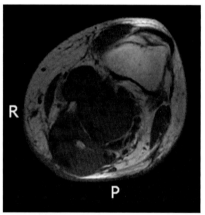

Figure 13-2. Axial T1-weighted knee MRI.

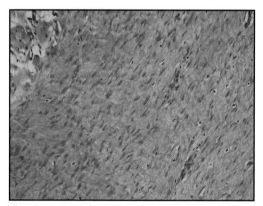

Figure 13-3. High-power photograph of the biopsy specimen (200× magnification).

▶ *What is the diagnosis?*

▶ *What are the treatment options?*

Vignette 13: Answer

Aggressive fibromatosis, or a desmoid tumor, is an infiltrative neoplasm arising from the deep soft tissues. It is a benign entity, without potential for distant metastasis, but it can be extremely aggressive locally with a high recurrence rate after attempted excision. In some cases, local extension can result in the need for amputation and even death. The tumors can present at any age (test questions often describe a patient between the teenage years and 40 years old). In patients between puberty and 40 years old, the incidence is 2 to 3 times higher in females, and the abdominal wall is a common site. In older adults, the tumors are split equally between abdominal and extra-abdominal sites of disease. The most common extra-abdominal locations are the shoulder, chest wall, back, thigh, and head and neck. Some associated conditions include palmar and plantar fibromatosis (ie, Dupuytren's and Ledderhose, respectively).

Clinically, these present as slow-growing, deep, usually painless lesions. They often feel as hard as a rock on palpation and may be varying sizes. Typically, the borders of the mass are poorly defined on exam. The tumors are occasionally multifocal. Rarely, patients will have neurological compression or reduced joint motion depending on the location of the lesion. Women can have new lesions present during pregnancy or in the first year after childbirth.

There are many factors that may be associated with desmoid tumors. Evidence for a genetic component (possibly a trisomy of chromosomes 8 or 20) to the disease is suggested by familial cases and their association with Gardner's syndrome (a variant of familial adenomatous polyposis). Endocrine factors, specifically high estrogen levels, likely contribute to their appearance around gestation and response to hormonal therapy. Posttraumatic responses and prior surgery are also thought to contribute.

Radiographically, a desmoid tumor usually presents as a multilobulated soft tissue mass that has a heterogeneous low signal on T1- and T2-weighted sequences. There are occasionally areas of relative T2 hyperintensity. They often infiltrate between and around structures, such as muscle, tendon, nerves, and vessels, making treatment difficult. Because they tend to be slow growing, they usually do not instigate a significant inflammatory reaction.

Histologically, the microscopic borders of the tumor are poorly defined due to its infiltrative nature. The spindle cells are uniform, lack atypia, and are found in a collagenous stroma. The lesions can be quite cellular and often have a storiform, whorled appearance over a collagen stroma. The tumors stain strongly positive for vimentin, beta-catenin, and estrogen receptor-beta.

Treatment is required in progressive lesions and tumors that threaten vital structures (brachial plexus, spinal cord). Some tumors may be slow growing or have an extended period of latency, necessitating minimal intervention other than continued monitoring. In active lesions, surgical excision, chemotherapy, hormonal treatment, and radiation therapy are all viable options. There is no agreed-upon regimen for the treatment of desmoids, but a multidisciplinary approach is recommended. The poorly defined clinical and histological borders translate into difficulty with complete surgical excision. An attempt at wide margins can cause significant morbidity and result in a high rate of local recurrence. Over time, the indications and recommendations for an extensive, disfiguring surgery have diminished. When lesser margins are obtained, typically to preserve vital structures or overall function, radiation is typically used in addition to surgery. Radiation treatment alone has also been shown to have similar local control rates to surgery and to surgery plus radiation in some studies. Medical management focuses on interventions that are well tolerated with an acceptable response. Options include low-dose chemotherapy, hormonal therapy (tamoxifen), and NSAIDs (through cyclooxygenase inhibition). Regardless of the treatment, most reported local control rates for nonrecurrent disease are 70% to 80%.

Why Might This Be Tested? This is a painless tumor that grows rapidly at times. When described in vignettes, it can easily be mistaken for a malignant tumor. The association with Dupuytren's and familial adenomatous polyposis allows for a good tie for a vignette.

Here's the Point!

Fibromatosis is a benign, aggressive tumor with no risk of metastasis or malignant transformation. It is typically a rock-hard, enlarging, palpable mass. Wide resection is typically chosen for surgical management with adjunctive radiotherapy. Nonoperative treatment can be tamoxifen and NSAIDs.

Vignette 14: I Think I May Have a Baker's Cyst

A 32-year-old female presents with a painless mass in her posterior thigh. She first noticed it 4 months ago and thinks that it has enlarged. She has no history of trauma or previous injuries. She has no systemic symptoms (weight loss, fevers, chills, etc). This was discovered when clothing was noted to be tighter on one leg compared with the other. MRIs and a histology image of the mass are shown in Figures 14-1 to 14-3.

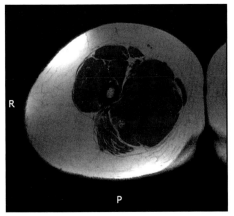

Figure 14-1. Axial T1-weighted MRI showing the thigh mass.

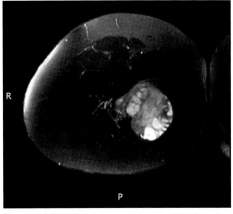

Figure 14-2. Axial T2-weighted MRI showing the thigh mass.

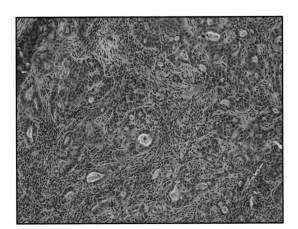

Figure 14-3. Histological specimen of the tumor (200× magnification).

▶ *What is the differential diagnosis?*

▶ *What are the treatment options?*

▶ *Compare and contrast pre- and postoperative radiation therapy.*

Vignette 14: Answer

Soft tissue sarcoma is estimated to affect more than 10,000 people in the United States each year, with the majority of these occurring in the extremities. Although the prognosis depends on stage and grade, roughly one-third of all patients will die from the tumor. The most common site of spread is to the lungs, representing around 80% of all distant metastases. Most sarcomas occur spontaneously, but exposure to external beam radiation increases the risk of the formation of a secondary sarcoma in the irradiated field.

Most patients present with a history of a painless enlarging mass, with 60% of lesions found in the extremities. Soft tissue sarcomas, such as undifferentiated pleomorphic sarcoma and liposarcoma, usually involve older adults, whereas rhabdomyosarcoma is common in children. Synovial sarcoma and epithelioid sarcoma typically affect young adults.

These patients are best treated with a systematic approach to diagnosis. Initially, a physical exam is necessary to determine mass size (< or >5 cm), depth (above or below the investing muscle fascia), and character (firm, tender, soft, fluctuant) and whether the mass is fixed to the bone. By having the patient actively move the limb, the clinician may tell the depth of the lesion. A superficial tumor will not move as the muscles are engaged, whereas a deep lesion may move or become less prominent. Red flags concerning for a malignancy are size larger than 5 cm, deep to the muscle fascia, painful, and growing. Tumors may be distinguished clinically from hematomas by the absence of ecchymosis (tumors are typically contained, whereas hematomas spread out of and around tissue planes). Abscesses can have a similar presentation; they are commonly painful, erythematous, and fluctuant. There is often a history of fever, constitutional symptoms, or penetrating trauma. Location of the tumor can help with the diagnosis because alveolar cell sarcoma is more commonly found in the anterior thigh and synovial cell sarcoma in the posterior region.

X-rays of the area may be helpful in certain types of tumors. Synovial sarcoma can present with calcifications in roughly 20% of cases. Hemangiomas may display characteristic calcified phleboliths. Extraosseous osteosarcoma and chondrosarcoma (CHS) are rare, yet they also display radiographic findings consistent with mineralization. The most detailed and helpful study is MRI with and without contrast. Most malignancies will be bright on T2 sequences, relatively darker on T1 sequences, and enhanced in postcontrast images. Areas of heterogeneity are worrisome because they are indicative of hemorrhage and necrosis characteristic of more aggressive pathology.

The most common soft tissue tumor is a benign lipoma. This can be easily diagnosed on MRI because each sequence (including fat suppression) has the appearance of subcutaneous fat and is completely homogeneous. When the tumors grow to larger than 5 cm, they appear identical to well-differentiated liposarcoma and should be excised or watched closely. Needle biopsy has little use in homogeneous, lipomatous neoplasms.

The staging of soft tissue sarcoma consists of some type of pulmonary imaging, usually with a CT scan in higher-grade lesions. Lymph nodes should also be examined, although lymph node spread is not typical for most sarcomas. The exceptions include synovial sarcoma, epithelioid sarcoma, angiosarcoma, rhabdomyosarcoma, and clear cell sarcoma (vignettes often include these data to help guide your diagnosis in tumors that spread to the lymph nodes). Myxoid liposarcoma has an unusual pattern of metastasis to the bone and retroperitoneum, and some advocate bone scans and CTs of the chest, abdomen, and pelvis on these patients.

The final step in diagnosis is a tissue biopsy. This can be performed as a core needle or open biopsy, but in either case, it should be performed in line with the incision for a definitive resection so it may be easily excised without compromising the limb. Fine-needle aspiration is usually not sufficient for diagnosis. Referral to a tertiary care center should be made prior to biopsy of a suspected malignancy, whether it is bone or soft tissue.

The hematoxylin-eosin stain for this case (synovial sarcoma, the most common sarcoma of the foot) shows a biphasic population of atypical spindle cells and epithelial cells forming glands with central lumina. The epithelial cells have ovoid nuclei with abundant cytoplasm. Synovial sarcoma is associated with a translocation at X:18 (found on cytogenetic analysis), producing the proto-oncogene SYT-SSX. Go ahead, try to memorize that!

Chemotherapy is controversial for many soft tissue sarcomas, but it is considered for synovial sarcoma in large lesions and healthy patients. External beam radiation is a mainstay of treatment in large, deep, high-grade sarcomas when a wide excision is not possible or desired. For example, when a major peripheral nerve is immediately adjacent to the tumor, a wide excision would require resection of the nerve and compromise the function of the limb. Radiation can be delivered pre- or postoperatively. There has never been any proven significant difference in local recurrence or survival between the 2 methods. Preoperative radiation uses a smaller dose and field, but it is associated with a substantially higher rate of wound complications. Postoperative radiation is associated with more long-term local consequences, such as limb edema and joint stiffness. Surgical resection, with or without adjuvant therapy, is the accepted treatment of nonmetastatic soft tissue sarcoma.

Prognosis of stage I disease (low grade) is good, with a 90% 5-year survival. Stage II and III (high-grade) have 5-year survivals closer to 50% to 70%. Stage IV (metastatic disease) has a 5-year survival of 15%. The treatment of choice of an isolated pulmonary metastasis is surgical excision because there is a survival benefit if the lesion can be completely excised. Chemotherapy and radiation may be used in palliation.

Why Might This Be Tested? Soft tissue sarcomas are often on the tests because there is much overlap between the various entities. Furthermore, there is a systematic approach to diagnosis, treatment, and overall prognosis of these tumors.

Here's the Point!

Soft tissue sarcomas often metastasize to the lungs and have a high mortality rate. Correct diagnosis, staging, and management will afford the best chance for survival. Synovial cell sarcoma is a highly malignant tumor that typically arises outside of the adjacent joint (despite its name implying it is an intra-articular structure). It typically has a biphasic histologic appearance, 30% to 60% will metastasize, and treatment is wide surgical resection and radiotherapy.

Vignette 15: What's Wrong With My Kid's Posture?

A 15-year-old female who started menstruating 1 year ago presents after a school physical that noted a little curve in her back. Her mom has noticed that her posture has changed over the past few years, and the patient states that her breasts are asymmetric, which has bothered her. She reports back pain when she carries her backpack and has even switched to using a rolling backpack at times. She has no family history of scoliosis, has no other medical problems, and has met all developmental milestones on time. Upon consultation with a spine surgeon, a full radiographic series of her spine was conducted. An AP x-ray is shown in Figure 15-1. The patient and her family want to know about the risk of progression and the treatment that you recommend.

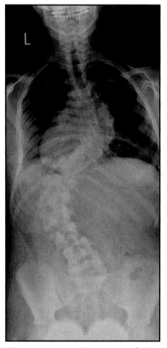

Figure 15-1. AP x-ray of the thoracolumbar spine.

▶ *What is the recommended treatment at this time?*

Vignette 15: Answer

Children are typically screened during well exams or for sports physicals, with a good screening tool being the scoliometer (threshold of 7 degrees). Things that typically warrant referral are shoulder elevation, trunk shift, limb-length inequality, rib hump, and asymmetry of the hips at the waist. Natural history studies of adolescent idiopathic scoliosis have been reported in the literature. Progression is defined as a 5- to 10-degree increase in deformity from time of presentation. The highest risk for progression is during the peak growth spurt. In girls, the peak growth spurt occurs around Tanner stage 2, which typically occurs around age 10 to 12 years. Menarche occurs 1.5 to 2 years after the onset of this growth spurt. In boys, the onset of this rapid growth spurt occurs during Tanner stage 2 or 3, which correspond to the chronological age of 11 to 15 years.

Lonstein and Carlson[39] correlated Risser stages with rates of curve progression. Risser sign is assessed radiographically by looking at the ossification of the iliac apophysis. Ossification occurs in a lateral-to-medial direction. Stage 1 is when 25% of the bony cap has formed, stage 2 is when 50% has formed, stage 3 is when 75% has formed, stage 4 is when 100% has formed, and stage 5 is when the space between the cap and the pelvis fills in completely with bone.

For curves of 20 to 29 degrees in a child with Risser sign 0 or 1, the risk of progression was 68%. For curves less than 19 degrees with Risser 2 or more, the risk was 1.6%. For curves less than 19 degrees in children with Risser 0 or 1 and in children with Risser 2 or more with curves 20 to 29 degrees, the risk of progression was approximately 22% (Table 15-1).[39]

Table 15-1.		
RISSER STAGES		
Risk Progression	*Risser 0 or 1*	*Risser 2 or More*
20 to 29 degrees	68%	22%
0 to 19 degrees	22%	1.6%

Because of this fact, the treatment algorithm of adolescent idiopathic scoliosis depends on risk of progression. For patients at Risser 0 or 1 and curves between 10 to 20 degrees, close observation is warranted. X-rays should be obtained every 6 to 12 months until skeletal maturity to detect progression. Curves between 20 and 30 degrees should be followed more closely, with x-rays being taken more frequently. Bracing is indicated for skeletally immature patients with curves between 30 and 45 degrees or an immature patient with a curve greater than 25 degrees but with documented progression. Bracing may be less beneficial in adolescent males than females, most likely due to poor compliance. The goal of bracing is to minimize curve progression to hopefully less than 5 degrees. Part-time bracing can be effective in some patients, but, in general, full-time bracing has better published results (the more you wear the brace, the better!).

Surgery is indicated in idiopathic scoliosis in progressive curves greater than 40 to 45 degrees in growing children, failure of bracing, and progressive curves beyond 50 degrees in adults. In this case, the patient was recommended for surgery.

Beyond the scope of this question is classification of idiopathic scoliosis. The old classification, King classification, has been replaced by the Lenke classification.[40] There are 6 major types. Type 1 is a main thoracic curve, type 2 is double thoracic, type 3 is double major with the thoracic greater than lumbar, type 5 is thoracolumbar, and type 6 is a double major with the lumbar curve greater than the thoracic. The typical double major curve is a right thoracic and left lumbar curve. If a patient has the opposite, it may warrant a spine MRI to rule out any pathological condition, such as tethered cord or congenital abnormalities.

Why Might This Be Tested? Understanding the natural history of scoliosis is important in order to develop an intelligent and rational treatment program. This is a common disorder, and the algorithms for management are relatively set in stone. You just have to know this material.

Here's the Point!

Predicting the risk of progression determines the treatment of idiopathic scoliosis. Typically, curves progress the most during rapid adolescent skeletal growth. Structural curves may require frequent radiographic follow-up, while others require bracing to control the curve or surgical fusion. Criteria used to decide if surgery is warranted relates to the Weinstein et al[35] landmark study, which found that curves tended to progress if greater than 50 degrees in the thoracic or lumbar spine.

Vignette 16: Middle-Aged Man With a Crooked Knee

A 57-year-old male presents with chronic right knee pain. About 25 years prior, he underwent a procedure to remove torn cartilage. This procedure provided him with several years of relief, until about 4 or 5 years ago when he began having medial-sided pain with strenuous activity. Over the past year or so, the pain has become constant, worse with prolonged standing, walking, and ascending/descending stairs. The pain is now diffuse in nature and is most severe on the medial side of his knee. About 1 year ago, his primary care physician administered an intra-articular corticosteroid injection that resulted in about 3 months of partial relief. Two weeks ago, he was given a repeat injection that worked for only a couple of hours. Figure 16-1 shows the latest x-rays taken in the office.

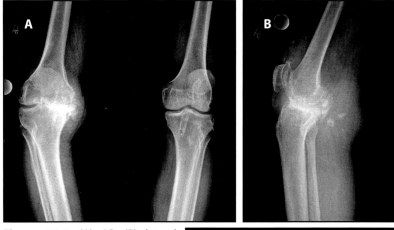

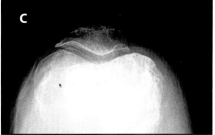

Figure 16-1. (A) AP, (B) lateral, and (C) Merchant's views showing advanced OA with a varus malalignment.

▶ *What is the diagnosis?*

▶ *What nonoperative treatments are available?*

▶ *What are potential surgical options?*

▶ *What sequence of steps should be performed to create coronal balance of a varus knee when performing TKA?*

▶ *What is the best fixation option for components in this case?*

Vignette 16: Answer

This patient has tricompartmental knee OA, most severe on the medial side, with a varus coronal plane deformity. Varus deformities are the most common anatomic deviation encountered in TKA and are generally defined as an anatomic coronal alignment of less than 4 degrees of valgus (neutral being 4 to 9 degrees of valgus). He most likely had a prior open medial meniscectomy, which has been associated with accelerated medial compartment arthritis (as has ACL insufficiency).[41]

The AAOS has established guidelines for the nonoperative treatment of OA of the knee.[42] The authors note sufficient data to support the use of acetaminophen, NSAIDs, and corticosteroid injections for temporary pain relief. Corticosteroid injections have been shown to have decreasing efficacy with repeat injections. The fact that this patient received a couple of hours of relief is important in that it confirms intra-articular placement of the injection. Other nonoperative interventions recommended include weight loss in patients with a BMI greater than 25 kg/m^2, low-impact aerobic exercises, aquatic exercise, and quadriceps strengthening.[42,43] Additional guidelines have conditionally recommended the following to manage osteoarthritic pain: medial wedge inserts (valgus), subtalar strapped lateral inserts (varus), patellar taping, walking aids, hot/cold therapy, and psychosocial interventions.[43]

TKA is the only surgical procedure that is indicated for this patient. Arthroscopy in the setting of advanced arthritis is ineffective.[44] UKA is contraindicated given the degree of lateral and patellofemoral arthritis present.[45] The generally accepted sequence to balance a varus knee involves the following:

1. Removal of osteophytes from proximal medial tibia and distal medial femur
2. Deep MCL release
3. Semimembranosus release (posteromedial release)
4. Superficial MCL release
5. PCL release (may contribute to the deforming force)

More recently, the possibility of "pie crusting" the MCL has been evaluated in 65 cases. The authors found adequate correction (2 to 4 mm and 2 to 6 mm of correction in extension and flexion, respectively) in 95% of cases.[46]

Despite the young age of the patient, the gold standard at this time remains a cemented TKA. Recent strategies using highly porous metal structures have been used to emphasize the potential benefits of cementless TKA, which include a simplified surgical procedure, bone conservation, biologic fixation, limited third-body debris, and decreased operative time. Morbid obesity, osteoporotic bone, loss of early fixation, and residual coronal deformity can lead to early failure of cementless TKAs. Careful patient selection and surgical technique are required to make cementless TKA successful. Traditionally, the tibial component has been the culprit for early failure; however, recent concerns have been raised regarding femoral fixation with certain implant designs (do not coat pegs of the femur that can cause anterior stress shielding).

Why Might This Be Tested? Varus DJD is the most common deformity TKA surgeons face. Accepted forms of nonoperative management are becoming more important prior to replacement with current state legislation. In addition, modern techniques for medial release are being explored.

Here's the Point!

Varus knee alignment often leads to subsequent TKA. Cemented TKA is the gold standard for primary surgery at this time. Medial release can be managed systematically or via a "pie crusting" technique.

Vignette 17: Hey Doc, What's the Best Implant for My TKA?

A 67-year-old male with advanced DJD and varus deformity of his right knee presents to your office for a second opinion for a TKA. The patient is well educated and has conducted a substantial amount of research on the currently available options for knee replacements. As a mechanical engineer by trade, he is interested in the specific mechanics and kinematics of the implant designs and has a significant number of questions regarding his potential upcoming surgery. The following are a series of questions proposed by the patient that he would like to review prior to considering having a TKA.

▶ *What's the PCL and what does it do?*

▶ *What are the differences between posterior-stabilized (PS) and cruciate-retaining (CR) TKAs?*

▶ *What are the common arguments for retaining the PCL?*

▶ *What are the common arguments for substituting for the PCL?*

▶ *Have there been conclusive data to support one design (PS or CR) over another in standard primary TKA?*

Vignette 17: Answer

What's the PCL and what does it do? The PCL has a fan-shaped origin on the femur extending from the anterolateral aspect of the medial femoral condyle. The insertion lies on the posterior tibial plateau and extends along the posterior proximal tibia for about 1 cm. The PCL functions as a restraint against posterior translation of the tibia.[47] There are 2 bundles associated with the PCL: the anterolateral portion is tight in flexion and the posteromedial fibers are tight in extension. In conjunction with the ACL, the 2 cruciate ligaments guide femoral rollback in the native knee.

What are the differences between PS and CR TKAs? In a CR TKA design, the PCL becomes taut in flexion and causes the femur to roll back on the tibial component, allowing flexion past 90 degrees by preventing impingement of the posterior femoral cortex on the posterior tibial plateau. However, in the absence of an ACL, some of this motion is a sliding force, not just pure rolling. Initial designs used a flat polyethylene surface to accommodate this motion. Unfortunately, the flat polyethylene surface led to small femoral-polyethylene contact areas and subsequent high-contact stresses (an important concept—the lower the total area of contact the greater the forces generated in the specific area being loaded). More congruent polyethylene designs have been developed, and although there is increased constraint inherent in such a system, the contact stresses are lower, and the PCL is more a static stabilizer.

In a TKA in which the PCL has been removed, there are 2 implant designs that can be used: a substituting and nonsubstituting TKA. With a PS (substituting) design, the surgeon sacrifices the PCL and replaces it with a polyethylene component with a post. A polyethylene tibial post engages a cam on the femoral component, creating a mechanical source of femoral rollback. This mechanical rollback allows a more conforming polyethylene and lower contact stresses. In cases of PCL sacrificing but no substitution, an ultracongruent polyethylene is used to direct rollback. In such cases, the advantages of sacrificing the PCL are realized without the downsides of having a cam-post mechanism (post fracture/wear, caused by hyperextension with a flexed femoral component; jumping the post, knee dislocation from being too loose in flexion).[48]

What are the common arguments for retaining or substituting the PCL? Proponents of the CR design often report evidence of improved motion, proprioception, and a more natural-feeling knee. In addition, there is less stress transfer to the tibial component (possibly lower long-term rates of loosening), it is more bone preserving, and avoids complications associated with a tibial post. A report suggested that CR knees may have an improved survival rate.[49] Proponents of a PS design point to conflicting data that demonstrate no improvement in ROM or proprioception and some studies that have demonstrated more consistent and reproducible mechanics in the PS design. The knee is easier to balance without the PCL, it is an easier approach to teach, and there is no concern about late PCL rupture. In addition, 3 scenarios exist in which a PS is the answer you are being guided toward on the test (despite being challenged clinically at this time and not necessarily espoused by the author): prior patellectomy patients, inflammatory arthropathy, and absence of an intact PCL.

Have there been conclusive data to support one design (PS or CR) over another in standard primary TKA? The choice to use a CR or PS TKA design remains controversial without conclusive evidence in support of either design.[50-52] If placed in satisfactory alignment with good balance in the correct patient, either design will work quite well.

Why Might This Be Tested? Management of the cruciate has long been debated, and there are several good topics to question in this genre. Despite the controversy, there are several pathways for questions to head with this topic.

Here's the Point!

The PCL functions to aid in femoral rollback and prevent anterior translation of the femur on the tibia. There are 3 options with TKA: CR, PCL sacrificing, and PCL substituting. All work well when the surgical technique is meticulous.

Vignette 18: I Saw This Ad for a THA, and I Want That One!

An 85-year-old female presents to your office with progressively worsening right hip pain. She has tried all forms of nonoperative management over the last 5 years, and her activities of daily living are severely limited by the pain. She is set on having a right THA at this time and wants to discuss her options and what type of implants you use. She has seen several advertisements for recalled components and she specifically wants to understand your technique. Her medical history is significant for hypertension and osteoporosis. A preoperative x-ray is shown in Figure 18-1.

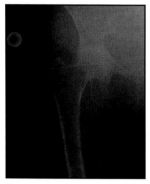

Figure 18-1. AP x-ray of the right hip.

▶ *How would you classify her bone quality/structure?*

▶ *Based on her history and bone structure, what type of THA is best indicated?*

The patient undergoes a successful THA (Figure 18-2).

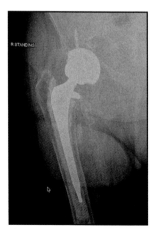

Figure 18-2. Postoperative x-ray after successful THA.

▶ *Describe the evolution of cementation in THA.*

▶ *How would you grade this cement mantle? Is this an important finding?*

Vignette 18: Answer

Using the Dorr classification (A, champagne flute proximal femur; B, funnel-shaped bone morphology; and C, cylindrical or stove pipe appearance), this bone can be described as a type C.[53] Furthermore, the bone quality appears osteoporotic (looks weak and osteopenic), with thin cortices noted preoperatively. With thin, osteoporotic bone in the proximal femur, the choice of a cemented stem is reasonable; on the cup side, cementless acetabular components are favored (so-called *hybrid technique*). Excellent results have been reported with hybrid THA, whereas fully cemented surgery has fallen out of favor. The shear forces on the acetabulum and difficulty in getting a dry bed of bone led to early failure of cemented acetabuli, particularly metal-backed cemented cups (when you see this on x-rays, the cup is always loose!).

Bone cement is composed of polymethylmethacrylate and was championed by Charnley in the 1960s. The cement acts only as a grout and really has no adhesive properties (essentially, the stems are loose in the cement mantle and are held axially and rotationally stable by the cement mantle). The process of cementing a component in place has evolved through various generations:

- First generation: Finger packing of cement, no canal preparation, sharp edges on stem, and no pressurization

- Second generation: Cement gun, canal prepared (cleaned and dried), cement restrictor, round stem edges

- Third generation: Vacuum mixing, cement pressurization, stem centralizer used

    o Vacuum mixing reduces porosity and has fewer voids; however, early on, the cement may reduce in volume compared with hand mixing. The long-term benefit of reduced porosity outweighs the early volume contraction.

    o Cement should be inserted into the canal as soon as it is manageable to inject, then it should be pressurized, and the stem should be inserted when the cement becomes more viscous (this has produced the best results and mantles).

- Fourth generation: Preheating the stem (has to be to at least 44°C), improved shear strength and porosity

When good cement technique is used, this method of fixation has excellent results, and the purported advantages include the ability to add antibiotics to the cement and to match offset and head height by adjusting component size and depth of penetration, that it is easy to adjust anteversion for stability, and that immediate weight bearing is not a concern. The overall cement technique can be graded based upon the system developed by Barrack et al.[54] Grade A is described as a complete "white-out" with a uniform mantle noted on x-ray. Grade B is reported to have a slight lucency at the cement-bone interface, whereas grade C is when there is radiolucency involving 50% to 99% of the cement-bone interface. Grade D is when the metal component is touching the bone, 100% of the cement-bone interface is compromised, or the tip of the stem is not covered. Grades C and D are associated with higher rates of failure, and it is generally recommended to achieve a uniform 2- to 3-mm cement mantle around the component. It is also important to understand the integrity of the cement mantle at the time of revision because a useful technique is to tap out a cemented stem (helps exposure and allows adjustment of head height and offset) and recement a smaller prosthesis back in.

Concerns with cement fixation stem from the lack of adaptability of this bond because it is likely to loosen over time as the bone remodels around it. Furthermore, there is concern that during cementation, relative hypotension may occur and marrow and fat emboli are being introduced into the bloodstream. The cement monomer is thought to cause the hypotension, and emboli can cause hypoxia. This combination can lead to death and the need for greater resuscitative measures in the operating room. For this reason, cementing THAs has become less prevalent. A less worrisome issue with cementing is that cement fixation leads to distal loading of the bone and proximal stress shielding akin to that of an extensively coated, distally fixed stem.

Other cemented THA facts include the following: most stems are made of a stiffer material (cobalt-chromium); the components are typically of a matte finish or highly polished; cement mantle defects are a concern, so mixing antibiotics into cement needs to be done carefully; and Palacos cement (Zimmer) has been shown to superior antibiotic elution properties. When using cement in the setting of a fracture or trochanteric osteotomy, it must be kept out of the bone interfaces so as not to prevent healing. Loose cemented stems (will see subsidence or cement mantle fracture) will typically remodel into varus and retroversion.

Why Might This Be Tested? Cemented THA is a good lead-in for many types of questions regarding antibiotics, revision surgery, and material properties. Often on tests, cemented components are pictured to be loose or associated with periprosthetic fractures. Such issues are typically related to the bone quality (Dorr classification) and cement technique (Barrack grading system and generation used).

Here's the Point!

Cement is a grout, not an adhesive. Generally, it loosens as the bone remodels around it. However, good third- or fourth-generation cement techniques can lead to excellent outcomes. Beware cemented implants on a test; look for loosening and/or remodeling because this may direct treatment.

Vignette 19: Finger vs Circular Saw

A 28-year-old male carpenter was using a circular saw 2 hours ago when he suffered a complete amputation through the MCP joint of the nondominant thumb (Figure 19-1). Emergency medical services placed the part in saline-soaked gauze, then in a separate plastic bag, which was placed in ice water. He has no other history of trauma or conditions to this extremity. The emergency department has given him appropriate antibiotics and updated his tetanus.

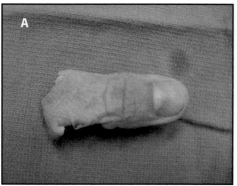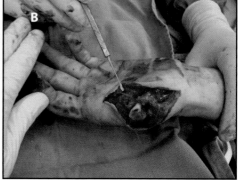

Figure 19-1. (A) Clinical photograph of the amputated thumb. (B) Intraoperative photograph depicting complete amputation through the MCP joint.

▶ *Is he a candidate for replantation?*

▶ *What are some common indications and contraindications for replantation?*

At 10 hours postoperatively, the fingertip begins to take on more of a purplish coloration with swelling but has capillary refill unchanged from postoperatively.

▶ *What is likely occurring?*

▶ *What are treatment options?*

Vignette 19: Answer

A complete amputation of the thumb in an otherwise healthy young individual is a clear indication for replantation given the severe functional limitations incurred by absence of a thumb.[55] All attempts should be made at replanting a thumb whenever possible. Other factors favoring replantation in this case include the small zone of injury imparted on the digit by a saw in comparison with a larger zone of injury, such as in a crush or avulsion injury, favors replantation. Replantation of a crushed or avulsed digit risks poor vessel quality in the part and decreases survivability. Also, this patient has a cold ischemia time of just 2 hours. Acceptable warm ischemia time is 12 hours for a digit and 6 hours for a major limb replantation (a part with significant muscle content). This increases to 24 and 12 hours, respectively, with appropriate cooling of the digit, as in this case. Placing the digit directly on ice must be avoided.[56]

In addition to the thumb, replantation is also indicated in the setting of multiple digits, as well as any level through the palm or more proximal, given the severity of the functional loss if not replanted.[57] Almost any amputated part should be replanted in a child due to the many years of productivity that lie ahead and the child's ability to functionally adapt. Be aware that failure rates after replantation are higher in children, likely due to wider indications, smaller vessels making the procedures more technically demanding, and increased spasm postoperatively. In general, the priority for replantation is as follows: thumb, long, ring, small, and then index finger.

Contraindications include a single-digit amputation through flexor tendon zone II (between the start of the flexor sheath proximally and the flexor digitorum superficialis [FDS] insertion distally) since the PIP joint becomes predictably stiff and the finger functions poorly.[58] Replantation may also be contraindicated in injuries due to crush or avulsion, self-inflicted amputations, and amputations in elderly or low-demand patients. The medical morbidity of undergoing replantation can be high risk in an elderly patient who may not benefit as much functionally from replantation as a young patient would.[56]

The second portion of the vignette describes signs of venous failure of a replantation. A swollen, purplish digit with capillary refill suggests venous engorgement with poor outflow. The dressings should be immediately loosened to be sure there is no undue compression. Assuming the symptoms do not rapidly improve, the principle options include leech therapy (to produce the anticoagulant hirudin; infection with *Aeromonas hydrophila* is a risk with leeches) or removal of the nail with regular scraping of the nailbed and placement of heparin pledgets to maintain outflow. Not infrequently, the latter leads to significant blood loss over a period of days, often necessitating transfusion. If the digit does not improve with this treatment, a return to the operating room is indicated to inspect the anastomosis.

Arterial failure typically presents with a cool and pale digit. Any potentially constrictive dressings should be loosened. Heparin bolus followed by therapeutic infusion can be considered with early signs, but a low threshold should be maintained for a return to the operating room for evaluation of the anastomosis. Early failure is most likely from vasospasm of the vessel. Successful replantation can lead to restoration of half of the normal ROM and 10 mm of 2-point discrimination. The most common complications are infection and cold intolerance.

Why Might This Be Tested? The indications and contraindications for replantation are well established and frequently tested. Most replantation questions will assess indications, but knowing management of the failing replant is important as well.

Here's the Point!

Rules for replantation, in general: (1) yes—sharp cut, major limb, child, thumb, multiple digits, maybe single digit distal to zone II; (2) no—single digit in zone II, crush or avulsion mechanism, maybe elderly, self-inflicted, or single digit (especially border digit).

Vignette 20: My Child Is Missing a Thumb

A 2-month-old male without other known medical problems is referred for left arm deformity. His physical exam reveals absence of a thumb, severe radial deviation of the digits, and carpus in relation to the forearm. This deviation is passively correctable to within 20 degrees of neutral. His forearm has an overall foreshortened appearance. He demonstrates good active flexion and extension of the digits and responds to noxious stimuli throughout the hand. The other upper extremity is normal. His x-ray is shown in Figure 20-1.

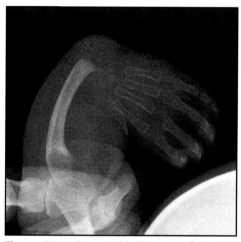

Figure 20-1. Attempted AP x-ray of the left forearm and hand.

▶ *What is the patient's underlying diagnosis?*

▶ *What is the classification of this injury?*

▶ *What conditions/syndromes are associated with this patient's deformity?*

▶ *What is the recommended treatment?*

Vignette 20: Answer

The underlying diagnosis in this case is radial deficiency, also known as radial club hand. It is rare, with an incidence of 1 in 30,000 live births, but it is the most common longitudinal deficiency (bilateral in approximately 50% to 70% of cases). This condition has been classified by Bayne and Klug.[59] Type N has only a hypoplastic or absent thumb with a normal carpus and radius. Type 0 has a normal distal radius but also has carpal hypoplasia, proximal radioulnar synostosis, or radial head dislocation. Type 1 has a distal radius with more than 2 mm of shortening but relatively normal morphology. Type 2 has a truly hypoplastic distal radius with a physis. Type 3 has a hypoplastic distal radius but no physis. Type 4 has an absent radius.[59] Type 4 can be differentiated from thrombocytopenia absent radius syndrome by the presence of a thumb in thrombocytopenia absent radius.[60,61] Based on this patient's x-rays, this is a type 4.

This patient has no known medical problems, but radial deficiency is commonly associated with several syndromes, including vertebral, anal, cardiac, tracheoesophageal, renal, and limb defects; Fanconi's anemia; trisomy 13 and 18; and Holt-Oram syndrome (cardiac defects). Spine x-rays, echocardiography, and renal ultrasound are recommended in patients with radial deficiency. Genetic counseling for Fanconi's anemia should be considered if no other syndrome is present to confirm whether pancytopenia is present.[60,61]

Treatment is different depending on the type. Any patients with radial deviation contractures should undergo serial long-arm casting or soft tissue distraction with an external fixator to get as close to neutral as possible before undergoing open corrective surgery. Once this is achieved, stretch to at least neutral must be maintained regularly until 1 year of age, when the first stage of surgery is typically performed. This includes centralization of the hand and carpus over the ulna. Performing centralization typically requires elevation and release of the contracted radial capsule and remnant of the radial wrist extensors. The carpus is then freed from the volar capsule, centralized over the distal ulna, and held in place with a transfixion pin from the third metacarpal across the carpus into the ulna. The extensor carpi ulnaris should be transected distally, shortened, and advanced back to its insertion on the fifth metacarpal base under appropriate tension. If the radial wrist extensors are not too hypoplastic, they can be transferred to the extensor carpi ulnaris. Excess skin and soft tissue from the ulnar side may need to be excised.[59,61] The absence of a thumb will typically be addressed with pollicization as a second stage once the wrist centralization has stabilized.[62]

Why Might This Be Tested? Although uncommon overall, radial deficiency is the most common longitudinal deficiency with well-established syndrome associations and a well-defined treatment algorithm, especially for the common type 4 variant.

Here's the Point!

Know the associated syndromes! Type 4 is most likely to be tested. Patients should undergo soft tissue stretching right away until close to 1 year of age and then undergo centralization. Pollicization will typically be performed as a second stage.

Vignette 21: My Expensive Shoes No Longer Fit!

A 48-year-old female business executive presents with a history of worsening medial forefoot pain and increasing deformity over a course of many years. She states that the "bump" has substantially increased in size over the past year. She reports difficulty with closed-toe shoewear and is unable to tolerate wearing high heels. Her pain has persisted despite attempts at activity and shoe modifications. She is ultimately diagnosed with a hallux valgus deformity by her local orthopedist.

▶ *What is the natural history of a hallux valgus deformity?*

▶ *What effect does this condition have on the rest of the forefoot and lesser toes?*

On physical examination, she is noted to have a large, swollen, prominent medial eminence of the hallux. Her first ray is hypermobile. A large painful callus is present on the plantar aspect of the second metatarsal head. She has flexible hammertoe deformities of toes 2 and 3.

The patient is scheduled for reconstructive surgery to address her pathology.

▶ *What physical exam findings may influence the surgeon's choice for surgical management?*

▶ *What radiographic parameters help guide surgical decision making?*

Vignette 21: Answer

The term *hallux valgus* refers to a lateral subluxation of the great toe caused by a medial subluxation of the first metatarsal. The notion of shoewear as the chief external contributor to the development of bunion formation has been well substantiated in the literature. Another extrinsic cause of hallux valgus is amputation of the second toe. Likewise, the concept of a hereditary predisposition to developing hallux valgus has been supported by 5 different adult studies showing a positive family history in 58% to 88% of patients with hallux valgus. Other intrinsic causes include pes planus, hypermobility of the first ray (tarsometatarsal [TMT] joint), ligamentous laxity, and forefoot pronation. Systemic conditions, such as inflammatory (RA) arthritis or neuromuscular conditions (cerebral palsy, cerebrovascular accident), are also risk factors for development of hallux valgus. The incidence of bilaterality has been reported to be as high as 84%.

The key to high-yield mastery of this condition is a basic knowledge of the pathoanatomy of bunion formation and an understanding of the broad surgical algorithm for correction of hallux valgus. Because there is no muscular insertion on the metatarsal head, the metatarsophalangeal (MTP) joint is particularly vulnerable to outside forces. When the metatarsal is destabilized, it will drift medially, while the muscles (adductor hallucis) and ligaments (MTP capsule, sesamoid ligaments) pull laterally. The result is an attenuation of the medial MTP capsule, contracture of the lateral MTP capsule, and lateral displacement of the sesamoids into the first webspace. As the sesamoid sling gradually slides beneath the metatarsal head, the hallux pronates and the medial eminence becomes more prominent. What is important to grasp is that as the ability of the first MTP joint to function as the principle weight-bearing focus of the forefoot diminishes, the result is a transfer of the weight to the lateral aspect of the foot, causing development of transfer metatarsalgia (and callus formation) underneath the second or third metatarsal head. As the severity of this deformity progresses, transfer lesions and lesser toe deformities (hammertoes) are likely to develop.

Weight-bearing x-rays are critical to the formulation of a treatment strategy for symptomatic bunions. Important measurements include hallux valgus angle (HVA), 1st-2nd intermetatarsal angle, and distal metatarsal articular angle. Congruency of the MTP joint (vs subluxation) is also an important consideration with implications for treatment options. Other x-ray considerations include first metatarsal length (the shorter the hallux metatarsal, the more likely the presence or development of a transfer lesion), hallux valgus interphalangeus (presence of a laterally oriented proximal phalanx will confer a more significant cosmetic deformity and may require a second osteotomy to achieve a better surgical outcome), joint congruity (an incongruent joint can be corrected by surgically rotating the proximal phalanx on the metatarsal head), and first TMT instability (plantar gapping of this joint on the lateral image is telling of significant hypermobility of the first ray).

While classification of hallux valgus deformities does not strictly guide treatment, it is helpful to broadly classify this condition in order to develop an approach to surgical planning. In grade I, or mild, deformity, the intermetatarsal angle is 11 degrees or less, HVA is 20 degrees or less, and MTP joint is typically congruent. In grade II (moderate) hallux valgus, the intermetatarsal angle is 11 to 16 degrees, HVA is 20 to 40 degrees, and the joint is subluxed, unless the distal metatarsal articular angle is abnormal (greater than 6 degrees), and is therefore the cause of the angulated articular surfaces. Grade III (severe) deformity boasts an intermetatarsal angle greater than 16 degrees, HVA greater than 40 degrees, significant subluxation of the MTP joint, and, oftentimes, an overriding or underriding deformity of the hallux on the second toe.

Conservative treatment (wide toe box shoes [aka "orthopedic shoes"], bunion night splints, etc) is adequate to curtail symptoms in most patients. When this approach fails to yield relief or in the setting of increasing deformity, surgery should be pursued. In juvenile hallux valgus, surgery should typically be delayed until skeletal maturity if possible. With more than 100 surgical procedures described to correct the hallux valgus deformity, no single procedure will adequately address all types of deformity. Therefore, an algorithm that distinguishes between a congruent, incongruent, or degenerative MTP joint will most adequately guide treatment and, more importantly, help answer questions on your exam.

In a congruent joint, one attempts to correct the deformity through an extra-articular repair in order to preserve the congruency of the articular surfaces. Options include distal metatarsal osteotomy (chevron), proximal phalanx osteotomy (Akin) with medial eminence resection, and double first-ray osteotomy (proximal and distal). In an incongruent joint, the procedure of choice must move the proximal phalanx back onto the metatarsal head in order to reestablish congruency of the joint. Here, the degree of the deformity (grade I, II, III) plays into the decision-making process. For grade I, a distal chevron osteotomy, midshaft metatarsal osteotomy (scarf), or distal soft procedure (+ or – proximal metatarsal osteotomy) is preferred. With moderate deformity, a midshaft osteotomy or distal soft tissue procedure with proximal osteotomy is done. In severe deformity, a distal soft tissue procedure with proximal osteotomy, fusion of the MTP joint, or fusion of the TMT joint (Lapidus procedure, in cases of hypermobility) are the options. Significant arthrosis of the MTP precludes most osteotomy procedures, and arthrodesis of the joint achieves the goal of a stable, painless outcome. MTP joint prostheses are not recommended as a long-term treatment option.

Common complications after bunion correction surgery include recurrence of deformity (juvenile hallux valgus), MTP joint stiffness (unrecognized arthrosis, realignment of a congruent joint, or overlengthening of the metatarsal in opening-wedge osteotomy), entrapment of dorsal or plantar cutaneous nerve to hallux, hallux varus (overcorrection), avascular necrosis (distal metatarsal osteotomy), transfer metatarsalgia (shortening of the hallux metatarsal can occur after distal chevron), nonunion (arthrodesis of MTP or TMT), malunion (poorly tolerated in any plane for MTP fusion, troughing of a scarf osteotomy is common with osteopenic bone), and cockup deformity (resection arthroplasty).

Why Might This Be Tested? Hallux valgus is the most common forefoot deformity seen in the office setting. Bunions are not preventable, and the deformity will slowly, but invariably, progress, altering the mechanics of weight bearing and wreaking havoc on the rest of the forefoot (hammertoes, transfer metatarsalgia, crossover toes).

Here's the Point!

Never operate on an asymptomatic bunion. However, when indicated, consider the severity of the deformity, the congruency of the MTP joint, and the presence/absence of hypermobility when determining your surgical plan.

Vignette 22: Foot Injury After Fall From a Ladder

A 48-year-old male contractor sustained an injury to his left foot when he lost his footing and fell 8 feet from his ladder. As he struck the ground, his foot was plantarflexed and his MTP joints were flexed. He complained of severe midfoot pain upon presentation to the emergency department. He was found to have an avulsion fracture at the base of the second metatarsal and was discharged in a nonweight-bearing splint. Upon follow-up in the office setting 2 days later, he was noted to have a markedly swollen foot and plantar ecchymosis of the midfoot and forefoot.

▶ *What anatomical considerations factor into the management of this injury?*

▶ *How is stability of the midfoot determined?*

The patient was scheduled for surgical stabilization of the injury.

▶ *What factors influence the decision to fix (ORIF) or fuse (primary arthrodesis)?*

Vignette 22: Answer

Injuries to the TMT joints are referred to as Lisfranc injuries. Greater awareness of the potential for long-term disability resulting from even subtle Lisfranc joint injuries has led to increasing attention to this spectrum of injuries. An understanding of the basic anatomy is critical to grasp the pathology of midfoot injuries. An important premise to understand, which is critical in guiding treatment of Lisfranc joint injuries, is that very little motion is present through TMT joints 1 through 3 in the coronal and sagittal planes. The Roman arch configuration of the metatarsal bases imparts rigidity and stability to the anatomy by preventing plantar displacement of the transverse arch (hail Caesar!). The plantar ligaments are significantly substantially stronger than the dorsal ligaments, featured by the Lisfranc ligament, which anchors the second metatarsal base to the medial cuneiform. Therefore, displacement of the metatarsals occurs in a dorsal direction in the vast majority of injuries.

A high index of suspicion for Lisfranc injuries should be maintained with all foot injuries; it should be the one injury you always rule out and do not miss. While severe injuries with wide displacement are usually obvious, subtle injuries are often missed. The plantar ecchymosis sign is often indicative of a TMT injury and must not be ignored. In the radiographic evaluation of a midfoot injury, several contiguous lines between the borders of the metatarsal and cuneiform bones are evaluated on the AP and oblique views to determine the presence of instability. A small bony avulsion fragment from the base of the second metatarsal (fleck sign) is considered pathognomonic for a Lisfranc injury. Stress abduction x-rays (or weight-bearing AP films) are also recommended, in the clinic setting or under anesthesia, to determine whether instability of the TMT complex is present. In subtle Lisfranc injuries, a stress x-ray or MRI are critical in determining the extent of the damage.

Lisfranc injuries are classified as type A (homolateral, total incongruity, all 5 metatarsals displace dorsally as a single unit), type B (homolateral incomplete; partial incongruity; some, but not all, of the metatarsals are displaced), and type C (divergent, medial and lateral metatarsals are splayed in opposite directions). This classification is not particularly useful in guiding treatment but is commonly asked about in fracture conferences.

Once instability of the Lisfranc complex has been established, there is no role for nonoperative treatment because the natural history of missed or malaligned injuries to the Lisfranc complex is invariably that of posttraumatic arthritis of the midfoot. The goal of surgical intervention, therefore, is the restoration of a stable midfoot with an anatomic reduction of the TMT articulations 1 through 5. Although there is uniform agreement among authors that the prognosis of surgical management is closely correlated to the accuracy of reduction, controversy exists in the recent literature surrounding the surgical plan of attack. A better understanding of the sequelae of missed, subtle Lisfranc instability has guided the trend toward open (rather than percutaneous) treatment and more rigid fixation constructs (screws rather than K-wires).

The single greatest point of controversy in the active literature involving the operative treatment of Lisfranc injuries surrounds the decision to fix the fracture (ORIF) or perform primary fusion (TMT 1 through 3, not 4 and 5). Although primary fusion was once reserved for cases with extensive comminution, preexisting arthrosis, or neuropathic joints, the literature now firmly supports this option in the treatment of acute Lisfranc injuries (bony or ligamentous). In several studies comparing injuries treated with ORIF vs fusion, the 2 groups showed equivalent outcome scores, whereas the fusion group had significantly lower reoperation rates.

Why Might This Be Tested? Injuries to the TMT joints are uncommon, but when missed, they lead to considerable long-term disability (posttraumatic arthrosis).

Here's the Point!

The diagnosis of Lisfranc injuries is often delayed or missed altogether. A high index of suspicion should be maintained by mechanism of injury and upon the finding of plantar ecchymosis on examination. Outcome is tied to the ability to achieve an anatomic reduction of the TMT joints. Fusion, once reserved as a salvage option, has emerged as a viable alternative for management of acute injuries.

Vignette 23: Hey Doc, What Kind of Stuff Are You Putting Into Me?

A 60-year-old male presents to the clinic with severe degenerative OA of his hip. He has exhausted all conservative measures and is a suitable candidate for a THA. He is a retired metallurgist and has questions regarding the materials used for THA and orthopedics in general. He has heard about several recalls and wants to know more about the material properties of the implants you will be using.

▶ *How are the properties of these materials characterized?*

▶ *Which materials are the strongest?*

▶ *When metals are used, what concerns are there for corrosion, fatigue, failure, and modulus of elasticity?*

Vignette 23: Answer

In the context of medicine, biomaterials are substances that interact with the human body, and regarding orthopedic surgery, they commonly include metals (titanium alloys, stainless steel, tantalum, and cobalt alloys), nonmetals (polyethylene, polymethylmethacrylate, ceramic, silicone), and biologic materials (bone, cartilage, tendon, ligament). The properties of these materials are typically described by plotting a curve with strain (change in length/original length) on the x-axis and stress (force/area) on the y-axis (Figure 23-1). Young's modulus of elasticity is a measurement of the slope of this curve, with a steeper slope indicating a stiffer material. With low strain, a material is in the elastic zone of the curve, undergoes elastic deformation, and will return to its original shape when the stress is released. With increasing strain, the material enters the plastic zone of the curve, undergoes plastic deformation, and does not return to its original shape when the load is removed. The transition point is known as the yield point, with yield stress being the amount of stress necessary to produce a permanent deformation. Other important points on the curve include ultimate strength, which is the point at which the material is loaded to failure, and the breaking point, which is the point at which the material breaks. Toughness is the area under the curve, which is the amount of energy a material can withstand prior to failure. Creep (aka, cold flow) is the tendency for a solid to permanently deform under mechanical stresses, often seen with polyethylene deforming through screw holes in an acetabular component.

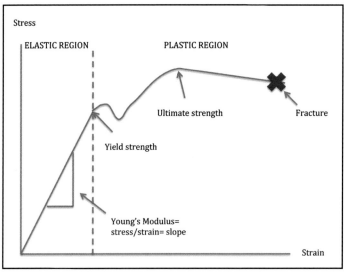

Figure 23-1. Typical stress-strain curve with appropriate regions and points on the curve labeled. Note the steeper the curve, the greater the modulus of elasticity and the more brittle the material.

The most common metals used in orthopedic surgery include stainless steel, titanium alloys (often titanium-aluminum and vanadium or niobium, tantalum), and cobalt alloys (usually a combination of cobalt, chromium, and molybdenum). These materials must be biocompatible and elicit minimal local responses when implanted within the body. The key to this compatibility is the formation of a self-passivation layer on the surface. This surface oxide is protective and prevents early degradation. Furthermore, metals are typically ductile, which means they undergo plastic deformation prior to failure. This property is in contrast to brittle materials, which undergo minimal plastic deformation and have a linear stress strain curve with failure as soon as plastic deformation begins (like ceramics). Metals will typically fail by fatigue, which is failure due to repetitive loading below the ultimate strength (this is a key property in implant failure [ie, if a fracture does not heal, a plate will typically break, just like a femoral stem potted distally without proximal support]). The endurance limit is the stress limit at which fatigue failure does not occur regardless of the number of cycles. Metals also undergo creep and can deform under stress, which may have grave implications depending on the application.

It is also important to understand the most common types of corrosion associated with orthopedic implants. Galvanic corrosion is due to electrochemical reaction between 2 different metals (from almost a battery effect). Fretting corrosion is due to micromotion at the contact surface of 2 metals. This has become a large concern with tapers and modular junctions in THA. It is felt that fretting can lead to fracture of the self-passivation layer of a metal. When this happens, the metal undergoes another self-passivating process and consumes oxygen. The local microenvironment can be drastically altered and, with continued fretting, can lead to extensive corrosion. Crevice corrosion will occur in cracks in the metal due to differential oxygen tension. In combining these processes, we can see mechanically assisted crevice corrosion, junctional fretting, taper fractures, and local adverse tissue reactions.

Regarding specific metals, titanium has a modulus of elasticity closer to bone then cobalt alloys (~100 vs 200 GPa), is highly biocompatible, and is relatively resistant to corrosion. Tantalum is a similar transition metal with similar properties for use as a standalone material or coating in orthopedics. The downside to these softer metals is that they are less wear resistant and therefore are not used as bearing surfaces.[63] Stainless steel is an alloy of primarily carbon and iron that has the advantage of being stiff and unlikely to break. However, the stiffness comes at a cost of stress-shielding bone (in the setting of a cylindrical stem in THA, the stiffness is related to the radius of the implant to the fourth power). This is the property of the metal in which it bears most of the stress and shields the bone, creating an osteoporosis type of picture. Also, stainless steel tends to corrode more than the other metals. Cobalt alloys are typically composed of cobalt, chromium, and molybdenum and are very strong and stiff. However, there is some concern over toxicity of the wear products of cobalt alloys, particularly with metal-on-metal articulations. A final nonmetal biomaterial to be familiar with is ceramic. The substance is very wear resistant, has a high wettability, and is noncompressible but has the downside of being more brittle and prone to fracture (particularly based on design).[64] Ceramics are harder than metals, and when they come into contact, the metal scratches, not the ceramic surface.

These properties truly come into play in orthopedics because stress shielding is important to recognize as a sign of a well-fixed cementless femoral component. Fatigue fracture is a common sign of a nonunion or failure of fixation of an implant. Adverse local tissue reactions are a sign of corrosion and/or excessive wear of an articular surface. While basic science is painful to learn, it is well rooted in Board and OITE questions.

Why Might This Be Tested? It is important to understand the properties of materials that are implanted into the body during orthopedic surgery. Therefore, these are testable concepts in many different arenas.

Here's the Point!

In terms of orthopedic standardized testing, the concepts that are most commonly tested include stress strain curves, basic definitions about material properties, and characteristics of commonly used metals. Just know them!

Vignette 24: Bone Disorders

An 82-year-old male presents with worsening left hip pain over the past 6 months. AP and lateral x-rays of the left hip show a loose femoral stem with cortical perforation (Figure 24-1). He underwent a cementless right THA 10 years ago and a hybrid replacement 5 years ago on the left side. The patient initially recovered completely without pain or limitation. Over the past year, he has developed thigh pain, difficulty hearing out of his left ear, and multiple areas of musculoskeletal pain.

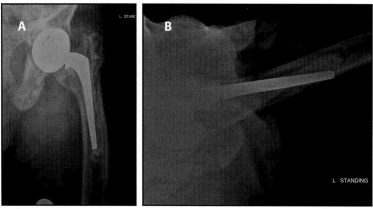

Figure 24-1. (A) AP x-ray of a hybrid THA. (B) Shoot-through lateral of the left femur/hip.

▶ *What is the patient's underlying diagnosis?*

▶ *What is the pathophysiology of this disease process?*

The patient was eventually diagnosed with aseptic loosening of the femoral component. He subsequently underwent isolated revision of the femoral component under a regional anesthesia.

▶ *What complicating factors can be expected during the surgery?*

▶ *How does the patient's underlying disease impact the long-term success of this treatment?*

Vignette 24: Answer

The underlying diagnosis in this case is Paget's disease of bone, which is a chronic, nonmetabolic bone disorder. Paget's disease may be found in up to 3% of people older than 60 years and is more commonly found in men.[65] The hallmark of the disease is a loss of balance in bone formation and resorption with subsequent development of osseous deformities and structural abnormalities.[65,66]

The etiology of Paget's disease is unclear, with proposed theories including viral, genetic, and environmental causes. Viral inclusion bodies have been found in osteoclasts of patients with Paget's disease, and paramyxoviruses have been implicated in this process.[65,66] The pathophysiology appears to be centered around abnormal function of osteoclasts, which tend to be abnormal in size, quantity, and activity. In conjunction, osteoblasts are recruited and rapidly create new bone in an unorganized manner, leading to the formation of woven and weaker bone. Paget's disease follows 3 phases: (1) resorption phase, (2) mixed phase, and (3) sclerotic phase. Clinically, the disease can be seen on x-rays with patchy areas of sclerosis and lucency; it may be monostotic (25%) or polyostotic (75%). Paget's disease most often affects the pelvis, spine, femur, and tibia.[65] Warmth over the involved bones is common due to hypervascularity, and deafness may occur if the petrous temporal bone is affected and compresses the auditory nerve. Osteoarthritis of the hip is commonly found in patients with Paget's disease, as is coxa vara of the femoral neck and acetabular protrusio. Lab tests can help confirm this disease, with serum total alkaline phosphatase usually being markedly elevated. An elevated ESR may indicate malignant transformation (most commonly osteosarcoma [1% of cases]), while urinary and serum deoxypyridinoline, N-telopeptide, and C-telopeptide may be used to monitor a patient's response to treatment.[65]

Medical management typically consists of using bisphosphonate medications and calcitonin to control pain and attempt to normalize serum alkaline phosphatase levels. When surgical management is required, as in this case, it is important to have a thorough cardiac workup because patients with greater than 15% bony involvement may develop shunting and cardiac enlargement (buzzwords are *high-output heart failure*).[65] In addition, pagetoid bone has the propensity for a significant amount of bleeding, and blood salvage options should be explored because higher-than-normal estimated blood loss can be expected. This higher level of bleeding may make it more difficult to obtain an optimal environment for cementing components in these patients (as evidenced by increased rates of early aseptic loosening [9% to 15%]).[65] As seen in this patient's x-rays, Paget's disease often causes bowing of the long bones; corrective osteotomy may be necessary during primary and revision surgery. Delayed healing of these osteotomies through affected bone can be anticipated and may slow down the postoperative recovery period.

Postoperatively, there is a relatively high risk of developing HO (23% to 52%).[65] Pre- or postoperative radiation (1-time 700 cgy dose) or prophylactic oral medications (indomethacin 75 mg daily) should be prescribed in these patients within the first 72 hours of surgery to help minimize the risk of developing symptomatic HO. Despite the high potential for complications, recent data suggest that cementless THA may provide good intermediate to long-term management for Paget's disease affecting the hips.

Why Might This Be Tested? Paget's disease is a commonly selected nonmetabolic bone disease that often appears on standardized tests. There are many arenas from which questions may be derived (ie, basic science, x-ray findings, laboratory values, treatment options, and possible complications).

Here's the Point!

Paget's disease typically occurs in those older than 50 years. X-rays are often all that is needed to make the diagnosis and look for a markedly elevated alkaline phosphatase. Make the diagnosis first, and always beware the 1% malignant transformation in patients older than 70 years.

Vignette 25: Doc, I Have a Pain in the Neck!

A 50-year-old male presents with a 3-month history of neck and right arm pain. A full course of non-operative management was followed, including physical therapy with manual traction, NSAIDs, and pain medication. He subsequently underwent a transforaminal epidural injection 6 weeks ago, with relief of approximately 50% of his symptoms. Two months postinjection, the pain has now returned to preinjection levels. Mild objective weakness and sharp pain with provocative maneuvers are now evident on physical examination. A T2-weighted axial MRI was ordered (Figure 25-1).

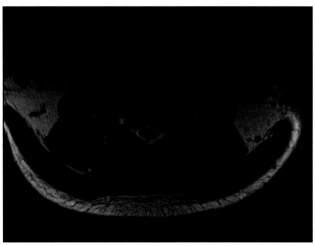

Figure 25-1. T2-weighted axial cervical MRI.

▶ *What level is the disk pathology if the following deficits are present (Table 25-1)?*

Table 25-1.			
DISK PATHOLOGY			
Level	*Sensation*	*Motor*	*Reflex*
A	Medial forearm	Hand intrinsics	
B	Radial forearm to the thumb	Biceps and wrist extensors	Brachioradialis diminished
C	Lateral arm to the elbow	Deltoid	Bicep diminished
D	Ulnar forearm to little finger	Intrinsics and finger flexor	
E	Radial forearm to middle finger	Triceps, finger extension, and wrist flexion	Triceps diminished

▶ *What are the treatment options?*

Vignette 25: Answer

Answers to Table 25-1: A: T1 thus T1-T2 disk; B: C6 thus C5-C6 disk; C: C5 thus C4-C5 disk; D: C8 thus C7-T1 disk; E: C7 thus C6-C7 disk.

Cervical radiculopathy classically presents with pain radiating from the neck into a dermatomal distribution. Associated sensory, motor, and reflex disturbances are typically present, but not always. In the cervical spine, there are 8 nerve roots, which exit through a separate foramen. C1 exits above the C1 vertebrae, C2 above C2, etc. The C8 root exits above the T1 vertebrae. Because the nerve roots exit quickly after branching from the spine, any disk pathology usually affects the exiting nerve root. Thus, at the C2-C3 level, the herniated disk compresses the C3 nerve root, while at the C6-C7 disk level, the C7 nerve root is affected. Sorry, but please memorize the following!

- C4 pathology results in weakness of the scapular muscles and sensory loss over the lateral neck and shoulder.

- The C5 root has a sensory distribution involving the lateral arm to the elbow. There is some contribution to the biceps reflex; however, the biceps reflex can also be innervated by the C6 root. Motor function is to the deltoid.

- C6 sensation involves the radial forearm to the thumb. The brachioradialis and biceps reflex are innervated by the C6 nerve root, whereas the biceps and wrist extensors can be tested for motor function. Extensor carpi radialis longus (ECRL) and brevis are both innervated by C6.

- C7 innervates the midradial forearm to the middle and parts of the index and ring fingers. The triceps reflex is primarily a C7 reflex, whereas motor function involves triceps and wrist flexion. Finger extensors are also part of the C7 distribution.

- C8 extends along the ulnar forearm to the little and ring fingers for sensation. There is no associated reflex, while the intrinsics and finger flexors are from its innervation.

- T1 innervates the medial (ulnar) forearm. There is no associated reflex, and the hand intrinsics are innervated by this nerve root.

Some anatomy facts about the cervical spine include the following:

- The cervical cord is typically compressed when the diameter is reduced to less than 13 mm.

- Neck extension often reduces the effective canal diameter, whereas flexion increases it, often contributing to the loss of the normal cervical lordosis.

- Disk herniation typically occurs in a posterolateral direction between the uncinate process and the posterior longitudinal ligament.

Physical exam findings include the following:

- Neck pain or occipital headache

- Positive Spurling test (rotation and lateral bend with compression of the neck produces pain in the ipsilateral extremity)

- Nerve deficits as described above. Myelopathy hallmarks are bilateral hand numbness, decreased manual dexterity (finger escape sign), weakness (upper greater than lower extremities), ataxic gait, spasticity, and urine retention (occurs late).

- Upper motor neuron signs can be differentiated with findings of hyperreflexia, Hoffmann's sign, clonus, or Babinski's sign.

In general, most acute cervical radiculopathy has a self-limited clinical course, and nonoperative management is the most appropriate initial approach for most patients.[67] Surgery is warranted if nonsurgical treatment has failed or in patients with a significant or progressive neurological deficit. In this case, the patient has failed a complete course of nonoperative management, including immobilization, traction, medication, cervical manipulation, therapy, and injection. None of these measures have reached Level I recommendations, and there are no well-done studies demonstrating their effectiveness.

Specific indications for surgery include myelopathy with motor or gait impairment and radiculopathy with persistent pain. The 2 common surgical approaches include ACDF and posterior laminoforaminotomy. The advantages of anterior surgery include direct removal of the pathology without neural retraction, bone graft restores disk height and provides indirect decompression, fusion prevents recurrent compression, and the fact that it is a muscle-sparing approach. Posterior surgery avoids fusion and can be done with a minimally invasive approach. Disadvantages for the anterior approach include fusion-related issues, nonunion, plate complications, dysphagia, and, theoretically, acceleration of adjacent-level degeneration. The posterior approach does not directly address symptoms occurring at the level, and removal of anterior pathology would require neural retraction. Anterior cervical diskectomy and fusion is the gold standard, but laminoforaminotomy has success rates up to 91.5% (complications include pseudarthrosis, neurologic injury, and dysphagia [greater with plate fixation of ACDF]).[68] Success rates in the literature for motor and sensory function improvement range from approximately 80% to 90%.

Of note, disk replacement technology has been emerging. The theoretical advantages of replacement include maintenance of motion, avoidance of nonunion, and avoidance of plate and screw complications, esophageal erosion, and periplate ossification. Currently, most Food and Drug Administration indications are for one-level disk and for radiculopathy or myelopathy.[69] A recent randomized, controlled trial reported similar results with ACDF and disk arthroplasty for a single level with lower dysphagia scores, higher satisfaction, and better ROM.[70]

Why Might This Be Tested? Many spine questions on the Boards are related to understanding the spinal anatomy cold. Understanding what nerve roots are affected by herniated disk pathology and what the related dermatomal sensory, motor, and reflex exam involves are critical in answering these questions.

Here's the Point!

Memorize the motor, sensory, and reflexes associated with the cervical nerve roots and remember that the herniated disk affects the exiting nerve root in the cervical spine. ACDF and disk arthroplasty are nearly equivalent in outcomes, with higher rates of dysphagia and less motion with the former.

Vignette 26: Knee Pain—Look Out for the Snowboarders!

An 18-year-old female twists her knee and hears a pop while avoiding a downed snowboarder on the double black diamond course. She is seen by the ski patrol, who are unable to range her knee and note a large effusion. She has difficulty bearing weight on the lower extremity and is taken by ambulance to the nearest hospital.

▶ *What is the most likely diagnosis?*

▶ *What is the differential diagnosis for acute-onset knee pain with immediate hemarthrosis?*

▶ *What are the most common mechanisms of injury?*

▶ *What is the relevant pathoanatomy?*

▶ *Why may women be more susceptible to this type of injury?*

▶ *What are useful physical exam tests to help confirm the diagnosis?*

▶ *Are x-rays helpful in aiding the diagnosis?*

Vignette 26: Answer

The most likely diagnosis based on this history is an ACL tear. The keys to the diagnosis in the vignette are 2-fold: immediate hemarthrosis and the sensation of or hearing a pop. The hemarthrosis in an ACL tear is acute, usually within 2 hours, and is due to vascular disruption within the ligament itself (if a blood vessel is ruptured, it will bleed!). Approximately 70% of patients with an acute hemarthrosis will have an ACL tear. In the skeletally mature patient, the midsubstance or femoral insertion is most often completely disrupted. In addition, almost 70% of all ACL tear patients will have a popping sensation or sound at the time of injury.

The ACL is the most common ligament torn in the knee; however, its relative incidence (1:3500) is relatively uncommon.[71] Although contact injuries in these type of patients certainly can produce an ACL tear, more often the injury is noncontact related and associated with cutting or pivoting. Female athletes are 2- to 8-fold more likely to sustain a noncontact ACL tear compared with their male counterparts.[72]

The ACL is composed of 2 principal bundles: a small anteromedial band and a larger posterolateral portion. The ACL arises from the posteromedial corner of the medial aspect of the lateral femoral condyle in the intercondylar notch and attaches to the fossa in front of and lateral to the anterior tibial spine. The ACL is the primary restraint to anterior translation of the tibia relative to the femur and acts as a restraint to internal-external rotation and varus/valgus stressing. A key to the function of the ACL is that the anteromedial bundle is tight in flexion and the posterolateral bundle is tight in extension. The ACL itself is innervated by the tibial nerve and derives its blood supply from the middle geniculate artery.[73,74]

This type of injury is more common in female soccer and basketball players than in male athletes (2.7 and 3.5 times greater risk, respectively).[75] Although subject to debate, some factors that may predispose female athletes to injury include ligamentous laxity, increased Q angle, knee recurvatum, decreased femoral notch size, geometry/size of the ACL, estrogen effects on the ligament, and BMI.[72] However, there appears to be a significant reduction in ACL injuries in female athletes who undergo proprioceptive and neuromuscular training.

An orthopedic surgeon evaluating the patient in this vignette may have a difficult time performing a comprehensive physical exam of the knee given the patient's acute pain and hemarthrosis. However, a thorough exam is a must given that ACL injuries rarely occur in isolation. Frequently, the MCL can be sprained or completely torn, depending on the mechanism of injury. Fortunately, the posterolateral/lateral elements usually remain uninjured. Furthermore, a concomitant injury of one of the menisci can occur in up to 15% to 40% of patients. A thorough physical examination will necessitate careful palpation of the insertion of the MCL on the femur to pick up on subtle sprains and mild injury. Stressing the knee in full extension and 30 degrees of flexion should afford an accurate assessment of varus and valgus stability. ACL injuries can be easily confused with extensor mechanism disruption (ligament tear or patella fracture); therefore, one must determine the patency of the patellar or quadriceps tendon. As we all see on television, the most sensitive exam for an acute ACL tear is Lachman's test (what the trainers/doctors do on the field). The examiner places the knee at 30 degrees of flexion and secures the distal femur with one hand while the other hand anteriorly translates the tibia. If the ACL is injured, there is forward translation and lack of endpoint.[74]

Although imaging is not truly necessary to diagnose an ACL tear, obtaining orthogonal x-rays is essential to rule out a fracture that may be associated with the tear. Looking at the location of the patella (baja or alta) may help direct your physical exam and differential diagnosis (quadriceps or patella ligament tears). There are 2 important fracture patterns that may suggest a torn ACL. The Segond fracture is a small avulsion fracture of the proximal lateral tibial condyle just below the joint line, which represents excessive varus force and internal rotation of the tibia. In the skeletally immature patient, a tibial intercondylar eminence fracture may also represent an ACL injury.

An MRI is useful in determining other concomitant injuries, such as meniscal pathology, ligamentous sprains, and subchondral fractures. There are several characteristic MRI findings that point to a diagnosis of an ACL tear, besides seeing the ACL tear sagittally or coronally. The classic edema pattern, or bone bruising, is often seen in the posterolateral tibial plateau and the anterolateral femoral condyle (near sulcus terminalis). These patterns represent subchondral fractures.

Why Might This Be Tested? ACL tear is a very commonly tested topic. With the recent interest in ACL footprint anatomy, the discussion on anatomic ACL reconstruction has received considerable interest.

Here's the Point!

Noncontact knee injury with an audible pop and an acute hemarthrosis is an ACL tear until proven otherwise. Check by using Lachman's test, and always assess for concomitant meniscal and ligamentous injuries.

Vignette 27: I Was Lifting This Chair and Now My Elbow Is Incredibly Painful

A 58-year-old female reports pain in her elbow over the past 6 weeks. She had a recent increase in the pain 2 days ago after lifting a chair in her living room. Past medical history includes borderline hypertension and hyperlipidemia. She has lost 20 lb of weight unintentionally over the past 4 months. An x-ray and histology slides can be seen in Figures 27-1 to 27-3.

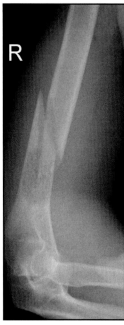

Figure 27-1. Lateral x-ray of the right humerus.

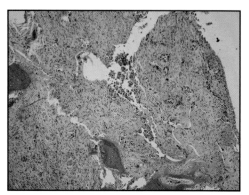

Figure 27-2. Biopsy specimen (100× magnification).

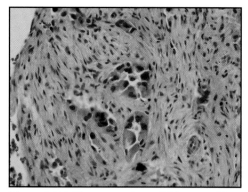

Figure 27-3. Biopsy specimen (400× magnification).

▶ *What is the diagnosis?*

▶ *What additional studies are indicated?*

▶ *What is the definitive treatment?*

Vignette 27: Answer

Metastatic carcinoma and multiple myeloma must be considered in the workup of any patient older than 40 years with a new presentation of a destructive lesion of bone (always think mets, myeloma, lymphoma!). In this age group, metastatic disease and myeloma are 2 orders of magnitude more common than a lymphoma or primary sarcoma. Even so, the potential diagnosis of a sarcoma must be considered because the treatments for metastatic disease and sarcoma are vastly different. The goals in metastatic disease are pain control and improving or maintaining function. For nonmetastatic sarcoma, en bloc resection in an attempt to eradicate the cancer is warranted. A worst-case scenario is treatment of a presumed carcinoma with an IM device and subsequent pathology consistent with sarcoma. In this hypothetical circumstance, a previously limb-salvageable extremity may have to be amputated to gain oncologic control.

A complete history and physical exam are important. Specifically, patients should be asked about a previous history of cancer and smoking. A complete description of axial and appendicular pain is necessary to determine all sites of concern. A history of pain with weight bearing is especially worrisome because this may imply an impending pathologic fracture. The common sources of primary tumors are lung, breast, kidney, prostate, thyroid, and GI. Prostate carcinoma metastases are typically blastic (as are approximately 60% of breast cancer mets). The other common tumors to metastasize present as lytic lesions (lung, thyroid, and renal). Think like a doctor, not an orthopod; ask questions pertaining to these tumors that commonly metastasize.

The initial imaging studies should consist of orthogonal plain x-rays of the entire affected bone. This will characterize the lesion, determine the extent, and assess for disease elsewhere in the bone. In the case of fractures, the x-rays should be analyzed with a high index of suspicion if the mechanism of injury is a lesser force than what is normally expected. Additional staging studies include chest, abdomen, and pelvis CT scans to search for a possible primary tumor (lung, kidney, colon) and visceral metastases (lung, liver, spleen). A bone scan helps determine if there are any other sites of osseous disease. The most common site of metastasis is the thoracic spine (remember Batson's vertebral plexus—a means for mets to gain access to the axial skeleton via this valveless venous plexus). Areas of increased uptake on bone scan must be investigated with plain x-ray to ensure that they are not structurally significant lesions. Bone scans can be negative in multiple myeloma, and a skeletal survey may be used in its place. A full set of laboratory values are obtained because patients may have anemia, hypercalcemia, or renal failure. A serum protein electrophoresis is often drawn if a diagnosis of multiple myeloma is suspected (serum protein electrophoresis and urine protein electrophoreses—think Bence Jones proteins).

After the staging studies are completed, a tissue biopsy is required for the definitive diagnosis. The diagnosis must be made prior to stabilization. It is common practice to plan for stabilization immediately following confirmation of metastatic carcinoma or myeloma with a frozen section. It is imperative to consider the approach that would be used for excision if the lesion is found to be a sarcoma. The biopsy should be in line with this approach and transverse incisions should be avoided (very important concept; in general, don't biopsy if you aren't going to do excision). If surgical stabilization is not needed, needle biopsies can be very accurate in this scenario and do not require general anesthesia.

Histologically, carcinoma appears as atypical glands with a surrounding desmoplastic response interspersed between bony trabeculae. At higher power, the glands are composed of atypical cells with increased nuclear:cytoplasmic ratios and hyperchromatic nuclei characteristic of metastatic adenocarcinoma. Multiple myeloma (and plasmacytoma) appears as sheets of homogenous small, round, blue cells in a mosaic pattern.

Sites of metastatic disease and multiple myeloma are treated with radiation for disease control and pain relief. Chemotherapy is usually palliative and given to reduce the burden of disease. Bisphosphonates are commonly used to decrease the incidence of future skeletal events by inhibiting osteoclastic activity. The mechanism of bone destruction in metastatic disease is not by the tumor, but by osteoclastic activation by the receptor activator of nuclear factor-$\kappa\beta$ (RANK) and RANK ligand interaction. Factors secreted by the tumor can directly and indirectly stimulate this pathway.

The consideration of stabilization of osseous lesions is dependent on the expected risk of pathologic fracture. The classic system to assess this is Mirel's criteria (Table 27-1).

Table 27-1. MIREL'S CRITERIA			
	Points		
Criteria	3	2	1
Location	Peritrochanteric	Lower extremity	Upper extremity
Lesion type	Lytic	Mixed	Blastic
Pain	Functional	Moderate	Mild
Cortical erosion	>2/3	1/3 to 2/3	<1/3

Lesions with a total score of 9 or more have an unacceptably high rate of fracture without stabilization and should be fixed. Scores of 7 or less should be observed. Vascular lesions, such as renal cell carcinoma, should be considered for preoperative embolization to reduce blood loss at the time of surgery.

A goal of surgical stabilization is to protect the entire bone in case of tumor growth or metastasis to a noncontiguous site in the same bone. The femoral neck should always be stabilized when possible, and all IM devices should be locked for rotational control. For large periarticular lesions, replacement with an arthroplasty is usually more appropriate and definitive.

Why Might This Be Tested? Metastases are much more commonly seen by orthopedic oncologists than primary bone tumors. These can come from many sites and often present differently. This genre of questions is frequently touched upon because it requires the orthopedist to think more like a doctor and assess the whole-body situation.

Here's the Point!

Metastatic disease is frequently encountered and has to be high on your list for patients older than 65 years with pain and a lesion on plain x-rays (in this group, always think mets, myeloma, and lymphoma). It is important to obtain a firm diagnosis and prognosis prior to operative management. Stabilization of the whole bone is imperative when prophylactically managing an impending pathological fracture.

Vignette 28: I Fell on My Arm and Now I Can't Extend My Wrist

A 68-year-old, right-hand-dominant female arrives in the emergency department after a ground-level fall. She is otherwise healthy with no history of prior fractures. She takes a baby aspirin, multivitamin, and calcium/vitamin D daily and denies smoking.

Physical examination reveals gross deformity of the right arm with no open lacerations or wounds. The patient has 2+ radial pulses bilaterally and less than 2-second capillary refill to the fingers. Full motor and sensory exam exhibits absent sensation over the dorsoradial surface of the right hand. Furthermore, the patient displays 0/5 strength in wrist extension, MCP joint extension, thumb extension, and thumb abduction. The rest of the upper extremity motor and sensory exam is normal, as is the remainder of the patient's complete general and musculoskeletal exam.

AP and lateral x-rays show a mid-diaphyseal, oblique fracture of the right humerus with roughly 30 degrees of varus and 20 degrees of apex posterior angulation, along with 4 centimeters of shortening. The fracture does not extend proximal or distal to the diaphysis and displays minimal comminution. X-rays of the shoulder, elbow, and forearm show no other osseous abnormalities. A coaptation splint is applied in the emergency room without change in neurovascular examination. Postsplint x-rays show angulation improved to 20 degrees of varus, minimal AP angulation, and 1.5 cm of shortening (Figure 28-1).

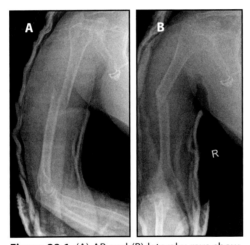

Figure 28-1. (A) AP and (B) lateral x-rays showing the right humerus post-reduction with the splint in place.

▶ *What are the generally accepted parameters for nonoperative treatment of a humeral shaft fracture (ie, varus/valgus angulation, AP angulation, and shortening)?*

▶ *What nerve was injured in this patient, and what is the prevalence of injury to this nerve in the setting of a diaphyseal humeral shaft fracture?*

▶ *After initial triage in the emergency room, how should this patient's fracture and nerve palsy be treated?*

▶ *With this treatment, what is the chance of nonunion?*

▶ *With this treatment, what is the chance of recovery of this nerve palsy?*

▶ *If recovery occurs, what 2 muscles would likely recover first?*

Vignette 28: Answer

Generally, up to 3 cm of shortening, 20 degrees of AP angulation, and 30 degrees of varus/valgus angulation are tolerable in the nonoperative treatment of individuals with a humeral shaft fracture. There are no current studies that correlate these parameters to acceptable functional outcomes; however, Klenerman found that 20 degrees of AP angulation and 30 degrees of varus/valgus angulation are necessary before clinical deformity is perceived by visual inspection due to the large soft tissue mass around these fractures.[76] Furthermore, this cohort of patients did not experience appreciable loss of function secondary to their deformity.

This patient experienced primary complete radial nerve palsy, which is commonly associated with a diaphyseal humerus fracture. A meta-analysis of 14 prior studies by Papasoulis et al[77] documented a 9.2% mean incidence of radial nerve palsy in the setting of diaphyseal humeral shaft fractures.

Although it is always imperative to discuss the risks and benefits with every patient and take into account personal preferences, given her history, physical exam, and x-rays, this patient is a candidate for functional bracing. As discussed below, complete, primary radial nerve palsy is not an indication for operative management without another relative indication. Common indications (while debatable, this is what you can expect on the current tests) for immediate surgical intervention include unacceptable fracture alignment following a trial of bracing, new-onset radial nerve palsy following closed reduction, multitrauma patients, segmental humerus fractures, floating elbow or ipsilateral arm injuries, pathologic fractures, vascular injury, obesity (inability to control the fracture with a brace), progressive radial nerve palsy, and a distal intra-articular fracture. Low-velocity gunshot wounds are not, in themselves, an indication for operative management, and a fracture brace or coaptation splint is recommended when there is minimal soft tissue injury and the fracture can be held in alignment.

In 18 prior studies involving 1550 patients treated with functional bracing of diaphyseal humerus fractures, the rate of nonunion ranged from 0% to 22.6%, with an overall rate of 5.3% (82 of 1550 patients).[77] A Cochrane review of previous randomized, controlled trials of operative fixation showed a nonunion rate of 6.1% (8 of 132) for plate osteosynthesis and 10.6% (13 of 123) for IM nail fixation rates comparable with, and possibly worse than, those seen in patients treated with functional bracing.[78]

Prior meta-analyses reveal a spontaneous recovery rate between 74.3% (397 of 534) and 86.2% (112 of 130); therefore, most authors agree that acute exploration of the radial nerve is not warranted if palsy presents before reduction or manipulation.[77] In 581 patients with primary radial nerve palsy undergoing expectant management, Shao et al reported that the average time to initial signs of spontaneous recovery was 7.3 weeks and the mean time to complete recovery was 6.1 months.[79] It is recommended that patients without signs of recovery by 4 to 6 months undergo electromyography (EMG) and, if there is no electrophysiological evidence of recovery, that late nerve exploration be performed.

The radial nerve emerges from the radial sulcus (also known as the radial groove) on the lateral aspect of the arm, pierces through the lateral intermuscular septum, and courses inferiorly between the brachialis and brachioradialis, where it innervates brachioradialis. As the nerve continues distally, it courses anterior to the lateral epicondyle, where it innervates the ECRL prior to splitting into the deep (posterior interosseous nerve) and superficial (superficial radial nerve) branches (the brachioradialis and ECRL would be first to come back).

Why Might This Be Tested? Humeral shaft fractures constitute nearly 3% of all bony injuries.[80] The incidence of humeral shaft fractures increases from 14.5/100,000 per year in the fifth decade to nearly 60/100,000 per year in the ninth decade. Although it is important to recognize concomitant nerve palsy, it is likewise imperative to understand the natural progression of the palsy when deciding on a treatment algorithm.

Here's the Point!

Humeral shaft fractures are common injuries, as are associated nerve palsies; we need to know how to optimize patient recovery in terms of the fracture and any associated neurologic deficits.

Vignette 29: Intramural Football Injury

A 21-year-old male describes a twisting injury to his knee while playing intramural football yesterday. He was able to finish the remainder of the game but noticed that his knee began to swell during the rest of the day. The following day while walking, he felt a catching sensation in his knee with a sensation of the knee wanting to give way. In addition, he was experiencing pain along the inside of his knee. MRIs are shown in Figure 29-1.

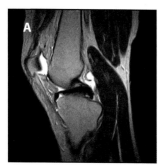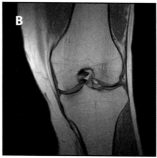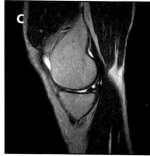

Figure 29-1. (A) Sagittal MRI of the right knee showing a double PCL sign from a displaced meniscus tear in the intercondylar notch. (B) Coronal MRI showing a displaced meniscus in the notch. (C) Sagittal MRI of the medial compartment showing deficiency in the posterior meniscus.

▶ *What is the most likely diagnosis?*

▶ *What is the essential pathophysiology regarding these injuries?*

▶ *What best aids with the diagnosis?*

▶ *What is the classification for this specific type of injury?*

▶ *What are the treatment recommendations?*

Vignette 29: Answer

The most likely diagnosis is an acute meniscal tear. Meniscal injuries represent some of the most common injuries presenting to orthopedic clinics annually. Meniscus tears occur in about 60 to 70 cases per 100,000 patients every year, with a significantly higher male:female ratio.[81]

The functions of the knee menisci are to provide shock absorption, stability, lubrication, and proprioception; disperse contact forces; and increase the articular surface.[82] The wedge-shaped meniscus is largely water by weight. However, its dry weight is predominately collagen, and its structure is integral to its complex functions. The collagen fibers are oriented in a mostly circumferential pattern with interspersed radial fibers. The circumferential fibers allow for compressive loads, whereas the radial fibers disperse longitudinal strain. Shear stress is reduced at the surface with a mesh configuration of the collagen fibers. In full extension, the menisci transmit 50% of load across the knee; the force transmission is 85% at 90 degrees of knee flexion.[82] Consequently, when the menisci are removed, the contact area is dramatically reduced while the contact stresses transmitted across the knee increase by 100% medially and 200% to 300% laterally.[82]

The menisci are largely avascular, with usually 25% of the outer rim vascularized by the superior and inferior branches of the medial and lateral geniculate arteries. It is this limited blood supply that limits the ability of the menisci to heal.

Meniscal tears can be diagnosed readily with a thorough history, physical examination, and certain diagnostic modalities. Usually, the patient reports localized tenderness to the posterior knee or the affected joint line. Usually, patients with acute meniscal pathology are teenagers and young adults who present after a knee twisting or pivoting injury. The knee gradually develops an effusion over hours (often delayed), as opposed to an ACL injury wherein an effusion develops within a couple of hours. Although a description of locking or clicking of the knee is a common complaint, such symptoms may be related to secondary pathology of the articular surface or ligamentous injury. A patient with a bucket handle meniscal tear may report a mechanical block to full extension. Patients with chronic tears may describe intermittent mechanical symptoms or joint effusions over a longer period of time.

On physical examination, the patient's ROM must be documented to ensure that there are no mechanical blocks to motion. Palpation and ligament stability should be routinely assessed to determine concomitant injuries. Although there are many physical exam findings that may aid in the diagnosis of meniscal pathology, such as the Apley or McMurray's tests, the only one to show a high sensitivity is joint line tenderness (74%).[83]

In addition to the history and physical exam, imaging is a key to diagnosis. Routine x-rays of the knee are used to assess joint space narrowing or other bony pathology. A 30- to 45-degree flexion weight-bearing view may be more sensitive than the standard AP knee x-ray.[82] In addition, a view of the patellofemoral joint (lateral or Merchant's) is helpful to evaluate joint space narrowing and tracking of the anterior compartment of the knee. An MRI is essential in the noninvasive diagnosis of meniscal tears. Only grade III changes represent tears (increase in signal that touches the articular surface of the meniscus).[84]

The classification of tears is based on the arthroscopic pattern seen and the underlying etiology. The location of the meniscus tear can occur in 1 of 3 zones corresponding to the blood supply: red-red zone, peripheral third; red-white zone, middle third; and white-white zone, inner third. The decision to repair the meniscus depends on the blood supply to the injured portion of the meniscus. The periphery of the meniscus is more vascular; therefore, it is more likely to heal after repair. The types of patterns seen during arthroscopy are vertical longitudinal, radial, bucket-handle, flap, horizontal cleavage, and complex. Vertical tears are associated with younger individuals and ACL tears. A bucket-handle tear is a vertical tear that displaces completely and usually starts in the posterior horn (Figure 29-2). Both of these tears may be repaired if the radial tear is located in the peripheral vascular zone and if the reduced bucket-handle tear is in reasonable condition. Radial or transverse tears propagate from a central to an outward location. If these tears proceed circumferentially, they become flap tears. These tears are usually arthroscopically debrided. Horizontal tears are usually age related and represent chronic injuries. They usually begin at the inner margin and propagate toward the capsule. These types of tears are usually debrided to a stable base.

The symptomatology and pattern of the tear influences the type of treatment. For chronic, degenerative-type meniscus tears, nonsurgical management includes activity modification, physical therapy, NSAIDs, and corticosteroid injections. Surgery is reserved for patients in whom nonsurgical management fails, symptoms affect the activities of daily living (mechanical issues, such as locking or buckling), and positive

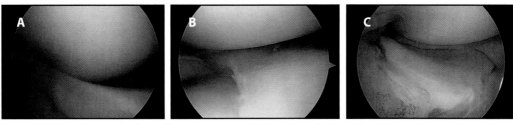

Figure 29-2. Arthroscopic views of meniscus tear showing (A) a displaced bucket-handle medial meniscus tear, (B) all-inside repair stitches, and (C) a repaired meniscus tear.

physical exam findings elicit pain. Surgery may entail arthroscopic debridement or direct repair. The goal for arthroscopic debridement includes resecting as little of the meniscus as possible to ensure a stable, well-shaped rim.

In the case presented, the patient describes knee pain after a twisting injury to the knee and having developed swelling and mechanical symptoms the following day. Surgical treatment would be recommended in cases of a displaced bucket-handle tear to provide the best opportunity for repair of the torn meniscus. There are 3 methods that have been described to repair the meniscus: inside-out repair, outside-in repair, and all-inside repair.

Why Might This Be Tested? The classification of meniscus tears is commonly tested because it serves as a guide for treatment.

Here's the Point!

Meniscus tears are very common injuries in the knee. Displaced bucket-handle tears should be repaired as soon as possible to allow for meniscus preservation.

Vignette 30: Shoulder Pain After a Spill Off of a Bicycle

A 22-year-old male professional cyclist presents to the emergency department after sustaining a fall off of his bicycle onto his left shoulder during a competition. On physical examination, the patient has severe pain throughout the anterior shoulder region and has a notable bony prominence over the middle third of his left clavicle, with tenderness to palpation and skin tenting. There is overlying ecchymosis over the prominence, with no signs of skin compromise. The patient denies any other injuries and is neurovascularly intact to motor and sensory function to his left upper extremity. Initial x-rays of the clavicle are obtained (Figure 30-1).

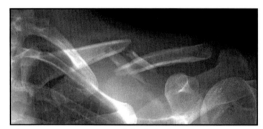

Figure 30-1. AP x-ray of the left clavicle after injury.

▶ *What is the diagnosis?*

▶ *What other aspects of the physical exam are important to note?*

▶ *What other tests should be ordered?*

▶ *What are the treatment options?*

Vignette 30: Answer

The diagnosis is a closed, comminuted, displaced midshaft clavicle fracture after a direct traumatic blow to the shoulder. Clavicle fractures account for 5% to 10% of all fractures and 35% to 45% of all shoulder girdle injuries. Midshaft fractures account for roughly 80% of all clavicle fractures, and these injuries are generally classified as lateral third, midshaft, or medial third fractures. Lateral third and medial third fractures make up 12% to 15% and 5% to 6% of total clavicle fractures, respectively. The clavicle is located subcutaneously and has a relatively small muscle and soft tissue envelope, which make it susceptible to injury. For those into orthopedic trivia, the clavicle is the last bone to ossify; the medial growth plate fuses in the early twenties.[85-92]

The most common mechanism of injury to the clavicle is from a direct blow to the anterior and lateral aspect of the shoulder or from a fall onto the lateral shoulder. During physical exam, it is important to assess for skin abrasions, skin tenting, signs of open fracture, soft tissue integrity, displacement of the shoulder girdle, and swelling. A small subset of clavicle fractures occurs in combination with more severe injuries, such as scapular fractures, rib fractures, pneumothorax, scapulothoracic dissociation, and/or brachial plexus injuries. Scapulothoracic dissociation is a serious complication that should be considered in cases of severe clavicle displacement. It is important during physical exam to perform a full neurovascular exam of the brachial plexus to determine any potential nerve injuries.

The following x-rays should be obtained during the workup of a clavicle fracture: AP view of the clavicle, 45-degree cephalic tilt view to look for superior vs inferior displacement (serendipity view), and 45-degree caudal tilt view to evaluate anterior vs posterior displacement. CT may be obtained to help determine degree of displacement, shortening, comminution, and articular extension. CT is particularly helpful for evaluating medial physeal fractures and sternoclavicular injuries.

There are distinct treatment strategies for each of the 3 types of clavicle fractures. Midshaft fractures can be largely treated nonsurgically with immobilization in a simple sling or figure-8 brace. Surgery is indicated for open midshaft fractures, displaced fractures with greater than 2 cm of shortening (see Figure 30-1), fractures associated with flail chest, and concomitant subclavian neurovascular injuries. Relative indications include criteria such as skin tenting and displaced fracture with an associated scapular neck fracture or scapulothoracic dissociation. The case presented here would meet indications for ORIF given the displaced fracture with greater than 2 cm of shortening, severe comminution, skin tenting, and high physical activity level of the patient (Figure 30-2). The amount of initial displacement correlates well with rates of healing. Studies have shown that fractures with 100% displacement and 2 cm of shortening have better results with ORIF. Contraindications to surgery are minimal fracture displacement and shortening, which should be treated nonoperatively. Surgical fixation can be achieved with ORIF using a plate and screws placed superiorly or anteriorly. Complications of surgery include neurovascular injury (supraclavicular nerves in particular), hardware failure, hardware irritation, infection, and nonunion (1% to 5%).

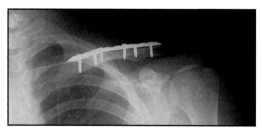

Figure 30-2. Plain x-ray after ORIF showing a midshaft clavicle fracture with plate fixation.

Lateral third clavicle fractures can be treated nonoperatively if there is minimal displacement. However, unlike midshaft and medial third fractures, displaced lateral third clavicle fractures are inherently unstable and prone to malunion or nonunion. Therefore, there is a lower threshold for surgical intervention with these types of fractures. Classification of lateral third fractures is based on the status of the coracoclavicular (CC) ligament complex. Fixation can be achieved with ORIF using plate and screws depending on the length or the lateral fragment. If the fragment is too short for a plate, CC fixation of the medial fragment with heavy sutures can be used. Alternatively, if the fragment is very small, it can also be excised with CC ligament reconstruction. Complications include acromioclavicular (AC) joint arthritis, nonunion, and hardware failure.

Medial clavicle fractures can be treated nonoperatively if there is minimal displacement. Surgery is indicated for these fractures with severe displacement, especially if displaced posteriorly because this can push fracture fragments into the critical structures of the lower neck and mediastinum. Complications include retrosternal and mediastinal injuries, neurovascular injury, and hardware migration and failure.

Why Might This Be Tested? Clavicle fractures are one of the most common fractures seen in orthopedics and have a well-defined clinical exam, workup, classification, and treatment paradigm based on location.

Here's the Point!

Establish the diagnosis, classify the fracture, and determine which treatment strategy should be used; know the indications, pros, and cons of each option. Remember that 80% of clavicle fractures are midshaft and most do well nonoperatively in a sling or brace. Recent clinical outcome studies have demonstrated improved outcomes after ORIF of clavicle fractures with 100% displacement and 2 cm of shortening.

Vignette 31: I Just Can't Shake This Tingling in My Arm

A 56-year-old male presents to your office with pain and tingling in his left lateral forearm for the past 2 months. His symptoms began insidiously and have been getting progressively worse. His pain involves his lateral hand and his left thumb and first finger. He denies trauma but reports intermittent neck pain and a history of a cervical disk herniation years ago. He has not noticed any frank weakness but has been having mild coordination problems with his left. An EMG/nerve conduction study (NCS) was obtained, and the results are as follows. The left median and ulnar sensory nerve action potentials were within normal limits. The left median compound motor action potential was reduced in amplitude, and 1+ fibrillations were present in the biceps and pronator teres muscles on EMG testing. A diagnosis of left C6 radiculopathy is made.

▶ *What are the typical electrodiagnostic study findings for radiculopathy?*

▶ *What are the different electrodiagnostic findings for a demyelinating lesion compared with an axonal injury?*

▶ *If he had been having his symptoms for only 1 week, how would the EMG/NCS results have likely been different?*

Vignette 31: Answer

EMG is a diagnostic study in which needles are used to assess the functionality of muscles. Nerve conduction studies are used to evaluate peripheral nerves and their sensory and motor function anywhere along its traversing path. Basically, you shock the person and record the conduction of the impulse with surface electrodes. With radiculopathy, the pathologic process affects nerves at the level of the root. Since it spares the dorsal root ganglion, the sensory NCSs are normal. The compound motor action potential is often reduced but may be borderline or normal if the injury is purely demyelinating or incomplete or if reinnervation has occurred. On needle EMG testing, varying amounts of fibrillations or positive sharp waves in 2 different muscles innervated by 2 different peripheral nerves but originating from the same root should be present. However, this part of the test can also potentially be normal in select cases, including once reinnervation has occurred or if missed by random sampling.[93,94]

A demyelinating lesion to a peripheral nerve can cause prolonged latency, increased temporal dispersion, and decreased conduction velocity (10% to 50%) on NCS due to the loss of myelin insulation, thus hindering salutary conduction. A decreased amplitude across the site of injury can also be seen. On EMG, insertional activity and motor unit action potentials are classically within normal limits, and decreased recruitment may be present.[93]

In contrast, electrodiagnostic testing after an axonal injury would typically demonstrate normal latency times, but decreased amplitude throughout the entire nerve and decreased conduction velocity on the NCS. On the EMG portion, abnormal insertional activity, positive sharp waves and fibrillations, decreased recruitment, and abnormal motor unit action potentials can all be seen.

Other nerve injuries include the following:

1. Anterior horn cell disease (polio, spinal muscular atrophy; AR disorder)
   a. EMG: Increased insertional activity, fibrillations, positive sharp waves, fasciculations, and large polyphasic potentials
   b. NCS: Normal latency and conduction velocities, normal or polyphasic evoked response with prolonged duration, and decreased amplitude
2. Myopathy (muscle injury/damage)
   a. EMG: Increased insertional activity, no fibrillations (normal), and small polyphasic potentials
   b. NCS: Normal latency and conduction; decreased amplitude of evoked response
3. Neuropraxia (transient episode of motor paralysis with little or no sensory or autonomic dysfunction, no disruption of nerve or its sheath)
   a. EMG: Normal insertional activity, no fibrillations (normal), and no contraction
   b. NCS: Latency, conduction velocity, and evoked response all normal distal to the lesion and absent proximally
4. Axonotmesis (destruction of the axons of nerve cells with preservation of the supporting structures, affording the possibility of regeneration)
   a. EMG: Increased insertional activity, fibrillations and positive sharp waves, and no contraction
   b. NCS: Latency, conduction velocity, evoked response all absent, except for evoked response distal to the lesion
5. Neurotmesis (worst injury with destruction of the nerve and sheath; full recovery is not possible)
   a. EMG: Increased insertional activity, fibrillations and positive sharp waves, and no muscle contraction
   b. NCS: Latency, conduction velocity, evoked response all absent

If the electrodiagnostic study had been done only 1 week after the initial nerve injury, the results would indeed be different and quite possibly normal. Initially, decreased recruitment in EMG in muscles innervated by the affected root level may be the only findings seen. Abnormal spontaneous activity, specifically positive waves and fibrillations, may start to be seen at around 1 week, occurring often first in the paraspinal muscles. Abnormal spontaneous activity in the limbs and abnormal motor unit action potentials may then start to be seen at roughly 2 to 3 weeks. Of note, in some cases it is difficult to determine the exact timing of nerve injury, or it may be the result of repetitive insults to the nerve, creating a more chronic injury and thus possible changing the pattern seen on electrodiagnostic testing.[93]

Why Might This Be Tested? Electrodiagnostic medicine can serve as an extension of the clinical exam and can provide additional information on the pathophysiology of a disease process. It can provide functional details regarding the location, duration, severity, and prognosis for a variety of conditions seen by orthopedic surgeons.

Here's the Point!

By combining data obtained from one's history and physical exam with those found on NCS and EMG testing, neuromuscular injury can be categorized based on certain patterns (eg, acute vs chronic radiculopathy and axonal vs demyelinating lesions).

Vignette 32: Pediatric Fall Onto an Outstretched Hand

A 9.5-year-old, right-hand-dominant female fell off her bike and sustained a midshaft radius and ulna fracture that underwent a closed reduction and splinting. The closed reduction was performed in the emergency room, and she was sent to you for follow-up and definitive treatment. She returned to the office after 2 weeks in the splint for follow-up. No new problems have occurred, and she has minimal pain. X-rays were obtained (Figure 32-1).

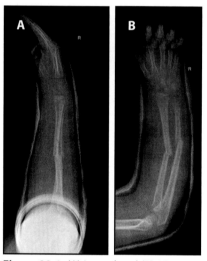

Figure 32-1. (A) Lateral and (B) AP x-rays showing the right forearm in a cast.

▶ *What is the next step in treating this fracture?*

Vignette 32: Answer

The fracture is a displaced both-bone forearm fracture. These fractures typically occur from an indirect trauma or fall onto an outstretched hand. Apex-volar fractures (more common, as in our case) tend to occur when the forearm is supinated during the injury, while apex-dorsal angulation occurs with the forearm pronated at the time of impact.[95]

The initial treatment for this fracture is a closed reduction and splinting in the emergency room with a good mold to the sugar-tong splint. Conversion to a cast or overwrapping the splint with a cast is acceptable at 2 weeks if reduction is well maintained. Fractures that are close to the physis have a high chance of remodeling, as do fractures in the plane of motion. This patient's fracture was reduced well, but it shifted in position during the 2 weeks in the splint (not well molded). This indicates that the fracture is unstable and has now shifted into an unacceptable position.

That being said, it is important to know what is acceptable for pediatric both-bone forearm fractures. Current textbooks indicate that, following closed reduction, the limits of acceptable angulation range from 10 to 20 degrees depending on the age of the child and the location of the fracture.[95-101] In adults, anatomic reduction is required; this is not the case for pediatric forearm fractures. For patients younger than 8 years, we can accept up to 20 degrees of angulation, complete displacement, and 45 degrees of malrotation. In patients who are older than 8 years, we can only accept up to 10 degrees of angulation, bayonet apposition, and 30 degrees of malrotation.[95]

In this case, the fracture has shifted into an unacceptable degree of angulation for a 9.5-year-old child, and ORIF with a flexible rod vs plates and screws will be the next step to improve the overall alignment. Advantages of IM nailing include small incisions, low infection risk, easy-to-remove hardware, and less surgical dissection. Typically, a 1.5- or 2.5-mm-diameter rod will be used, with the ulnar one entering proximally and the radial one distally. Plating can be done with compression plates and is the better option in cases of refracture.

A complication of these fractures, even with successful treatment and healing, is refracture. Parents need to be warned about this, and children should be splinted and protected from activities for several weeks after fracture union in an attempt to minimize this complication.

Why Might This Be Tested? It is important to be aware when a pediatric patient requires surgical vs non-operative management. It is also important to be aware of which fractures will remodel and can be observed. The forearm and distal radius are classic areas in which ages and degrees will be thrown at you to mix you up.

Here's the Point!

In patients younger than 8 years, up to 20-degree angulation, complete displacement, and 45 degrees of malrotation can be accepted with closed treatment. For older patients, these criteria become tighter, with only 10 degrees of angulation, 30 degrees of malrotation, and bayonet apposition being acceptable. Flexible nails or plates are used when surgery is necessary.

Vignette 33: Hey Doc, Can You Fix My Other Left Foot?

Ms. Lopez is a 46-year-old, Spanish-speaking female awaiting surgery in the preoperative unit. An orthopedic intern arrives and reviews her history and physical exam and confirms that she has consented to a debridement and groove-deepening procedure for a chronic left peroneal tendon dislocation. He verifies with the patient in limited Spanish that this is the correct procedure and signs his initials over the dorsum of her left foot. The senior resident had originally planned to do a hallux valgus case next, but because this patient has not yet arrived, Ms. Lopez's case is bumped into his operating room. The resident and anesthesia team wheel Ms. Lopez back to the operating room and begin setting up for her case. The attending is hurried because he is already behind schedule, and he comes into the operating room shortly thereafter. The circulating nurse asks for everybody in the room to state his or her name and title, which they do. The attending then speaks in Spanish with the patient to answer any final questions she may have, which the unilingual circulator mistakenly takes for a time-out. The senior resident shows the attending her markings for her planned incision and asks the attending for verification. The attending looks down briefly and confirms that she has marked out properly the landmarks for a distal metatarsal osteotomy. An incision is made and the procedure begins.

► *What has been done correctly so far in the preparation process?*

► *What mistakes have been made in the preparation process?*

The patient undergoes a successful distal metatarsal osteotomy for an incidental hallux valgus that was not causing her any discomfort. Her attending surgeon realizes his mistake when he is dictating the operative report later that afternoon. Ms. Lopez has already returned home by this point, but the attending calls her to explain the error and schedule her for the correct operation the next day. Frustrated with her team's seeming incompetence, Ms. Lopez tells him that she will be seeking her care elsewhere.

► *How common are wrong-site surgeries?*

► *What are the most common contributing factors to them?*

► *Where anatomically are wrong-site surgeries most common?*

Vignette 33: Answer

The orthopedic intern properly reviews the patient's history and physical exam and acts to confirm the proper surgery with the patient. However, with only limited Spanish, he should have used an interpreter to speak with the patient. One survey found that more than one-third of patients are not helpful when asked to identify their surgical site,[102] so it is crucial to have a systematic and thorough way of speaking with the patient and identifying the correct operation. In addition, the intern signed the patient's foot but did not sign over the planned incision site, as advised by the Sign Your Site initiative.[103] In spite of concerns about possible infection, preoperative signing over the surgical site has been shown not to compromise sterility.[104] When the intern updated his senior resident, he should not have relayed a transient characteristic, such as her bed number, but instead should have distinctly identified Ms. Lopez by her name and procedure. Similarly, the senior resident should have reviewed the patient's chart prior to starting her case. The circulating nurse correctly asked everybody to state his or her name and role in the procedure but should not have relied on the attending to perform a time-out in a language she herself did not understand. Finally, and most glaringly, the senior resident and attending mistook Ms. Lopez for one of many similar patients with surgeries scheduled later in the day.

Wrong-site surgery is included in the list of adverse outcomes known as *never events*, hospital-acquired conditions that are typically nonreimbursable. Orthopedic surgeons are responsible for the largest number of wrong-site surgeries, accounting for 68% of claims in the United States.[105] A study of 917 AAOS members[106] found that approximately 5.6% of reported medical errors were wrong-site procedures or wrong procedures. Seventy percent of these cases resulted in no adverse event or one with short-term morbidity, but 17% led to permanent morbidity or even death. Although equipment-related mistakes are the most frequent type of error in orthopedics, subanalysis has found that the leading factor contributing to wrong-site surgeries are communication errors. The most frequent anatomic locations of wrong-site surgeries are the knee and fingers/hand, accounting for 35% each. Formal time-out protocols have been established to eliminate wrong-site surgery, including all in the room agreeing on the correct operative site, confirmation with the consent form, rechecking that the leg is appropriately marked, confirming the position of the patient on the operating room table, assessing if DVT prophylaxis is needed/ordered, reviewing the patient's drug allergies, checking to see if use of a beta blocker medication is required, and ensuring that prophylaxis antibiotics were given in a timely manner. Such comprehensive checklists and protocols are crucial in preventing wrong-site surgery.

Why Might This Be Tested? The elimination of wrong-site surgery has been a priority of the AAOS and various specialty societies for more than 15 years with the Sign Your Site initiative and the North American Spine Society's Sign, Mark, and X-Ray program. The Joint Commission on the Accreditation of Healthcare Organizations has mandated the Universal Protocol, which focuses on patient identification, surgical site marking, and a time-out prior to incision.

Here's the Point!

Wrong-site surgeries are rare events and usually result in low morbidity, but they occur most frequently in the orthopedic community. The knee and fingers/hand are the most common sites, responsible for 70% of cases. You must do a thorough time-out prior to surgery.

Vignette 34: Doc, the Inside Part of My Knee Is Killing Me!

A 63-year-old male presents with approximately 2 years of isolated pain over the medial aspect of his knee. For a prior sporting injury, he underwent an open medial meniscectomy about 30 years ago. Examination reveals a mild varus deformity that does not correct past neutral, isolated medial joint line tenderness, a negative patellofemoral grind test, and a stable ligamentous exam. He has active ROM of 5 to 120 degrees of flexion. He has no significant adjacent joint complaints and has full ROM of his hips, ankles, and feet. The patient reports substantial disability and is looking to return to a more active lifestyle. X-rays of the affected knee are shown in Figure 34-1.

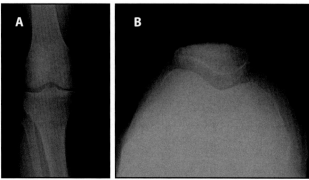

Figure 34-1. (A) AP and (B) Merchant's view x-rays showing medial compartment joint space narrowing.

▶ *What are potential treatment options for this patient?*

▶ *What unique potential risks are associated with UKA?*

▶ *What technical errors lead to progression of arthritis in the adjacent compartments?*

▶ *What are the classic indications for UKA?*

▶ *Describe the major design types of currently available UKA implants.*

Vignette 34: Answer

When a single compartment of the knee is affected and conservative management is no longer effective, there are 3 basic options for surgery. HTO is reserved for younger patients who are laborers and preferably have intact menisci. UKA is typically for elderly or younger patients not quite ready for a TKA. TKA is a reliable procedure but may be too much when only one part of the knee is diseased. In the setting of isolated unicompartmental arthritis, UKA allows for focal treatment of the disease while retaining uninvolved or minimally involved areas of the knee. In general, the surgery is less invasive and has a quicker recovery than TKA. In our case, the patient is no longer a young laborer with isolated disease, which would favor a UKA over HTO (higher reoperation rates, wound complications, and neurovascular injury) or TKA. Studies have demonstrated that patients with a successful UKA have a more normal-feeling knee, higher satisfaction scores, and 10-year survivorship of approximately 80% to 98%.[107,108] Most believe that these advantages are related to retention of the ACL, and gait analysis studies have demonstrated more normal knee mechanics after UKA when compared with TKA.[109]

Patients with partial replacements (UKA, patellofemoral arthroplasty, or bicompartmental arthroplasties) carry the unique risk of developing progressive arthritis in the unresurfaced compartments. The incidence of this complication has decreased with improvements in surgical technique. Care must be taken to not overstuff the resurfaced compartment and thereby shift forces to the adjacent compartment (overcorrection of alignment).[110] It is also important to avoid overhang of the femoral component anteriorly, creating patellofemoral impingement.[111] Despite good overall outcomes and survivorship, most studies and registry data note a higher revision rate for UKA compared with TKA.[112]

Revision of a UKA to a TKA can be straightforward, with results similar to that of primary TKA, or complicated, with results similar to that of revision TKA. Ultimately, the mode of failure and technical issues at the time of the index UKA (particularly the size of the tibial cut) will delegate the complexity of the revision.[113-115] However, in respecting modern principles of TKA and liberal use of stems and metallic augments, UKA conversion to TKA can be performed with a high level of success.

Although indications and contraindications for UKA are constantly evolving (some now suggest it is okay in the ACL-deficient knee and with moderate patellofemoral DJD), the classic criteria were initially described by Scott and Kozinn.[45] Patients are considered candidates for UKA if they meet the following criteria:

- Disease is isolated to only one compartment.
- The patient's weight is less than 180 lb (BMI < 35 kg/m^2). Although this is no longer strictly follow-up, it is where they will be leading you within a vignette. Obese patients have a higher failure rate, but there is no precise cutoff for BMI or weight.
- There is absence of a large coronal plane deformity (< 10 degrees of varus or < 15 degrees of valgus).
- There is less than a 10-degree flexion contracture.
- There is at least a 90-degree arc of motion.
- There is an absence of inflammatory arthritis.
- The cruciate ligaments are intact and functional.
- The patient has an average activity level and does not have the goal of returning to heavy labor or high-impact sports (typically older than 60 years). When the question writer mentions heavy laborer, he or she is typically pushing toward HTO vs arthrodesis.

The most common UKA designs can be divided into fixed and mobile bearing. The initial UKA designs were fixed bearing and performed poorly.[116] More recent fixed bearing designs implanted with improved surgical indications and technique have demonstrated survivorship of 90% to 98% at 10 years.[117] Mobile-bearing UKA consists of a polyethylene articular surface that is more conforming to the femoral component with a mobile articulation to a polished tibia baseplate. This provides the theoretical advantage of lower contact stresses with subsequent lower polyethylene wear rates, making this design more attractive for the younger patient population.[118] Although it is more technically challenging (increased risks for aseptic loosening, bearing dislocation, and arthritis progression) to implant than fixed-bearing UKA, specialized centers have reported equivalent survivorship rates of 95% at 10 years.[119,120]

Why Might This Be Tested? Partial knee replacements have been gaining popularity in the United States over the past decade. Improved surgical techniques and proper indications are important to understand and are commonly a source of test questions, as are associated complications with UKA.

Here's the Point!

With isolated unicompartmental disease in the setting of mild deformity and good ROM, UKA is an excellent option. Do not overcorrect the deformity, and remember that a well-done UKA has excellent results whether fixed or mobile bearing in nature.

Vignette 35: This Hip Is Killing Me Every Time I Stand Up!

A 73-year-old female presents with continued thigh pain after a primary THA. She reports pain with weight bearing, particularly when first getting up. She feels like she has to let her leg settle before she can start walking. Overall, there were no issues after her initial surgery, and she denies fevers or chills. There are occasional pains that start in the groin and radiate down the thigh. She is concerned something is wrong because all of her friends have had THAs and walk with no limp. Her AP hip x-ray is shown in Figure 35-1.

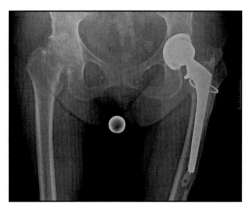

Figure 35-1. AP pelvis x-ray of a patient with worsening "start-up" left hip pain.

▶ *What is the diagnosis?*

▶ *Describe the bone defect classification systems associated with these findings.*

▶ *What are the treatment options?*

After undergoing hip revision, she feels great and refers her friend with continued groin pain after a THA to you. Her x-ray is shown in Figure 35-2. Infection workup is negative, and she is an otherwise healthy 70-year-old woman.

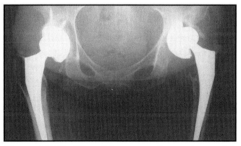

Figure 35-2. AP pelvis x-ray of a patient with continued left-sided groin pain.

▶ *What is the diagnosis?*

▶ *Describe the bone defect classification systems associated with these findings.*

▶ *What are the treatment options?*

Vignette 35: Answer

A 70-year-old patient with start-up pain (pain with initiating ambulation) in the thigh with a THA in place screams loosening of the femoral component. The vignette states no prior problems, fevers, or chills, which points to aseptic loosening. Figure 35-1 shows a serial x-ray (best test for loosening; 91% and 92% sensitive for the femoral and acetabular components, respectively) and shows subsidence of the cemented femoral component, cement mantle fracture, and proximal femoral remodeling. These are all criteria of loosening described by Harris et al (Table 35-1).[121]

Table 35-1.		
CRITERIA FOR DIAGNOSING A LOOSE CEMENTED FEMORAL COMPONENT		
Definite Loosening	Probable Loosening	Possible Loosening
• Continuous (new) radiolucent line at stem-cement • Fracture of the cement mantle • Fracture of the implant	• Continuous radiolucent line at bone-cement	• Radiolucent line around 50% to 100% of the cement-bone interface
Adapted from Harris WH, McCarthy JC Jr, O'Neill DA. Femoral component loosening using contemporary techniques of femoral cement fixation. *J Bone Joint Surg Am.* 1982;64(7):1063-1067.		

Additional criteria for loosening include component subsidence (often associated with a mantle defect) and debonding of the cement and femoral stem in the proximal femur (remember Gruen zones: 1 to 7 starting from the proximal lateral femur [zone 1] and extending around to the medial calcar area [zone 7]). There are 4 described modes of failure with cemented femoral stems: pistoning, medial midstem pivot, calcar pivot, and bending cantilever fatigue.[122] Cemented acetabular loosening can be diagnosed with a continuous radiolucent 2-mm line around the component (94% when in all 3 DeLee and Charnley zones and 71% in zones 1 and 2). Gross migration or change in the abduction angle are obvious signs of loosening.

It is also important to remember the signs of loosening of a cementless stem, which include component subsidence, presence of reactive lines adjacent to the component (okay to see these around smooth portion of the stem), distal canal expansion around a proximal fit stem, bead or porous surface shedding, presence of a bone pedestal (shelf at the end of the stem indicating vertical instability), and absence of spot welds (look for these at the point where the coating ends on the stem) or proximal stress shielding/calcar atrophy.[123] Fibrous stable implants can be seen with reactive lines in the porous coating area that are nonprogressive in the setting of a component that has not migrated. On the acetabular side, loosening is seen with screw breakage, shedding of the porous surface, and migration or change in angulation of the implant.

Bone defect classification systems exist for the femur and the acetabulum and can be used to direct treatment at the time of revision surgery. The 2 more common classification systems for both are the AAOS[124,125] (Table 35-2) and Paprosky[126,127] (Table 35-3) classifications.

For the first patient, this is a type IIIB (trust me, there is just under 4 cm of isthmus despite the limited x-ray) femur. For types I and II, it is possible to use a standard proximally coated stem, a cylindrical fully coated distal fixed stem, or a long tapered distal fit stem (modular or nonmodular). In type IIIA, a cylindrical, fully coated stem is suggested unless it appears to be greater than 18 mm thick, and a tapered, distal fit stem (Wagner style) can be used to manage this bony defect. Type IIIB typically require a modular or monoblock tapered, distal fit stem. Type IV femurs require an allograft-prosthetic composite (APC) or tumor prosthesis reconstruction. Case 2 depicts a Type IIIB acetabular defect and will likely require a larger (or jumbo) cup with the possibility of a figure-7 allograft or metallic augmentation. A cup cage construct could be used but is likely not necessary because there is no pelvic discontinuity. Type I and II defects can typically be treated with standard porous acetabular components (with type IIC, you may want a cup that gets a

Table 35-2.

AAOS ACETABULAR AND FEMORAL DEFICIENCY CLASSIFICATION SYSTEMS

Acetabular Defects	Femoral Defects
Type I: Segmental Deficiency • Peripheral • Superior • Anterior • Posterior • Medial wall	Type I: Segmental Deficiency • Proximal • Partial • Complete • Intercalary • Greater trochanter
Type II: Cavitary Deficiency • Peripheral • Superior • Anterior • Posterior • Medial wall	Type II: Cavitary Deficiency • Cancellous • Cortical • Ectasia
Type III: Combined Deficiency	Type III: Combined Deficiency
Type IV: Pelvic Discontinuity	Type IV: Malalignment • Rotational • Angular
Type V: Ankylosis	Type V: Femoral Stenosis
	Type VI: Femoral Discontinuity
Adapted from D'Antonio JA. Periprosthetic bone loss of the acetabulum. Classification and management. *Orthop Clin North Am.* 1992;23(2):279-290 and D'Antonio J, McCarthy JC, Bargar WL, et al. Classification of femoral abnormalities in total hip arthroplasty. *Clin Orthop Relat Res.* 1993;(296):133-139.	

better rim fit, elliptical shape, and medial bone graft). Type IIIB acetabular defects are similar to type IIIA in management and will likely require some element of augmentation (allograft or metallic) and possibly cage support if there is a discontinuity. Keep in mind that acute pelvic discontinuities should be plated and then a cup should be inserted, whereas chronic ones can be managed with a distraction technique that relies on the strong pelvic ligaments to clamp the remaining bone down to the distracting acetabular component.

Why Might This Be Tested? Classification systems that specifically direct treatment are commonly used for test questions. The Paprosky classification for femoral and acetabular defects helps guide appropriate management. Just know it and the criteria for a loose component.

Here's the Point!

Serial x-rays are the most accurate in diagnosing aseptic loosening. For Paprosky type IIIA and IIIB femurs, a long tapered stem (modular or nonmodular) is appropriate. For acetabular defects, a jumbo cup is favored when possible for all types of defects; however, augments, allograft-prosthetic composites, and impaction grafting are alternatives as well.

Table 35-3.

PAPROSKY CLASSIFICATION FOR ACETABULAR AND FEMORAL BONY DEFECTS

Acetabular Defects	Femoral Defects
Type I: Intact acetabular rim that is supportive • No significant migration • No ischial osteolysis • No teardrop osteolysis • Kohler's line is intact	Type I: Minimal loss of metaphyseal bone with an intact diaphysis, often with implants with only a macro-texture coating (ie, low-demand hip fracture stems)
Type II: Acetabular distortion, yet enough bone remains to support a hemispherical cup, <3 cm proximal migration, minimal osteolysis • IIA: superior bone loss • IIB: defect is not contained, columns are intact, and less than one-third of superior rim is lost • IIC: Significant medial wall defect	Type II: Extensive metaphyseal bone loss with an intact diaphysis, often seen with stems that are in the early phase of loosening
Type III: Significant segmental defect that is unable to support a hemispherical cup, >3 cm migration proximal to the obturator line • IIIA: Up and out defect, one-third to one-half of the circumference of the cup is deficient, mild to moderate osteolysis • IIIB: Up and in defect, only 40% of host bone will contact the implant, extensive lysis expected, and component is medial to Kohler line	Type III: Compromised metaphysis partially intact diaphysis • Type IIIA: The metaphysis is severely compromised and nonsupportive; a minimum of 4 cm of intact cortical bone is present in the diaphysis • Type IIIB: Severe metaphysis damage and <4 cm of intact bone in the isthmus
	Type IV: Extensive metaphyseal and diaphyseal damage with a stove-pipe like femoral canal, neither the isthmus or metaphysis is supportive

Adapted from Paprosky WG, Perona PG, Lawrence JM. Acetabular defect classification and surgical reconstruction in revision arthroplasty: a 6-year follow-up evaluation. *J Arthroplasty.* 1994;9(1):33-44 and Della Valle CJ, Paprosky WG. The femur in revision total hip arthroplasty evaluation and classification. *Clin Orthop Relat Res.* 2004;(420):55-62.

Vignette 36: Crystalline Arthropathy

A 65-year-old male presents to the emergency room with an acute onset of right knee pain and swelling. He denies a history of trauma, and this is the first episode that he has had knee pain, but he has had similar experiences in his feet before. He currently is on a diuretic and antihypertensive agents for high blood pressure but is otherwise healthy. He drinks 2 glasses of wine daily with dinner and does not smoke or use illicit drugs. On physical examination, the patient is 5 feet 7 inches tall, weighs 260 lb, is afebrile, and has a significant right knee effusion and pain with knee ROM. There is obvious calor and erythema to the skin but no open sores or lesions.

▶ *What is the presumed diagnosis?*

▶ *What tests are required to confirm the diagnosis?*

▶ *What are the treatment options?*

Vignette 36: Answer

The presumed diagnosis in this case is a gout attack or gouty arthritis. The clues in the vignette are the daily consumption of wine, male sex (men are 4 to 9 times more likely to develop gout), diuretic management, obesity, history of foot pain, and being afebrile (beware—on rare occasions, gout can cause fever and leukocytosis). These key words and phrases scream some form of crystalline arthropathy, more specifically gout. The main distractors that are placed to confuse or mislead you are the poor ROM, erythema, calor, and acute-onset knee pain. The goal is to piece the data together and come up with a good initial assumption that this patient has gout. In order to make the correct diagnosis, one must know a little bit about the disease itself.

Gout is typically caused by the body's inability to appropriately manage the uric acid balance in the blood, leading to hyperuricemia (serum uric acid levels >6.5 mg/dL). This results in crystalline deposition of monosodium urate systemically in various joints (arthritis), soft tissues (tophi), and organs (urate nephropathy, nephrolithiasis [ie, kidney stones]). Hyperuricemia can be related to a hereditary predisposition (purine metabolism or uric acid excretion disorders), high-purine diet (fine cheese), alcohol use, diuretic therapy (thiazide group of diuretics), poor kidney function, hematological diseases (myelo- and lymphoproliferative diseases), and obesity. Uric acid levels greater than 8.0 mg/dL correlate strongly with the incidence of gout; but remember, hyperuricemia does not equal gout.[128,129]

The pathophysiology of the disease relates to how the body regulates the uric acid pathway. Urate is the final product in the metabolism of the building blocks called purines and is excreted primarily through the kidneys. The crucial enzyme to commit to memory is xanthine oxidase, which degrades xanthine and hypoxanthine. Similarly in the kidney, polymorphisms may lead to dysfunctional transporters (URAT1 and SCL2A9), leading to the accumulation of serum urate. Low-dose aspirin and diuretics also reduce the urate excretion by inhibiting the URAT1 transport system.[128]

Gout typically presents as a monoarticular arthritis at the MTP joint of the first toe, called podagra. This is typically very painful and may be triggered by excessive food (seafood and red meat) and alcohol consumption, pH changes (acidosis), dehydration, systemic infection, trauma/surgery, decreased body temperature, or, paradoxically, with the initiation of urate-lowering therapy. (This is why we do not use allopurinol in the setting of an acute gout attack; it may actually make the symptoms worse!) Ninety percent of people will experience recurrent attacks at other joints in the first 5 years after the initial episode.[128] The differential diagnosis includes chondrocalcinosis/pseudogout (calcium pyrophosphate dehydrate crystals), oxalosis arthropathies (often with those on dialysis, calcium oxalate deposits), septic arthritis, psoriatic arthritis, and hemochromatosis (Table 36-1).

Table 36-1.

CHARACTERISTICS OF COMMON JOINT CONDITIONS

Diagnosis	Commonly Involved Joints	Synovial Cell Count (per mm³)	Crystals	X-Ray Findings
Gout	First MTP, knee, ankle	2000 to 50,000	Needle, (-) birefringence	Periarticular erosions
Pseudogout	Knee, wrist, first MTP	2000 to 50,000	Rhomboid, (+) birefringence	Calcification of cartilage
Septic arthritis	Knee most common	>50,000	None	Normal
MTP = metatarsophalangeal.				

The diagnosis is typically made on a combination of the history, present risk factors, and the classic location of podagra. Elevated serum uric acid does not necessarily confirm the diagnosis of gout; however, if suspected, we should act like doctors and not "boneheads" and order a complete blood cell count (CBC) and chemistry panel to assure we are not missing infection, hematological causes, or renal concerns in relation to a first-time gout attack. In addition, a joint aspirate or tophi biopsy to assess for urate crystal deposition can confirm the diagnosis when possible.[128,129]

Acute gout attacks should be managed to initially control the pain using NSAIDs (ibuprofen or indomethacin) and colchicine (0.5 mg every 2 hours until pain is improved or GI side effects arise). Steroids may be used but should be a second-line agent to the above medications. Long-term treatment should be based on uric acid level reductions to include altering the diet, maintaining hydration, treating associated conditions appropriately, and using allopurinol (xanthine oxidase inhibitor).[128,129] Allopurinol must be dosed per renal function, and typical side effects include skin reaction, elevated liver enzymes, eosinophilia, and hypersensitivity.

Why Might This Be Tested? Gout is another great imitator, and it is commonly confused with septic arthritis. It also affects 1% to 2% of adults in industrialized nations, so it is commonly seen by doctors around the world.

Here's the Point!

Confirm the diagnosis of gout with an aspiration (negative birefringence), look for underlying causes of excessive urate production or poor excretion, and then treat the condition (colchicine and NSAIDs acutely and allopurinol chronically).

Vignette 37: Hope This Fall Didn't Ruin My THA

An 85-year-old female presents to the emergency room with left-sided groin pain after a slip and fall while walking in her apartment. She denies any preceding events, hip pain, or medical concerns prior to the fall. She was able to stand and ambulate in her apartment, but the pain in her groin with weight bearing was severe. Her family brought her into the emergency room for evaluation of the groin pain and difficulty ambulating. She had a history of low back pain, a prior distal radius fracture, bilateral hip replacements, and treated breast cancer. The remainder of her past medical history includes hypothyroidism, hypertension, and hypercholesterolemia. She is 5 feet tall and weighs 110 lb, and her physical exam reveals some mild pain with log rolling of the leg and compression of the pelvis. An AP pelvis x-ray is shown in Figure 37-1.

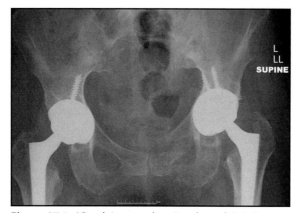

Figure 37-1. AP pelvis x-ray showing the pelvic injury.

▶ *What is the diagnosis?*

▶ *What is the underlying etiology of this injury?*

Vignette 37: Answer

The diagnosis is a fragility fracture of the pelvis, equivalent to a lateral compression type I pelvic fracture. The x-ray shows the obvious pubic rami fracture, and with close inspection, the contralateral sacrum has a compression fracture. The key to determining the etiology is the patient's age, sex, ethnicity, ability to ambulate, history of prior fragility fractures (wrist and vertebral body), and relative osteopenia on the x-rays. The distractors are the breast cancer history and the possibility of a hip fracture (ruled out by the x-ray). The bottom line is that this injury is related to osteoporosis.

Osteoporosis is an under-recognized condition, contributing to more than 2 million fragility fractures a year. The most common sites of fracture include the hip/pelvis, vertebrae, and wrist. In a nutshell, osteoporosis can be best described as a structural deterioration of the bony architecture related to low bone mass and an increased susceptibility to fracture. It is a quantitative and not a qualitative disorder of bone, meaning that the bone is normal but there is less of it. The mortality rate and morbidity associated with fragility fractures is significant, totaling more than $10 billion annually. Risk factors associated with fragility fractures include low body weight, history of fractures, family history, smoking, female sex, northern European background (fair skin and hair), early/postmenopausal (estrogen depletion), hyperthyroidism, medication use (corticosteroids, phenytoin, chemotherapy), and the natural aging process. There are 2 broad classifications: type I includes postmenopausal women and affects trabecular bone, namely in the vertebrae and wrist; type II is found in senile patients, is age related, and affects cortical and cancellous bone secondary to poor calcium absorption.[130,131]

Osteoporosis is diagnosed with a dual-energy x-ray absorptiometry (DEXA) scan because it is most accurate with the lowest radiation exposure. The World Health Organization (WHO) defines osteopenia as a T-score of -1 to -2.5, osteoporosis as a T-score of -2.5 or less, and severe osteoporosis as a T-score of -2.5 or less with a fragility fracture. The T-score is defined as the number of standard deviations below the average in healthy young women. Current indications for treatment include all postmenopausal women and in men 50 years and older with the following criteria:

- Any hip or vertebral fracture
- Other prior fractures and low bone mass
- T-score less than -2.5 after all secondary causes have been excluded
- Low bone mass (T-score between 1.0 and -2.5), plus the following:
  - Secondary cause associated with high fracture risk
  - WHO fracture risk algorithm, 10-year probability of hip fracture greater than 3%
  - WHO fracture risk algorithm, 10-year probability of any major osteoporosis-related fracture greater than 20%[130,131]

Current recommendations for maintaining optimal levels of vitamin D and calcium include 1200 mg of calcium for those older than 50 years and 1000 mg for those between 19 and 50 years. Similarly, the recommendation for those older than 50 years is to take 800 to 1000 IU of vitamin D. Bone health can also be improved by regularly participating in weight-bearing and muscle-strengthening exercise, minimizing risk factors for falling, and eliminating alcohol and tobacco use. Pharmacologic therapy includes hormone replacement (estrogen-progesterone) therapy if initiated in the first 6 years of menopause, calcitonin, raloxifene, parathyroid hormone, and the use of disphosphonates (oral or IV). Commonly used disphosphonates work by inhibiting osteoclast function and include alendronate, risedronate, ibandronate, and zoledronic acid. Transient side effects of the oral medications include GI upset, arthralgias, myalgias, and fever. ON of the jaw can occur with the use of disphosphonates and has been reported recently after IV administration. When taking these medications, one needs to have annual dental examinations and renal function tests periodically. Pharmacologic treatment has been successful in reducing hip and fragility fractures; however, recent reports of abnormal subtrochanteric femur fractures in patients on chronic disphosphonates have been described.[130,131]

Why Might This Be Tested? Osteoporosis and fragility fractures are regularly treated in practice and cover the upper and lower extremities, as well as the axial skeleton. Know the causes, diagnosis methods, treatments, and side effects associated with the currently available medications.

Here's the Point!

Osteoporosis is everywhere. We need to know how to maximize prevention methods and appropriately treat all those who meet the WHO criteria: osteopenia = T-score of -1 to -2.5; osteoporosis = T-score of less than -2.5; and severe osteoporosis = T-score below -2.5 and a fragility fracture.

Vignette 38: All of These Antibiotics—Which Do I Choose?!

A 45-year-old male presents for an elective TKA. The patient weighs 200 lb and is 6 feet 2 inches tall. He has a history of hypertension that is well controlled with diet and no other significant comorbidities or prior surgeries. Further discussion elicits a remote history of a rash after taking a penicillin variant as a child. He recalls no future reactions to antibiotics.

▶ *What are your options for antibiotic prophylaxis?*

The patient underwent a successful TKA and recovered without complication. At 3 months, the patient calls into the office to inquire about having some dental work performed because he vaguely recalls needing some sort of pretreatment.

▶ *What are the AAOS guidelines for prophylaxis prior to dental procedures?*

▶ *What other procedures necessitate the use of antibiotic prophylaxis after a TJA?*

▶ *What is the recommended duration that one requires prophylaxis after surgery?*

Vignette 38: Answer

Part I

The best management of surgical-site infections is prevention because this complication can hold grave consequences (particularly in TJA). The AAOS has created a set of evidence-based guidelines for antibiotic prophylaxis:

1. Choose antibiotic prophylaxis wisely, based on allergies and drug resistance. First-line agents include cefazolin and cefuroxime (dosed based on weight). For patients with a confirmed lactam allergy, vancomycin or clindamycin may be used. Patients colonized with methicillin-resistant *Staphylococcus aureus* (MRSA) should be treated with vancomycin as well.
2. Timing and dosing should optimize the efficacy of the antibiotics. The goal is to have therapeutic levels of systemic antibiotics by the time of skin incision, and it is recommended to give the antibiotic dose within 1 hour prior to surgery for cefazolin, cefuroxime, and clindamycin. For vancomycin, the infusion time is longer and should be started 2 hours prior to surgery (tourniquet inflation). For larger patients, dosing should be adjusted accordingly. Similarly, if the surgery is lengthy or substantial blood loss is incurred, redosing may be necessary: cefazolin should be given every 2 to 5 hours, cefuroxime every 3 to 4 hours, clindamycin every 3 to 6 hours, and vancomycin every 6 to 12 hours.
3. Antibiotic prophylaxis should conclude within 24 hours of the end of surgery.

In this case, due to a remote penicillin allergy, the options include a preoperative test dose of cefazolin, cefuroxime, or clindamycin. Due to his weight, doubling the routine dose would be suggested with redosing according to the schedule above. He has no history of prior infections or hospitalizations, so vancomycin is not indicated for his procedure. Routine nasal swabs are becoming more prevalent in practice, and antibiotic choice based on these findings has been suggested to improve clinical outcomes.

Although not specifically related to this question, it is important to know the mechanism of action of antibiotics because this is often tested (Table 38-1).

Why Might This Be Tested? AAOS guidelines are important to know and frequently appear on standardized tests. The use of antibiotic prophylaxis is crucial to all surgeons and should be well known and followed. Mechanism of action of antibiotics seems to show up on these tests as well, so just know it!

Table 38-1.

MECHANISM OF ACTION AND COMPLICATIONS OF ANTIBIOTIC CLASSES

Antibiotic Class	Mechanism of Action	Complications
Penicillins/ cephalosporins	Inhibits penicillin-binding proteins on the surface of cell membranes	Hypersensitivity/ drug resistance
Aminoglycosides	Inhibits protein synthesis by binding to ribosomal RNA	Auditory, vestibular, and renal toxicity
Macrolides and clindamycin	Binds to 50S-ribosomal subunit to inhibit dissociation of peptidyl-tRNA from ribosomes	Ototoxic/pseudomembranous enterocolitis
Quinolones	Inhibits DNA gyrase	Tendon ruptures
Vancomycin	Blocks the glycan subunit insertion into cell walls	Ototoxic, red man syndrome (rapid administration)
Daptomycin	Disrupts the bacterial membrane through the formation of transmembrane channels	Myopathies and increased creatine phosphokinase
Rifampin	Inhibits RNA synthesis in bacteria	Alters color of urine
Tetracyclines	Inhibits protein synthesis (70S and 80S ribosomes)	Stains teeth/bone

Here's the Point!

Make sure appropriate antibiotic prophylaxis is given, choose the correct antibiotics, make sure it is administered in the correct time frame, and confirm its completion within 24 hours of the procedure.

Part 2

The American Dental Association and the AAOS have developed recommendations for patients undergoing dental or other invasive procedures with an indwelling TJA. While these recommendations serve as guidelines, prophylaxis is indicated for all dental procedures, particularly in high-risk patients (inflammatory arthropathies, immune compromise, type 1 diabetes mellitus, TJA within 2 years, hemophilia, and malnutrition). Other procedures that require preventative antibiotics include all dental (extractions, gum manipulation, cleanings, orthodontic band placement, etc), GI, genitourinary, dermatology, and gynecological procedures that may cause bleeding. The current choice of antibiotics includes the following:

- Oral medications: cephalexin, cephradine, or amoxicillin: 2 gm orally 1 hour prior to procedure

    o Those allergic to penicillin may take clindamycin 600 mg 1 hour prior to the procedure.

- IV medications (those unable to take oral medications): cefazolin 1 g or ampicillin 2 gm intramuscular/IV 1 hour prior to procedure

    o Those allergic to penicillin may take clindamycin 600 mg IV 1 hour prior to the procedure.

Patients should follow these guidelines for at least the first 2 years after their TJA. Although acute hematogenous infections are rare (range, 0.5% to 17%[132,133]) late infections after dental and invasive procedures, they can be quite devastating. Early recognition of these infections is crucial because treatment may be successful in at least 50% of these cases.[134] Late hematogenous infections are typically more susceptible organisms, such as group B *Streptococcus*, and they can often be treated with an attempted irrigation and debridement with component retention. Although success rates are not optimal, these type III infections (type I acute infection, type II chronic infection, and type III acute hematogenous infection) warrant an attempt at retaining the initial implants with a modular component exchange.

Why Might This Be Tested? Prophylactic antibiotic guidelines have been established and should be well known. Appropriate management of hematogenous infections may be tested as well.

Here's the Point!

Antibiotic prophylaxis is indicated for at least 2 years after a TJA. Know the options and how to treat hematogenous infections if they develop.

Vignette 39: I Twisted My Knee a Week Ago and Now It's Swollen

A 53-year-old female presents to the emergency room with a 1-day history of progressive pain, swelling, and inability to bear weight on her right knee. She denies any history of recent trauma but says that she twisted her knee approximately 1 month ago. She also denies previous episodes of similar pain, prior knee surgery, sick contacts, or recent travel. She reports associated fevers and chills for the past 24 hours and says that she is getting over a cold. Her medical history is remarkable for non–insulin-dependent diabetes mellitus and hypertension. On physical examination, she is 5 feet 6 inches tall, weighs 140 lb, is febrile to 102.3°F, and has a heart rate of 112 bpm. There is a mild left knee effusion with overlying warmth and erythema, and the patient has pain with short arcs of passive flexion and extension. The ligamentous examination is stable, and her straight leg raise is intact. There are no open wounds or lesions. Serum laboratory values are notable for WBC of 18,000 cells/uL, with a differential of 96% PMNs, ESR of 63 mm/hr, and CRP of 92 mg/L; blood cultures are pending. X-rays are negative for fracture, dislocation, or foreign body but show a moderate knee joint effusion.

▶ *What is the presumed diagnosis?*

▶ *What tests are required to confirm the diagnosis?*

▶ *What are the treatment options?*

Vignette 39: Answer

The presumed diagnosis in this case is septic arthritis. The clues in the vignette are the acute presentation, history of non–insulin-dependent diabetes mellitus, fever, examination findings, and elevated WBC (including elevated neutrophil differential), and inflammatory markers. These key findings should shout infection to you, until proven otherwise. The main distractor here is her relatively recent history of trauma (twisting her knee). The goal is to piece the data together and presume that this patient has acute septic arthritis.

Acute septic arthritis is a surgical emergency most often caused by bacterial seeding of a joint, although viruses and fungi can alternatively be involved. The most common affected joints include the knee, hip, elbow, ankle, and sternoclavicular joint. Septic arthritis can occur in 1 of 3 ways: direct inoculation from trauma or surgery, contiguous spread from adjacent osteomyelitis, or in the setting of bacteremia (more common in immunocompromised patients and hospitalized individuals). Recently, several cases of septic arthritis following corticosteroid injection, as well as hyaluronic acid injection, have been reported. Bacterial seeding of a joint causes irreversible articular cartilage damage, often within 8 hours of inoculation, due to release of proteolytic enzymes from host PMNs and from the bacteria itself, as well as from a concomitant direct pressure effect.[135,136]

The most common pathogen responsible for causing septic arthritis is *S aureus*, which accounts for more than 50% of all reported cases. Other common pathogens include *Staphylococcus epidermis* and *Neisseria gonorrhea* (most common in otherwise healthy sexually active young patients, can be migratory). Less common, but still important, pathogens to be aware of include *Salmonella* (often seen in patients with sickle cell disease), *Pseudomonas aeruginosa* (often seen in patients with a history of IV drug use), *Pasteurella multocida* (encountered after an animal bite), and *Eikenella corrodens* (encountered after a human bite). *Streptococcus* species can also be seen, but they are more common in children than in adults (see www.wheelessonline.com/ortho/bacterial_menu for complete details).

Septic arthritis will typically present as an acute, monoarticular inflammation, most commonly affecting the knee joint. The differential diagnosis in these patients includes crystalline arthropathy (gout, pseudogout), inflammatory arthropathy (rheumatoid, psoriatic, reactive), and, less likely, tumor, occult fracture, and flare of OA. Patients with acute septic arthritis will have the acute onset of a warm, edematous, erythematous, and painful joint, often with inability to bear weight. Pain is typically diffusely throughout the joint (as opposed to localized to a single location); pain with passive ROM is a classic physical examination finding. X-rays are typically unremarkable but will often show the joint effusion.

Serum laboratory findings are extremely useful in the workup of patients with presumed septic arthritis. Patients will most often have an elevated WBC with a left shift, as well as elevated ESR and CRP (cutoff values depend on the laboratory because various ranges of normal exist). An elevated WBC count with a left shift is indicative of infection, but the absence of an abnormal WBC does not rule out infection. Inflammatory markers, including ESR and CRP, can be elevated in the settings of infection and inflammation. The ESR will remain elevated for up to 3 to 4 weeks, while the CRP typically normalizes within 1 week of appropriate treatment; however, the values can vary depending on the success of the treatment regimen and other concomitant conditions.

Aspiration of joint fluid remains the gold standard for the diagnosis of acute septic arthritis.[137,138] Every attempt should be made to aspirate the joint in an area away from any erythema or open wounds so as to avoid contaminating the joint. Joint fluid should be analyzed for cell count with differential, Gram stain, aerobic culture, anaerobic culture, and crystal analysis. If there is a clinical concern for atypical pathogens, such as *Propionibacterium acnes* (shoulder) or *Mycobacterium tuberculosis*, fluid will need to be analyzed for longer periods of time (ie, 21 days for *P acnes*). Aspirations consistent with septic arthritis will often show a WBC greater than 50,000 cells/uL, but lower values are possible. The Gram stain is only able to identify the organism in approximately one-third of cases and is not a cost-effective test.

Acute septic arthritis is a surgical emergency because cartilage destruction can occur within 8 hours of bacterial inoculation. After obtaining samples for cultures from the joint aspiration, broad-spectrum IV antibiotics should be initiated. Antibiotics should provide coverage for gram-positive and -negative organisms until antibiotic choices can be narrowed based on culture results. Regimens in young, healthy adults should include coverage for *S aureus* and *N gonorrhea*, while coverage in immunocompromised patients should include *P aeruginosa*. Surgical intervention with open or arthroscopic debridement and irrigation should be performed as soon as possible, with a low threshold to return to the operating room for repeat procedures pending the clinical course.[139] When arthroscopic debridement is unsuccessful, open synovectomy and debridement are recommended. Patients too sick to go to the operating room may be treated with serial aspirations, although it is a less ideal form of management.

Why Might This Be Tested? Acute septic arthritis is a common diagnosis that can cause significant joint morbidity if not quickly identified and treated. There is some clinical overlap between infectious and inflammatory arthropathies, so understanding the key components of patient presentation, examination findings, laboratory findings, and aspirate findings is critical.

Here's the Point!

Confirm the diagnosis of septic arthritis with an aspiration (WBC > 50,000 and elevated PMNs), look for underlying risk factors, and then treat the condition (operative debridement and irrigation with IV antibiotics).

Vignette 40: Doc, Why Are Batters Hitting My Fastball?

A 19-year-old minor league pitcher has noticed a drop in his pitching velocity over the past 3 months. Over just the past 4 weeks, he has noticed mild discomfort at his dominant right medial elbow at the late cocking phase of his throwing but not during follow-through. He denies any history of trauma and mechanical symptoms and has no symptoms unless he is throwing. He has no evidence of neurologic symptoms. His physical examination demonstrates painless elbow ROM from 0 to 145 degrees on the left and 10 to 145 degrees on the right, with no pain at terminal extension. He is tender over the medial epicondyle and the path of the MCL. Resisted active wrist flexion causes no symptoms, but he has asymmetric laxity on stress testing of the MCL with a positive moving valgus stress test. Neurologic examination demonstrates no focal deficits or abnormalities. Plain x-rays show a well-reduced ulnohumeral articulation without degenerative changes or loose bodies. An axial x-ray shows no posterior ulnohumeral abnormalities.

▶ *What is the most likely diagnosis? What is on the differential diagnosis?*

▶ *What advanced imaging may be helpful?*

▶ *Describe the soft tissue anatomy that creates stability against valgus stress.*

▶ *What are the principal surgical treatment options?*

▶ *What can be expected as far as clinical outcome and return to sport?*

Vignette 40: Answer

This patient presents with insufficiency of the MCL of the elbow. This is likely in the form of attritional insufficiency secondary to overuse as a high-level throwing athlete given the lack of trauma. His history and occupation make this diagnosis likely, as does his physical exam pattern of laxity. The moving valgus stress test is believed to be the most sensitive and specific exam for this diagnosis, and it is performed with the patient upright and the shoulder abducted 90 degrees. The elbow is quickly extended from 120 to 30 degrees of flexion while applying a valgus load, which should cause medial elbow pain.[140] The differential diagnosis in such a case must also include medial epicondylitis, which would also present with tenderness at the medial epicondyle but should have pain with resisted wrist flexion but no signs of laxity. Ulnar neuropathy or a subluxating ulnar nerve must also be evaluated for. Neuropathy will usually present with complaints of numbness and tingling and cold intolerance with hand weakness, and a subluxating nerve will typically rest in the ulnar groove in extension but subluxate anterior to the epicondyle in flexion. Advanced imaging is typically indicated because the diagnosis is sometimes unclear. MRA is now preferred, with the greatest sensitivity and specificity for diagnosing complete and partial tears, and can also help assess for other pathology. (This vignette is primarily for the MCL, but one cannot talk about MCL injuries without evaluating the ipsilateral shoulder, especially assessing for a glenohumeral internal rotation deficit [GIRD]. This discussion should be done to include in the initial physical exam. If GIRD is not corrected, MCL reconstruction will likely fail.)

The medial elbow has dynamic and static soft tissue restraints. The primary dynamic restraint is the flexor pronator mass, especially the flexor carpi ulnaris and FDS. The primary static soft tissue restraint is the MCL, which serves overall as the primary restraint to valgus load, even more so in flexion than extension. Although the MCL is composed of 3 bands (anterior, posterior, and transverse), the anterior is the primary restraint and is reconstructed surgically.[140] The anterior band originates on the anteroinferior medial epicondyle, inserts on the medial ulna at the sublime tubercle, and is most taut in mid-range flexion (30 to 90 degrees).[140,141]

A complete symptomatic tear in a high-level thrower who is eager to return to sport is typically treated with reconstruction using palmaris longus autograft or hamstring allograft or autograft through bone tunnels in the medial epicondyle and medial ulna. Every effort is made to create anatomic restoration of the anterior bundle of the MCL. Ulnar nerve decompression is required to access the insertion site, and formal transposition is recommended. There are several acceptable fixation options, but a detailed description of the surgical technique and fixation options is out of the scope of this vignette.

The original Jobe technique for reconstruction required complete release of the flexor pronator mass and ulnar nerve submuscular transposition, which resulted in ulnar nerve complication rates between 20% and 30%. This technique typically had return to sport rates of 60% to 70%. The docking technique described by Altchek[142] has become the preferred technique for many surgeons, allowing less invasive single-tunnel placement in the humerus and fine tensioning of the graft. Series using this technique report greater than 90% return to sport and decreased ulnar nerve complications.[141]

Why Might This Be Tested? The anatomic support of the medial elbow is well known, and insufficiency of the MCL presents classically in throwing athletes. MCL insufficiency is likely to be encountered by many general, sports medicine, and upper extremity surgeons, and the operative indications, surgical principles, and expected outcomes should be known.

Here's the Point!

Unlike LCL insufficiency, MCL insufficiency typically presents with a stable elbow that is largely asymptomatic at rest but demonstrates medial elbow pain and decreased throwing velocity in throwing athletes. Be aware of the classic physical exam maneuvers for MCL insufficiency. MCL reconstruction with tendon allograft is the preferred technique for athletes who plan to resume throwing, with return-to-sport rates of approximately 90% in most series.

Vignette 41: Why Does My Hip Snap After My THA?

A 65-year-old female returns to your office 12 months post primary THA with persistent groin pain. She reports that the groin pain is worse with climbing stairs and getting up from her car seat. Two weeks ago, she noticed a snapping sensation about her hip. On physical examination, gentle passive ROM is painless and she ambulates with a relatively normal gait. Resisted hip flexion is painful. A postoperative x-ray is shown in Figure 41-1.

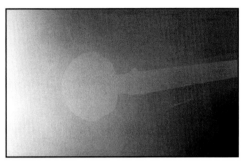

Figure 41-1. Shoot-through lateral x-ray. Notice the position of the acetabular cup and its relationship to the anterior aspect of the bony acetabulum.

▶ *What is the most likely diagnosis?*

▶ *What are some additional causes for persistent pain after a primary THA?*

▶ *What is the relevant pathoanatomy?*

▶ *How does one go about diagnosing this condition?*

▶ *What are the nonoperative and surgical options?*

Vignette 41: Answer

The patient in this vignette has anterior iliopsoas impingement/tendonitis after a primary THA. This poorly understood etiology for persistent pain after a primary THA has a low incidence of 4.3%, while the true incidence following a revision surgery remains unknown. Factors that may predispose a patient to develop this impingement include excessive offset, limb-length discrepancy, malpositioned acetabular component (see Figure 41-1), long screws, retained cement, or acetabular cage/reinforcement ring. Other common causes for persistent pain following a THA include infection, aseptic loosening, referred pain, bursitis, and HO.[143-145]

The iliopsoas musculotendinous unit is a convergence of the psoas and iliacus muscles, which originate from the T12, L1-L5 vertebral bodies, and iliac fossa of the pelvis, respectively. They join at the level of the inguinal ligament to insert onto the anteromedial aspect of the lesser trochanter. After a THA, the once extra-articular ligament may now be intra-articular if the anterior capsule was opened.

Patients usually report anterior groin pain that is persistent and exacerbated with activities that require resisted hip flexion, such as entering/exiting an automobile, walking up stairs, and rising from a chair. Only rarely do patients describe a sensation of clunking or snapping. On physical examination, the patient may have a slight antalgic gait. Pain may be reproduced or made worse with a straight leg raise or resisted seated hip flexion. Pain may occur with passive hyperextension or active external rotation and extension of the hip.

One must rule out infection, component loosening, adverse local tissue reaction, or periprosthetic fracture (often pubic rami). Laboratory results (ESR, CRP) and technetium Tc-99m scintigraphy will be normal in this case. Serial x-rays remain the most important imaging study (including preoperative films). If tests are normal, further imaging is warranted.

AP, frog, lateral, and cross-table lateral views of the hip should be evaluated for component positioning, retained cement, osteolysis, and intrapelvic screws. The lateral view may show prominence of the acetabular component relative to the bony rim (retroversion or prominence associated with a large cup). If the x-rays are equivocal, a CT scan may be useful to determine cup version, anterior uncoverage, and iliopsoas tendon or bursal hypertrophy. MRI is less useful given the scatter; however, recently metal artifact reduction software MRI have been able to pick up pathology around the hip in a more sensitive manner. Ultrasound is a useful modality in that the tendon can be visualized as it is displaced by the cup anteriorly or medially.

A useful technique that confirms the diagnosis of impingement is an image-guided diagnostic injection of contrast material, local anesthetic agent, and/or corticosteroid. A temporary relief of pain confirms the diagnosis. One must make sure that the tendon sheath is injected and not the joint or surrounding neurovascular structures (could lead to quadriceps weakness).

Conservative treatment for impingement after THA consists of NSAIDs, physical therapy, rest, and pain medication. An injection of a local anesthetic and corticosteroid may provide permanent relief for symptoms, but this is rare (particularly if mechanical cause of the syndrome is present).

Surgery offers the best chance for permanent relief from impingement. The procedures that have been considered successful include iliopsoas tendon release or lengthening, removal of excessively long screws or retained cement, and acetabular component revision with or without iliopsoas release. Acetabular revision is recommended when the preoperative x-rays or CT scan demonstrate that the anterior edge of the acetabular component protrudes in front of the anterior rim.

Why Might This Be Tested? Component malposition after THA is not very forgiving, and you must know the sequelae. Although soft tissue impingement may seem minor, the means for resolution may require a major revision procedure.

Here's the Point!

Retroverted and excessively large acetabular components can lead to anterior overhang and iliopsoas impingement. Symptomatic treatment often helps temporarily; however, a permanent solution may require component revision and correction of any malpositioned components or prominent hardware.

Vignette 42: Pediatric Atraumatic Limp

The parents of an 8-year-old male bring their child in for evaluation of a painless limp that they have noticed for the past 6 months. Initially, they thought the limp would go away; however, it has become more pronounced over the past 2 to 3 months. There is no history of traumatic injury. He has minimal pain but limited rotational motion of the hip (particularly abduction and internal rotation) and appears to be younger than his stated age. An initial AP x-ray of the hip is shown in Figure 42-1.

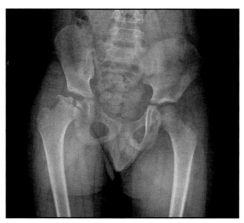

Figure 42-1. Initial AP hip x-ray.

▶ *What is the diagnosis?*

▶ *What are the bad prognostic indicators of this disease/injury?*

▶ *What are the current treatment options?*

Vignette 42: Answer

The diagnosis is Legg-Calvé-Perthes disease, which is a childhood disorder that affects the hip. The disease most commonly occurs in children aged 5 to 8 years, with a male:female ratio of 5:1. There is a 10% to 15% incidence of bilateral disease, and children often appear to be younger than their chronological age.[96] Legg-Calvé-Perthes disease is essentially an unknown cause for ischemic necrosis of the femoral head. Modern proposed etiologies include type II collagen mutations (missense mutation glycine for serine codon replacement of COL2A1) and inherited thrombophilia (factor V Leiden, increased protein C or S, and deficient antithrombin III).[96] Although Legg-Calvé-Perthes disease is often well tolerated at a young age, it is estimated that more than 50% of patients will develop disabling hip arthritis in the sixth decade of life.[96] Physeal changes are often found in the anterior part of the femoral head.

Waldenstrom reported 4 x-ray stages for Legg-Calvé-Perthes disease: initial (seen as early femoral head opacities), fragmentation (1 year long), reossification (3 to 5 years long), and healed. Stulberg classified femoral head shape in correlation with future radiographic signs of OA at maturity for patients with Legg-Calvé-Perthes disease: type I, normal hip (low risk of OA); type II, spherical head with enlargement, short neck, or steep acetabulum (16% with radiographic evidence of OA at 40-year follow-up); type III, nonsperhical femoral head (58% with radiographic findings of OA); type IV, flat femoral head (75% with radiographic findings of OA); and type V, flat head with incongruent acetabulum (78% with radiographic findings of OA).

Other classification systems to describe the femoral head and prognosis include the Catterall classification, which includes the following groups: group I (anterior head involved only), group II (anterior head involved only with a sequestrum), group III (only a small part of epiphysis not involved), group IV (total head involvement). Catterall head-at-risk signs include lateral subluxation, lateral calcification, diffuse metaphyseal reaction, horizontal growth plate, and Gage sign (v-shaped defect at lateral metaphysis). The last classification system is the lateral pillar (lateral 15% to 30% of femoral head)/Herring classification: group A (little head involvement and good outcome), group B (>50% of lateral pillar height maintained leads to good outcome in those younger than 6 years), and group C (<50% of lateral pillar maintained yields poor prognosis in all age groups).

When Legg-Calvé-Perthes presents in a child younger than 6 years, the long-term results are typically good with nonoperative management. Bad prognostic indicators include age older than 8 years, lateral head subluxation, metaphyseal cysts, group C lateral pillar classification, 2 or more head-at-risk signs, female sex, poor ROM, and premature physeal closure.

Initial treatment depends on the age of presentation and radiographic findings. A child who presents at age 9 years typically undergoes a more aggressive approach than a child who presents at age 4 years. The mainstay of management is nonoperative treatment for children younger than 6 years; children aged 6 to 8 years are in a gray zone, and children older than 8 years will require surgery (femoral and/or acetabular osteotomy). In our case, the child is presenting at 8 years old, and consideration for containment of the head should include femoral or acetabular osteotomy vs bracing, physical therapy, and close monitoring. The main goal is containment of the hip, so regardless of the age of presentation, surgical intervention is recommended if the hip begins to show signs of subluxation. In addition, pain relief and restoration of motion are paramount to a successful outcome. Again, in a child who presents at younger than 6 years of age, surgery is almost never performed.

You will never see bilateral Legg-Calvé-Perthes in the same stage. One hip may be in the fragmentation phase while the other is in the reossification phase. If you see bilateral Legg-Calvé-Perthes disease in the same stage, be aware of the diagnosis of multiple epiphyseal dysplasia.

Why Might This Be Tested? Legg-Calvé-Perthes disease is a common cause for a painless limp in a child. A common answer for this disease management is nonoperative treatment, and the question writers love this option. There are distinct prognostic indicators; bad prognostic indicators include age older than 8 years, group C lateral pillar classification, 2 or more head-at-risk signs, female sex, poor ROM, and premature physeal closure, making this an ideal topic for questions.

Here's the Point!

Patients younger than 6 years will not require surgery and will have a good prognosis, whereas ages 6 to 8 years is a gray zone and patients older than 8 years will need surgery. Know the Catterall, Stulberg, and lateral pillar classification schemes. The key for management of Legg-Calvé-Perthes disease is containment of the femoral head in the acetabulum.

Vignette 43: "Funny Looking" Walk

A 19-month-old female is brought to the office because her parents have noticed a limp developing. She was the result of a normal vaginal delivery. Her milestones were all met within an age-appropriate time frame. The parents had brought her to the pediatrician for evaluation when she began walking at 13 months of age because of a "funny looking" gait. They were told not to worry at that time because her gait should improve over time.

When she returned to the office, she was average height and weight. She had a limb-length inequality (left shorter than the right) and ambulated with a significant limp (best described as an antalgic gait). An AP pelvis x-ray is shown in Figure 43-1.

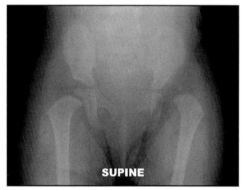

Figure 43-1. AP pelvis x-ray.

▶ *What is the diagnosis?*

▶ *What are the treatment options?*

▶ *How would the treatment differ if the patient were a newborn?*

Vignette 43: Answer

The patient has a unilateral hip dislocation with developmental dysplasia of the hip (DDH). These patients typically present with a limb-length inequality, abnormal gait, or limp. They will have asymmetrical hip abduction. When there is a unilateral hip dislocation, there will be an apparent limb-length inequality, asymmetric hip ROM, asymmetric skin folds, and limp (if the child is ambulatory). Risk factors for this condition include breech positioning, female sex, positive family history, and being the first-born child.[146] It is more commonly found on the left side and is associated with other packaging disorders, such as metatarsus adductus (10%) and torticollis (20%).[147]

This condition is associated with pathologic conditions leading to a shallow acetabulum, capsular laxity, and overgrowth of the pulvinar. There is delayed ossification of the acetabulum (deficient anterolaterally) and femoral head (small and exaggerated femoral anteversion). Radiographic findings of DDH often include a discontinuous Shenton's line, delayed or small femoral head ossific nucleus, and acetabular inclination angles of greater than 24 degrees at 2 years old and greater than 28 degrees at 3 months old.

The treatment in this patient (19 month old with chronic dislocation) requires an open hip reduction, possible adductor tenotomy, femoral shortening, and possibly an acetabuloplasty (Salter, Dega, or Pemberton). Typically between 12 and 18 months, a closed reduction can be attempted, and open procedures can be reserved for those who have an obstruction to a concentric reduction. In children older than 18 months old, an open reduction is the treatment of choice. Patients diagnosed after the age of 8 years will often not undergo open reduction because acetabular remodeling is not likely to occur.

If the patient were a newborn, initial treatment would be a Pavlik harness; however, Pavlik harness treatment protocol varies. When placing the harness, one needs to avoid excessive abduction in the harness because it can lead to ON, while excessive flexion can lead to a transient femoral nerve palsy. An ultrasound is usually done at 4 weeks to ensure reduction. If the hip is not relocated in the harness by 4 weeks, the Pavlik harness is discontinued so as not to cause Pavlik harness disease. If relocation is successful, length of treatment varies and should be maintained until the ultrasound is normal.

Patients older than 3 months for whom the ultrasound doesn't show reduction need to undergo closed vs open reduction and casting. An arthrogram is performed at the time of casting. If the medial dye pool is less than 5 mm, a closed reduction, possible adductor release, and casting is all that is needed. However, if it is greater than 5 mm, open reduction and casting is required. The open reduction should be done via a medial approach. Patients older than 1 year usually require an open reduction via an anterior approach (± acetabular and/or femoral osteotomy). All known causes inhibiting concentric reduction can be addressed with a medial open reduction, except performing a capsulorrhaphy. This can only be addressed with an anterior approach.

Obstruction to reduction can be intrinsic or extrinsic to the hip[147]:

- Extra-articular
    - Tight iliopsoas tendon (creates hourglass narrowing of capsule)
    - Adductor muscle contractures
- Intra-articular
    - Joint capsule contracture
    - Pulvinar
    - Hypertrophied ligamentum teres
    - Infolded labrum
    - Hypertrophied transverse acetabular ligament

The complication of avascular necrosis is only a result of treatment. Osteonecrosis may occur after Pavlik use (excessive abduction), after being placed in a spica, or after surgery. Osteonecrosis is not seen in hips that are left untreated. Bilateral hip dislocations are treated in a similar fashion, unless the child is older than 8 years. In patients older than 8 years with a unilateral hip dislocation, an attempt at a reduction may be performed; however, this would be an extensive surgery requiring femoral and acetabular osteotomies. If the patient is older than 8 years with bilateral hip dislocations, the hips should be left alone.

Why Might This Be Tested? The treatment is different depending on the child's age, which they love to test. Being able to identify the possibility of a hip dislocation via a clinical exam and history is crucial to not missing the diagnosis.

Here's the Point!

Newborn children are treated with a Pavlik harness (beware excessive flexion and abduction); for children aged 6 to 18 months, attempt closed reduction and move to an open procedure if concentric reduction is not obtained; and for children older than 18 months, it is more likely that an open reduction procedure will be needed. A medial approach for young children may be performed, whereas an anterior approach is reserved for those older than 1 year.

Vignette 44: Doc, Why Do I Keep Stumbling?

A 79-year-old female presents to the office with a 2-week history of mid-low back pain. She denies any falls or trauma but has noticed balance problems and occasional tripping over the past several months. She has many medical problems but is not sure of any specific diagnoses except for arthritis and does not know her current medications. She lives alone and rarely sees a physician. She denies any previous fractures, except for a broken wrist 26 years ago when she slipped on the ice outside her apartment building. She is currently taking acetaminophen for her pain but states that most of her daily activities are difficult to perform these days because they exacerbate the pain. X-rays show T9, T11, T12, and L2 compression deformities and multilevel degenerative changes.

▶ *What further workup may be considered?*

▶ *Based on bone density measurements, how is osteoporosis defined? Who should be routinely screened?*

▶ *The patient states that she is not interested in any surgery, interventional procedure, or medication for treatment. What other options for pain control and bone health management can be offered?*

Vignette 44: Answer

Further workup in the setting of osteoporotic vertebral fractures is intended to confirm osteoporosis as the most likely etiology of her fracture, to evaluate her current bone health status, and to rule out any secondary causes of her osteoporosis. A detailed history and physical exam can help identify the presence of risk factors or medical conditions. More advanced imaging (MRI or CT) may be considered if, upon further questions, her presentation was atypical in nature or depending on her medical history. A DEXA scan, chemistry panel, CBC, and 25-hydroxy vitamin D level should also be checked to measure bone mass and to primarily exclude other diseases or to identifiably modifiable conditions. More extensive laboratory studies can also be performed, including markers for bone resorption and formation, but their interpretation can be difficult and of limited usefulness. For this specific patient, her recent balance issues may also warrant further evaluation and possible EMG/NCS to rule out neuropathy or neurology referral.

Bone density is routinely reported as a T-score, or standard deviations above or below the young adult mean, which is the expected normal value of the patient's peak bone density at about age 20 years compared with others of the same sex and ethnicity. Normal bone mass is within one standard deviation of the young adult mean, whereas a T-score of -2.5 or less (>2.5 standard deviations below the young adult mean) is defined as osteoporosis.[148] Osteoporosis can also be diagnosed clinically in the setting of a spinal compression fracture or hip fracture. The classification of osteopenia is for those bone densities with T-scores between -1.0 and -2.5. According to the National Osteoporosis Foundation, a bone density test is generally recommended for women aged 65 years or older, men aged 70 years or older, those with a fracture after age 50, women of menopausal age with risk factors, postmenopausal women younger than age 65 with risk factors, and men aged 50 to 69 years with risk factors. Z-scores, the number of standard deviations the patient's bone density values are from the values expected for the patient's age, are also regularly reported and can be used instead of T-scores, particularly for children, teens, women still having periods, and younger men.[148]

Other options for pain may include bracing, physical modalities, and activity modification. To address pain exacerbations and to decrease risk for future falls and fractures, physical therapy could be prescribed to assess for use of assistive devices, to strengthen the supporting muscles, to improve balance and flexibility, and for postural correction and proper body mechanics education. Transcutaneous electric nerve stimulator (TENS), acupuncture, and biofeedback could also be considered. Further options with regard to her osteoporosis could also include a home evaluation to assess her living conditions and any home modifications that may put her at further risk of fall or fracture. Depression is common due to pain and functional decline and warrants attention if applicable. Finally, postural training supports and therapeutic exercise, including aerobic, weight-bearing activities, and resistance training options, have been preliminarily supported in the medical literature, although evidence of specific and detailed recommendations has been more conflicted.

Why Might This Be Tested? Osteoporosis is a common disorder in the US and worldwide. Many manifestations can occur, and vertebral compression fracture is a common one. Diagnosing and managing these fragility fractures can be difficult, making them a favorite for testing.

Here's the Point!

Know the primary and secondary causes of osteoporosis and how to diagnose it. DEXA scans are recommended for women aged 65 years and older, men older than 70 years, those with a fracture after age 50 years, women of menopausal age with risk factors, postmenopausal women younger than 65 years with risk factors, and men aged 50 to 69 years with risk factors.

Vignette 45: Shoulder Arthritis

A 63-year-old, right-hand-dominant male presents to your office with right shoulder pain that has progressively worsened over the past several years. The pain is worse with activity and bothers him at night. He denies any previous history of trauma or surgical procedures. On examination, he is noted to have limited active and passive ROM, particularly in external rotation. He has significant crepitus and pain with ROM. Strength testing reveals an intact rotator cuff. X-rays are shown in Figure 45-1.

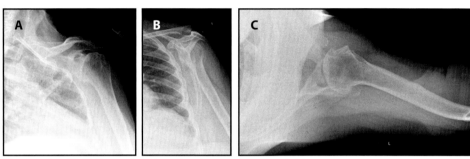

Figure 45-1. (A-C) X-rays showing glenohumeral osteoarthritis.

▶ *What is the most likely diagnosis?*

▶ *What radiographic features are characteristic of this disease?*

▶ *What other tests should be ordered?*

▶ *What are the treatment options?*

▶ *If this patient presented with similar complaints but a history of a massive rotator cuff and pseudo-paralysis on examination, how would this change your management?*

Vignette 45: Answer

The diagnosis in this case is primary shoulder OA. The patient demonstrates classic symptoms of OA, which is confirmed on exam and with imaging. He has no history of trauma, instability, or prior surgery that could cause secondary OA. History should also be obtained about any rheumatologic or systemic disorders that may suggest inflammatory arthritides. In OA, pain and crepitus on examination are characteristic. Due to posterior osteophytes, the anterior capsule can become contracted, leading to a significant decrease in external rotation.[149] The rotator cuff is typically preserved in patients with OA; only 5% to 10% have cuff tears.[149]

X-rays are diagnostic for OA and show joint space narrowing, subchondral sclerosis, and osteophyte formation. In OA, axillary views can demonstrate posterior humeral head subluxation and glenoid wear. This posterior subluxation can cause a false appearance of superior head subluxation on the AP image. Walch et al described the glenoid morphology in OA, classifying it into 3 types: concentric wear with no subluxation (type A), biconcave glenoid with posterior wear and subluxation (type B), and retroverted glenoid with posterior subluxation (type C).[150] In patients with RA, x-rays first reveal osteopenia, followed by erosions of the inferior humeral head and glenoid.[151] These erosions can progress and lead to significant medialization of the humeral head. If glenoid bone loss is ever a concern, then a CT scan is indicated for preoperative planning. MRI is used only if there is a concern about the rotator cuff. In patients for whom inflammatory arthritis is suspected, laboratory tests, including ESR, CRP, CBC, and rheumatologic laboratory tests, should be sent. An arthrocentesis with crystal analysis can also be performed to evaluate for gout or pseudogout.

Initial treatment options of shoulder arthritis are nonoperative. They include intra-articular corticosteroid injections, NSAIDs, and physical therapy. Surgery is indicated for patients who fail nonoperative therapy and continue to have significant pain and impairment in function. Arthroscopic debridement is controversial and is not routinely indicated, although it may be applicable in young patients. Hemiarthroplasty can be used in the setting of large rotator cuff tears or if insufficient glenoid bone stock exists to place a glenoid component (ie, RA with severe medialization). A concentric glenoid is key to success of hemiarthroplasty.[149] Total shoulder arthroplasty (TSA) is also a good option for the treatment of severe glenohumeral arthritis in patients who have an intact rotator cuff (Figure 45-2). Pain relief and ROM are typically significantly improved. A cemented polyethylene glenoid is the gold standard.[149] In patients with total shoulder arthroplasty and rotator cuff deficiency, glenoid loosening can occur from repetitive micro motion. However, a meta-analysis by Bryant et al of patients with OA revealed that TSA provided better functional outcome and ROM at short-term follow-up.[152]

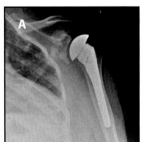
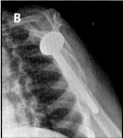
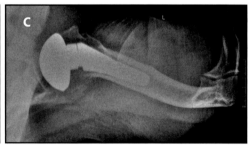

Figure 45-2. (A) AP, (B) scapular Y, and (C) axillary lateral x-rays of the left shoulder after TSA.

Patients with chronic massive rotator cuff tears can develop rotator cuff arthropathy. This form of shoulder arthritis typically affects the dominant hand and tends to have a female predominance. Examination will reveal muscle atrophy, pain with ROM, rotator cuff weakness, and possible anterosuperior escape of the humeral head with associated anterior prominence. Painful pseudoparalysis can be present at endstage rotator cuff arthropathy. The integrity of the deltoid should also be closely evaluated to help determine treatment options. X-rays can demonstrate superior migration of the humeral head, with bony changes termed femoralization of the head, and acetabularization of the acromion.[153] Peripheral osteophytes are less common. Nonoperative treatment is similar to OA. In patients for whom this fails and who demonstrate a functioning deltoid, then surgical intervention can be considered. Pseudoparalysis is an indication for surgery. The coracoacromial arch functions as the limit to superior migration of the humeral head in these patients and, consequently, must be carefully preserved during all procedures.[153] Treatment options include hemiarthroplasty or reverse TSA. Hemiarthroplasty provides pain relief but limited function. Reverse TSA places the center of rotation (COR) of the implant on the neck of the scapula (medial and distal), increasing the lever arm of the deltoid. For this reason, reverse TSA has the potential to improve pain and function. Good glenoid bone stock is required, and indications are typically limited to elderly patients. TSA is not indicated due to early glenoid failure.

Why Might This Be Tested? Differing forms of glenohumeral arthritis can present with different radiographic findings and different treatment principles. Glenoid erosion can change surgical planning and is a potential test topic. Some interventions are contraindicated in certain conditions, such as TSA in cuff arthropathy, or reverse TSA in the setting of deltoid dysfunction. Know the pathogenesis of OA, RA, and cuff arthropathy and the indications for intervention in each.

Here's the Point!

Establish the diagnosis of glenohumeral arthritis and determine which interventions are indicated. Shoulder OA with concentric glenoid = hemiarthroplasty; rotator cuff deficiency = reverse TSA; in between = standard TSA.

Vignette 46: My Neck Is Killing Me Since That Car Accident

A 35-year-old male is involved in a motor vehicle accident in the mountains and comes in 10 hours after the accident due to delay of transportation. A thorough neurological examination is performed in the trauma bay. The patient is unable to move his legs bilaterally and has no sensation from his neck down. On rectal examination at this time, no tone is noted. Plain x-rays and CT scans show a cervical burst fracture.

▶ *What type of spinal cord syndrome is this patient displaying?*

▶ *What signals the end of spinal shock?*

▶ *Are steroids indicated?*

After 36 hours, the patient is now out of spinal shock. Physical examination demonstrates loss of sensation in his legs and on the ulnar aspect of both hands. There is an absence of the triceps reflex and positive biceps and brachioradialis reflexes. On motor examination, he has 5/5 deltoid and bicep strength and 4/5 wrist extension.

▶ *What cord level is this patient?*

Vignette 46: Answer

In the setting of blunt trauma, cervical spine injuries can typically be found in 2% to 6% of cases and require a prompt diagnosis and timely management. One-third of all spinal cord injuries occur in the cervical spine region. The neck needs to be adequately immobilized for transport, and appropriate advanced trauma life support protocols, including neck x-rays (to visualize T1), should be performed. Recently, CT scanning has been implemented in place of plain x-rays because it is superior in diagnosing subtle fractures and provides better visualization of the craniocervical and cervicothoracic junctions. MRI is suggested for patients who are obtunded, comatose, or cannot provide a reliable physical examination.

In 1750, Whytt first described spinal shock as a loss of sensation accompanied by motor paralysis with gradual recovery of the reflexes. This phenomena occurs surrounding physiologic or anatomic transection of the spinal cord that results in temporary loss or depression of the majority or all spinal reflex activity below the zone of injury.[154] Neurogenic shock may also be accompanied by the loss of sympathetic tone, which results in hypotension and bradycardia. Spinal cord reflex arcs immediately above the level of injury may also be depressed.

The return of the bulbocavernosus reflex signals the end of spinal shock. This reflex is tested by eliciting rectal tone if the Foley catheter is gently pulled or the glans of the penis or the clitoris is squeezed. This typically returns within 48 to 72 hours after injury. Spinal shock does not apply to lesions below the cord (ie, cauda equina); therefore, if the bulbocavernosus reflex does not return, this may be due to cauda equina injury or a result of conus medullaris injury. Complete absence of distal motor function at recovery of the reflex indicates complete neurological injury, and the prognosis for function return is bleak. Other cord syndromes include the following:

- Posterior cord: Have bilateral vibration and proprioception deficits with preserved motor function (causes include tabes dorsalis, AIDS myelopathy, multiple sclerosis, and cervical myelopathy)

- Anterior cord: Have bilateral paraplegia, pain, and temperature sensory deficits and loss of sphincter control (causes include disk herniation, radiation myelopathy, and anterior spinal artery infarction)

- Central cord: Have bilateral motor weakness, arms greater than legs, with intact sensation above and below (causes include syringomyelia, tumors, and acute injury)

- Brown-Sequard: Have ipsilateral voluntary motor loss and lack of vibration and proprioception sensations with contralateral loss of pain and temperature function for 2 to 3 levels below the lesion (causes include knife or bullet injury and multiple sclerosis)

To determine level of function, the lowest segment where motor and sensory function is normal on both sides is designated as the cord level (Table 46-1). The motor level is considered normal at the level with 3/5 muscle strength just below the last level that is 5/5. The sensory level is the most caudal segment with normal light touch and pinprick sensation.

Table 46-1.	
FRANKEL GRADES	
Frankel Grade	*Motor/Sensory Function*
A	Complete paralysis
B	Sensory function is preserved below injury level but no motor function present
C	Incomplete, motor function is preserved below the neurological level with 1-2/5 strength
D	Incomplete, motor function is preserved below the neurological level with 3-4/5 strength
E	Normal motor and sensory function (5/5)

Acute management of spinal cord injury requires a multidisciplinary and multisystem approach. After appropriate in-field immobilization and treatment to prevent further damage, medical management is key in the acute postinjury period. Blood pressure management is critical to provide adequate oxygenation to the injury cord. Hypotension (systolic blood pressure < 90 mm Hg) and hypoxia (PaO$_2$ ≤ 60 mm Hg) have been shown to be independently associated with significant increase in morbidity and mortality following injury.[155] Close blood pressure monitoring is generally continued for 7 days postinjury.

Timing of surgery/decompression is still controversial. There is no Level 1 evidence to support early surgery, but most physicians would agree that emergent surgical decompression is indicated in patients with acute and progressive neurologic deficit in the presence of cord compression. Furthermore, there is a growing trend toward decompression of patients who present with complete neurological injuries.

Commonly discussed in the media today is the issue of hypothermia and steroids. Hypothermia is a condition in which the patient's temperature drops below what is required for normal metabolism. From a neuroprotective point of view, hypothermia reduces swelling and hemorrhage, potentially slowing the secondary injury cascade. Research into hypothermia emerged in the 1950s, but enthusiasm dwindled due to the complications such as atelectasis, pneumonia, and acute respiratory distress syndrome.[156,157] Hypothermia remains experimental. Steroid use is also a source of controversy. Steroid use in spinal cord injury has been tested in 3 independent trials. NASCIS I demonstrated no significant neuroprotective benefit with high- vs low-dose treatment. NASCIS II compared a high-dose steroid administered within less than 24 hours with placebo and naloxone. No significant benefit neurologically was found; however, post hoc analysis revealed neuroprotective potential if it was given within 8 hours of injury. However, the benefit was not of much functional gain but reflected more toward a rapid return of nerve root, rather than spinal cord function. NASCIS III compared steroids when administered less than 8 hours after injury. The study compared infusion at 24 vs 48 hours. Functional recovery was included for the first time as an outcome measure. No significant difference was found in neurological recovery. Post hoc analysis found improved function at 6 weeks and 6 months when initiated 3 to 8 hours after injury and continued for 48 hours. Because significant rates of sepsis, pneumonia, and death were found in the 48-hour-dose group, the 24-hour dose (30 mg/kg loading and then 5.4 mg/kg/hr) was recommended if it was started within 3 hours, and the 48-hour dose was recommended when it was started within 3 to 8 hours of injury. Because of the design of the trials and analysis of the data, the results and recommendation are questioned. Because of these factors, most physicians use steroids on a case-by-case basis, and many use them due to fear of litigation.

Ultimately, whatever treatment is offered, the physician should recognize that cord level is important because it helps determine patient independence status. Patients with C4 level are dependent for transfers with high head and back support. The patient can use puffer controls. C5 patients require assistance for most activities and can use hand control devices. C6 can use a manual wheelchair with a slide board, and they use a tenodesis grasp. C7 patients are independent with most activities of daily living and mobility. C8/T1 patients have bladder and bowel independence.

Why Might This Be Tested? Spinal trauma is common and creates a heavy financial burden to the medical system. A missed diagnosis can be devastating. In the trauma setting, a thorough physical examination and radiographic assessment must occur. One should recognize that knowing which cord level is intact is key in understanding the potential functional status the patient may have. Independent status is important for patients and is commonly tested on the Boards.

Here's the Point!

Make sure the patient is not in spinal shock before telling the patient and family the prognosis for recovery. Avoid hypotension and hypoxia in the postinjury time frame and use steroids judiciously to avoid the associated complications.

Vignette 47: Sacked!

A 21-year-old, right-hand-dominant college quarterback is sacked by a linebacker during a football game. His right shoulder is driven into the ground, with the linebacker landing on top of him. The quarterback is helped off the field and complains of pain over the "point" of his shoulder. As he is helped off the field, he is holding his arm at his side in an adducted, internally rotated position.

▶ *What is the most likely diagnosis?*

▶ *What is the differential diagnosis for acute-onset shoulder pain in an athlete?*

▶ *What are the most common mechanisms of injury?*

▶ *What is the most appropriate radiographic view to evaluate this injury?*

▶ *What is the classification of these lesions?*

▶ *What are the treatment options?*

▶ *What are the possible complications related to this injury?*

Vignette 47: Answer

The most likely diagnosis is an AC joint injury. AC joint injuries represent between 40% and 50% of athletic shoulder injuries and are often found in young males participating in contact sports such as football or wrestling. The differential diagnosis of shoulder pain in a traumatic athletic event includes glenohumeral dislocation, AC joint separation/dislocation, proximal humerus or clavicle fracture, rotator cuff tear, labral tear, muscle strain or contusion, and biceps tendon injury.[158-160]

The AC joint is a diarthrodial joint with less than 10 degrees of ROM. The upper extremity is suspended from the lateral clavicle by the CC (conoid and trapezoid) and AC ligaments, providing vertical and AP stability to the AC joint, respectively. The conoid ligament is stronger and inserts more medial than the trapezoid ligament. The AC capsule, deltoid, and trapezius act as additional joint stabilizers. Injury to any of these structures may confer instability to the AC joint.

An acute injury to the AC joint can occur through a direct or indirect mechanism. Direct injury is the most common, such as the case of the unfortunate quarterback, resulting from a fall onto the superolateral aspect ("point") of the shoulder. With the shoulder adducted, the impacting force drives the acromion inferiorly and medially while the clavicle is stabilized by the sternoclavicular ligaments, resulting in systematic failure of the stabilizing ligaments with propagation of energy first to the AC ligaments and capsule, followed by failure of the CC ligaments, and finally the deltotrapezial fascia. An indirect mechanism of injury, in contrast, is less common and usually results from a fall onto an outstretched arm or elbow with a superiorly directed force resulting in AC joint injury. Acromioclavicular dislocations can occur subsequent to a fracture at the base of the coracoid process, which is equivalent to CC ligament rupture.

A thorough history will give clues as to the mechanism and specific type of injury. On examination, the posture and contour of the shoulder in an upright position will give a hint as to the direction of displacement and, therefore, the type of injury. The mobility of the acromion relative to the lateral clavicle (and the contralateral side—always check both sides) and instability in the vertical and horizontal planes should be assessed (pain may limit thorough examination acutely). Often, those with an athletic injury will have pain with resisted adduction, abduction, and forward elevation. Fortunately, neurovascular compromise is rare during this type of injury; nevertheless, it is important to do a full neurovascular exam because the subclavian artery and brachial plexus are in close proximity.

Standard radiography is the only imaging modality required for diagnosis of a suspected AC joint injury. Routine x-rays for AC joint evaluation include true AP (preferably bilateral for comparison purposes), axillary lateral (required to diagnose type IV injuries), and Zanca views (10- to 15-degree cephalic tilt with 50% of standard AP shoulder penetration strength; Figure 47-1A) to give an unobstructed view of the AC joint. On the AP view, only about 33% penetration should be used to visualize the AC joint. Weighted stress views, although of historical value, are no longer routinely obtained.

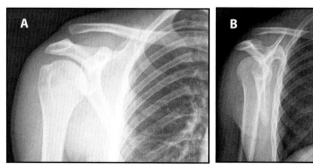

Figure 47-1. (A) Zanca and (B) scapular Y lateral x-rays showing a type III AC joint separation.

There are 6 types of AC joint injuries as defined by Rockwood. In a type I injury, a mild force applied to the point of the shoulder results in swelling or tenderness over the AC joint, but no disruption of either the AC or CC ligaments on normal x-rays. In a type II injury, a moderate to heavy force is applied to the point of the shoulder, disrupting the AC ligaments (with AP instability) but maintaining the integrity of the CC ligaments (vertically stable). X-rays may demonstrate a widened AC joint with little to no vertical displacement. Type III injuries occur with a severe force applied to the point of the shoulder, resulting in AC and CC disruption with horizontal and vertical instability and a superiorly displaced clavicle 100% to 300% on x-rays compared with the contralateral side (Figure 47-1B). In type IV injuries, both ligaments are disrupted and the distal end of the clavicle is displaced posteriorly into or through the trapezius muscle. Clinically, the anterior acromion may be prominent, the joint is irreducible, and the injury is best seen radiographically on the axillary view. Type V injuries require a violent force to induce rupture of the AC and CC ligaments, as well as disruption of the surrounding muscle attachments, creating a major separation between the clavicle and acromion with greater than 300% displacement. Clinically, the clavicle will lie subcutaneously with inferior displacement of the upper extremity, putting the patient at risk for development of a brachial plexus palsy. Finally, the rare, high-energy type VI injuries result in an inferior dislocation of the distal clavicle resulting from hyperabduction and external rotation, in which the clavicle is inferior to the coracoid process. Associated neurovascular and thoracic injuries are common.

Nonsurgical treatment, such as the use of a simple sling or shoulder immobilizer for comfort, is indicated for type I, type II, and most type III separations. After pain has subsided, ROM exercises are initiated, followed by a strengthening program. Most patients regain near-normal ROM, strength, and functional use of the arm within 6 weeks.

For type III injuries, treatment is controversial. Most studies show no significant difference in the clinical outcome between nonsurgically and surgically treated patients. In older patients, nonlaborers, or nonathletes, treatment should be nonoperative because results of surgical treatment have resulted in a higher complication rate and a longer recovery prior to return to sport/work, with equivalent functional results as nonoperative management. However, some studies have reported persistent disability, pain, and limitation of activities in high-level athletes undergoing nonoperative management of these injuries, so many surgeons will choose operative intervention in a subset of overhead athletes and heavy laborers requiring high-level function of the shoulder.

Surgery is indicated for all type IV, V, and VI separations with open reduction of the AC joint with or without distal clavicle resection and deltotrapezial fascia repair. A variety of surgical procedures have been described for the repair and/or reconstruction of the AC joint (Table 47-1), although as in many orthopedic treatment algorithms, there is no consensus on which technique to use. Recent studies have shown that the most important biomechanical factor to consider surgically is achieving an anatomic reconstruction that best restores native anatomy with vertical and horizontal stability of the AC joint. To date, many recommend anatomic CC reconstruction using free tendon graft with suture augmentation, which provides anterior, posterior, and superior stability as well as a biologic scaffold for revascularization. In contrast, distal clavicle resection is not recommended because the congruous bony surfaces may impart stability to the reduced AC joint.

The most common complications following nonsurgical management include late joint arthrosis, persistent instability, and distal clavicle osteolysis. Surgical treatment complications are technique related (see Table 47-1). Importantly, any technique that passes a graft or synthetic material medial to the coracoid process poses a risk to the suprascapular nerve and artery, brachial plexus, and axillary artery. Furthermore, wound infections, loss of fixation, persistent pain, recurrent instability, and posttraumatic arthrosis of the AC joint have been described in the aforementioned techniques.

Why Might This Be Tested? AC injuries are common in athletes with shoulder pain and usually show up on standardized tests. Test questions often focus on the proper radiographic imaging of the AC joint (Zanca view), as well as the controversial treatment of type III separations.

Here's the Point!

AC joint injuries are common in athletes, typically due to a direct fall onto the point of the shoulder, and diagnosed with plain x-rays, including the Zanca view to adequately visualize the AC joint. Nonsurgical management is indicated for type I and II separations, whereas surgical management is indicated for all type IV, V, and VI injuries. Management of type III injuries is controversial, but most patients should be treated nonoperatively, with surgery considered only for laborers or elite athletes.

Table 47-1.

SURGICAL TECHNIQUES FOR REPAIR OR RECONSTRUCTION OF THE ACROMIOCLAVICULAR JOINT

Technique	Method	Features	Complications
Primary acromiocla-vicular joint fixation	K-wires, hook plate	K-wires no longer used; requires plate removal	Pin migration into tho-rax; infection, plate/screw failure
Primary coracoclavicu-lar ligament fixation indicated for acute injury	Coracoclavicular screw, suture loop	Requires screw remov-al, passed via drill holes in clavicle around coracoids or fixed with suture anchor	Screw pullout; suture cutout through clavicle or base of coracoid
Coracoclavicular liga-ment reconstruction indicated for acute and chronic injury	Modified Weaver-Dunn Free tendon graft	Transfer of coracoacro-mial ligament to distal clavicle after distal clavicle resection with or without suture loop coracoclavicular aug-mentation; autogenous hamstring vs anterior tibialis allograft	Possible tunnel expan-sion, hardware failure Few long-term follow-up studies

Vignette 48: Nagging Groin Pain in a Young Athlete

A 25-year-old male who regularly performs martial arts presents with a 6-month history of nagging right hip pain. The pain is felt in the groin area, and he describes it as a muscle pull that has not gotten better. The patient reports significant pain with kicking maneuvers and prolonged sitting. He denies trauma or prior history of hip or knee pain. On physical examination, the pain is worse with flexion, adduction, and internal rotation, with 10 degrees of loss of internal rotation compared with the unaffected hip. X-rays taken in the office are shown in Figures 48-1 and 48-2.

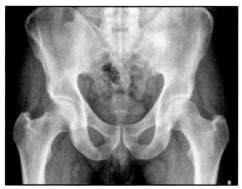 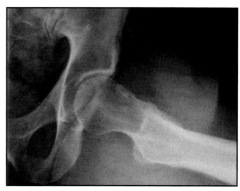

Figure 48-1. X-ray taken in the office.   **Figure 48-2.** X-ray taken in the office.

▶ *What is the most likely diagnosis?*

▶ *What specific physical exam will help elucidate this pathology?*

▶ *What are the key radiographic findings to confirm your diagnosis? What additional studies, if any, should you order?*

▶ *What are the treatment options?*

Vignette 48: Answer

The history, clinical examination, and imaging studies are consistent with combined-type femoroacetabular impingement (FAI). FAI is essentially a process in which abnormal morphology of the proximal femur and/or acetabulum leads to pathological contact between the 2 during terminal hip ROM.[161] This often leads to cartilaginous injuries and labral lesions. Most patients present with an insidious onset of groin pain that is worse with hip flexion and rotational maneuvers. The impingement test is positive when the patient has pain with flexion, adduction, and internal rotation. Cam lesions impinge with different provocative motions depending on the relative location (medial occurs with flexion, lateral with abduction, and centromedial with flexion to 90 degrees with internal rotation).[162] Patients with FAI may also have internal rotation asymmetry compared with the opposite hip. Cam-type impingement (common in young active patients) results from an aspherical femoral head with an increased radius, while pincer-type (common in athletic middle-aged women) is secondary to acetabular overcoverage (acetabular retroversion, coxa profunda, protrusion acetabuli). Most commonly, patients have a combination of the 2 types. Additional conditions in the differential diagnosis for cause of impingement symptoms include prior femoral neck fracture, periacetabular osteotomy, prior slipped capital femoral epiphysis, and residual Legg-Calvé-Perthes disease.[161] In addition, patients with an extensive hip ROM are prone to FAI symptoms.

Plain x-rays (AP pelvis, false profile, and lateral hip views) are the initial diagnostic imaging study to evaluation hip morphology. As seen in our patient, one should look for a crossover sign, which is visualized when the anterior wall of the acetabulum is more lateral than the posterior wall of the acetabulum. The alpha angle is the radiographic parameter that coincides with a loss of femoral head sphericity. An alpha angle greater than 55 degrees is consistent with cam impingement.[163] Currently, the most sensitive view to detect cam lesions is the Dunn lateral view taken at 45 degrees of hip flexion and 20 degrees of abduction, with the beam centered between the pubic symphysis and the anterior superior iliac spine.[164] MRA has been used by most orthopedic surgeons and has been shown to be most effective in detecting labral tears and chondral lesions.[161]

Nonoperative management consists of NSAIDs, restricted activity, and stretching exercises to maintain ROM. Early surgical intervention is suggested to prevent progression and further destruction of the hip joint. Surgical treatment was initially described with open dislocation of the hip with preservation of the blood supply to the femoral head (don't forget that the medial femoral circumflex artery is the critical blood source of the femoral head). The technique involves a trochanteric osteotomy with preservation of the medial femoral circumflex artery by an intact obturator externus muscle.[161] A femoral osteoplasty is performed, and the acetabulum is also inspected. Recently, however, hip arthroscopy for FAI has been used to address labral lesions and abnormal osseous morphology. The factor that has most commonly been associated with a poor outcome is joint space narrowing less than 2 mm or advanced joint degeneration. Arthroscopic treatment can include osteochondroplasty for the cam lesion, rim trimming of the pincer lesions, labral repair when possible, or resection if necessary. When appropriately indicated, results can reach 90% good to excellent at 5 years. Complications specific to hip arthroscopy include pudendal nerve palsy secondary to traction, femoral neck fracture (limit resection to > 30% of the diameter of the femoral neck), avascular necrosis of the femoral head, fluid extravasation into the retroperitoneal space, and postoperative instability.

Why Might This Be Tested? The number of hip arthroscopies and the diagnoses of FAI have been rapidly growing over the past 5 to 6 years. There has been significant interest in understanding the etiology, natural progression, diagnostic modalities, and clinical outcomes.

Here's the Point!

FAI is a popular recent clinical diagnosis. Appropriate radiographic studies to confirm the diagnosis include a true AP pelvis view, Dunn lateral view, false profile view, MRA, and CT scan with 3D reconstructions. Be aware of hip morphology that is amenable to hip arthroscopy and those that require open hip dislocation or pelvic or femoral osteotomies.

Vignette 49: Look Out for That Hay Swather!

A 61-year-old White male has been transferred to the emergency room from another institution one state away. He sustained multiple injuries after he was run over by a hay swather, a farm implement that cuts hay and forms it into a windrow. At initial evaluation, he is alert and oriented with normal vital signs; however, his condition deteriorates during transfer to your hospital. Upon initial assessment in the trauma bay, he is intubated for a GCS of 7 (E1 V1 M5) and inability to maintain a patent airway. Breath sounds are equal bilaterally and labored. Radial and dorsalis pedis pulses are 2+, and his extremities are warm and well perfused. Vital signs are as follows: blood pressure, 84/62; heart rate, 125; respiratory rate, 20; temperature, 35.5°C. A secondary survey reveals facial lacerations and swelling as well as a soft abdomen; FAST ultrasound is negative. Both a C-collar and a pelvic binder are in place. Following brief removal of the binder, visual inspection reveals no skin lacerations near the pelvis. Output through the Foley catheter shows gross hematuria. No gross deformities are present throughout the extremities; however, ecchymosis is noted at the right lateral ankle and above the left clavicle. Following log roll, no step-off or deformity is palpable throughout the posterior column of the spine. Rectal examination reveals no presence of blood; however, tone is decreased. Medical and surgical history is unknown.

Pertinent lab values are as follows: hemoglobin and hematocrit, 10.9 gm/dL and 31.7%, respectively; platelets, 95 k/uL; pH, 7.29; pCO_2, 45.1 mm Hg; HCO_3, 21.2 mEq/L; lactate, 1.8 mmol/L. He received 3 units of blood in the trauma bay. An AP x-ray of the pelvis and a single axial CT scan cut are shown in Figure 49-1.

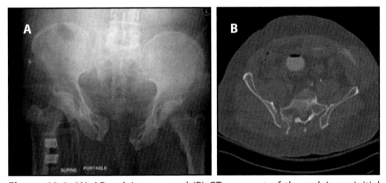

Figure 49-1. (A) AP pelvis x-ray and (B) CT scan cut of the pelvis on initial presentation.

The patient has also sustained the following injuries diagnosed via imaging: rib fractures, pulmonary contusion, grade 1 liver laceration, ruptured bladder, and fractures of his left clavicle and right lateral malleolus.

▶ *What is the diagnosis?*

▶ *When should definitive fixation be performed?*

Vignette 49: Answer

The diagnosis is a right posterior iliac fracture with symphyseal diastasis in excess of 2 cm and contralateral sacral diastasis. This injury pattern is most consistent with AP compression; without quantification of pelvic instability, the radiographs alone narrow the injury to either APC-II or APC-III predicated upon the degree of symphyseal diastasis. This patient's pelvis is both rotationally and laterally unstable and should be considered an APC-III "open book" injury fracture-variant. He was intubated on arrival per Advanced Trauma Life Support (ATLS) protocol due to difficulty protecting his airway in the setting of reduced mental status. In addition, he demonstrated labored breathing secondary to numerous rib fractures (possible flail chest), findings that present concern for inability to autoventilate. The hemodynamic instability, characterized by decreased blood pressure and tachycardia, was treated with rapid infusion of packed red blood cells in the trauma bay and further volume resuscitation with crystalloid solution.

The timing of definitive pelvic fixation to address the APC-III injury depends on the patient's physiologic state, which may be classified as borderline per guidelines described by Pape et al[165] (Table 49-1). Therefore, with hemodynamic stabilization, this patient may receive pelvic fixation acutely.

Table 49-1. ABBREVIATED CRITERIA FOR THE CLINICAL CONDITION OF MULTIPLE TRAUMA PATIENTS					
		Patient Status			
Factor	Parameter	Stable	Borderline	Unstable	In Extremis
Shock	Blood pressure (mm Hg)	≥100	80 to 100	<80	70
	Units pRBCs	0 to 2	2 to 8	5 to 15	>15
	Lactate (mg/dL)	Normal range	≈2.5	>2.5	Severe acidosis
Coagulation	Platelet count (/mm³)	>110,000	90,000 to 110,000	70,000 to 90,000	<70,000
Temperature	°C	>35	33 to 35	30 to 32	<30
Soft tissue injuries	Lung function (PaO₂/FiO₂)	350 to 400	300 to 350	200 to 300	<200
	Chest trauma	Abrasions	2 to 3 rib fractures	>3 rib fractures	Unstable chest wall
Treatment options	Level of care	Early total care	Resuscitate and reevaluate	Damage control procedures	Damage control procedures
	Location of care	Operating room	Trauma bay, then reassess	Operating room	Intensive care unit vs operating room

Trauma epidemiologic research identifies three distinct peaks in death rates as a function of time from injury. The first peak occurs within the first hours and is usually caused by massive hemorrhage or neurological injury. The second peak occurs over the next few hours and is characterized by airway, breathing, or cardiovascular insults. The final peak in mortality is delayed days or weeks and is often due to multi-organ system failure and sepsis. Patients who sustain traumatic injuries should undergo initial evaluation and management guided by the ATLS protocol to identify and treat conditions contributing to mortality in the second peak. The utility of fracture stabilization in polytrauma patients is not different than in patients with isolated fractures; proper treatment results in reduced pain, minimized incidence of fat embolization, and early patient mobilization. The severity of injuries to other organs may require temporary stabilization of fractures before definitive fixation to avoid increased physiological stress during the third peak of trauma mortality.

ATLS Protocol

The ATLS protocol begins with a primary survey to assess and guide management of a patient's airway status, breathing, and circulatory function. Inability to protect the airway, such as in patients with decreasing mental status, or anticipation of a worsening condition will result in intubation to control the airway. Poor breath sounds or labored breathing may indicate underlying thoracic injuries or responses to acid-base disturbances. Hemodynamic instability must be identified and controlled to maintain organ perfusion. Volume loss can be replaced with isotonic crystalloid solution and/or blood transfusion of O negative blood or typed and crossed blood. The average adult male carries approximately 5 L of blood in the circulatory system, while children carry 75 to 80 mL/kg of blood in circulation. Obese patients may have an expanded volume of blood reserves. This patient stayed in sinus rhythm; the discussion of arrhythmia management per ATLS is outside the scope of this vignette.

Shock

Shock is defined as the state of inadequate perfusion of oxygen to tissues, which can occur at systolic blood pressures below 90 mm Hg and heart rates over 120 bpm. Shock is classified by its causative pathway: hypovolemic, cardiogenic, neurogenic, or septic origins (Table 49-2). Shock is often masked in young patients due to strong compensatory responses. Cardiogenic shock is the result of pump failure, caused by extrinsic limitations such as tamponade or intrinsic myocardial dysfunction. Neurogenic shock is the result of disruption of the autonomic pathways within the central and peripheral nervous systems; decreased systemic vascular resistance results in poor blood return from the extremities. Septic shock is generally caused by the release of bacterial endotoxins resulting in systemic vasodilation, endothelial injury, and global hypoperfusion. The most common cause of shock in the trauma patient is hypovolemic shock resulting from hemorrhage, in which reduced preload to the heart results in decreased cardiac output. Hemorrhagic/hypovolemic shock is further classified by the quantity of blood lost as estimated by physiologic parameters (Table 49-3). Hypovolemic shock may also be caused by third-space fluid loss in the setting of extensive soft tissue injury.

Pelvic Hemorrhage

In any high-energy blunt trauma, the pelvis must be evaluated as a possible source of bleeding. Although the pelvis contains numerous vessels, angiography has a limited role in the management of patient with pelvic ring injuries. Most pelvic bleeding is venous in nature and generally comes from bony edges, the iliolumbar vein, or the sacral venous plexus. Large-vessel embolization is also known to cause extensive muscle necrosis of the hip abductors.

There are few predictors for the need for angiography. Hemodynamic instability associated with pelvic fractures without another known significant source of bleeding warrants the use of angiography. Contrast extravasation on CT has a sensitivity of 60% to 84% and a specificity of 85% to 95% for the need for pelvic embolization. Although some studies have established known associations between pelvic fracture pattern and blood transfusion requirement, fracture pattern alone has not been predictive of the need for angiography. The combination of age older than 60 years and major pelvic fracture (vertical shear, open book) is highly associated with the need for embolization, regardless of the patient's hemodynamic status.

Finally, of all pelvic ring injuries, APC-III fractures have the highest rate of blood loss, transfusion requirement, and mortality.

Methods of Resuscitation

The ideal treatment for hemorrhagic shock is to stop the source of bleeding and replace the lost fluid volume. Because these are not always simultaneously achievable, adequate resuscitation can maintain a patient's cardiac output until hemorrhage is appropriately controlled. Access is best achieved with 2 large-bore IV catheters to minimize line resistance. The initial crystalloid must be isotonic (Table 49-4) to maximize the volume of fluid delivered to the intravascular space. Even so, the delivery of 1 L of normal saline (0.9% NaCl) will result in an addition of 275 mL to the plasma volume and 825 mL to the interstitium. As fluid resuscitation continues, it

Table 49-2.

TYPES OF SHOCK

Type of Shock	Hypovolemic	Cardiogenic	Distributive	Obstructive	Neurogenic
Pre-load	Decrease	Increase	Either	Either	Decrease
Cardiac output	Decrease	Decrease	Either	Decrease	Decrease
Afterload (SVR)	Increase	Increase	Decrease	Increased	Decrease
Mixed venous O_2 saturation	Decrease	Decrease	Increase	Decrease	Decrease
Systemic O_2 consumption	Increase	Decrease	Decrease	Decrease	Decrease
Examples	Hemorrhage; burns; pancreatitis	Post-MI; arrhythmia	Sepsis; anaphylaxis	Tension pneumothorax; cardiac tamponade	Neurological injury/trauma
Treatment	Fluid resuscitate; control bleeding; splint fractures; conserve body heat, oxygen	Pending symptoms; bradycardia vs tachycardia; monitor fluids so as not to tax a weak heart; revascularization and ionotropes as needed	Bolus fluids; oxygen—secure airway; conserve body heat; for anaphylaxis—Epi, Benadryl, steroids, pending the cause; pressors as needed	Secure airway; relieve compression; bolus	Secure airway; spine precautions; bolus; steroid protocol—being questioned; pressors as needed

CVP = central venous pressure; MI = myocardial infarction; PAOP = pulmonary artery occulsion pressure; SVR = systemic vascular resistance.

is important to keep in mind that further fluid repletion will distribute along a sodium gradient, such that a hyperchloremic acidosis may result after large-volume resuscitation. Although not clinically deleterious, it prevents the ability to use pH as an indicator of lactic acidosis and tissue ischemia. Lactated Ringers solution (LR) contains lactate, which acts as a buffer, as well as potassium and calcium ions to match plasma ion concentrations. In order to meet electrical neutrality, sodium concentration is lower in LR. Chloride ions are also lower, which reduces the concern for acidosis after large-volume resuscitation. Although resuscitation with hypertonic solutions would certainly retain greater intravascular volume, use of these fluids is impossible in the rapid infusion trauma setting due to the predictable cerebral complications. For these reasons, initial resuscitation is done with 2 L of warm LR. Poor response warrants conversion to blood products in the form of O-negative blood until blood typing enables matched delivery.

Monitoring Resuscitation

The progress of resuscitation can be grossly monitored via accurate hemodynamic monitoring of pressures and heart rates and also through urine output. Classical guidelines indicate that urine output should stay above 0.5 cc/kg/hr (or 420 cc/12 hrs for a 70-kg man) in children and adults with appropriately perfused kidneys. However, kidney physiology is often deranged by the effects of trauma or is deranged at baseline,

Table 49-3.

CLASSIFICATION OF HEMORRHAGIC SHOCK

	Class I	Class II	Class III	Class IV
Blood loss (estimated mL)	<750	750 to 1500	1500 to 2000	>2000
% blood loss	<15	15 to 30	30 to 40	>40
Heart rate	<100	100 to 120	120 to 140	>140
Blood pressure	NL	NL	Decreased	Decreased
Pulse pressure	NL	Decreased	Decreased	Decreased
Urine output (mL/hr)*	>30	30 to 20	20 to 5	Negligible
Mental status	Anxious	Anxious	Anxious, confused	Confused, lethargic
Appropriate replacement fluid	Crystalloid	Crystalloid	Crystalloid and blood	Crystalloid and blood

*Normal values: adults, 0.5 mL/kg/hr; pediatrics, 1 mL/kg/hr; neonates, 2 mL/kg/hr.

Table 49-4.

COMPARISON OF PLASMA AND CRYSTALLOID SOLUTIONS

	(mEq/L)							(mOsm/L)
Fluid	Na	Cl	K	Ca	Mg	Buffers	pH	Osmolality
Plasma	140	103	4	5	2	Bicarb (25)	7.4	290
0.9% NaCl	154	154	-	-	-	-	5.7	308
Lactated ringers	130	109	4	3	-	Lactate (28)	6.4	273

and this guideline then becomes useless. Additionally, vital signs have been shown to poorly correlate with levels of blood loss and may not be the best measure of resuscitation. McGee et al demonstrated that supine tachycardia was absent in over 50% of patients who experienced moderate (450 to 630 cc) or severe (630 to 1150 cc) blood loss.[166] Hematocrit lab values are also inappropriate because this test measures the fraction of plasma to erythrocytes and can be confounded by the acute loss of blood or rapid introduction of crystalloid. Arterial lactate can be used as a surrogate for adequate tissue oxygenation because it quantifies the output from anaerobic cellular metabolism. Lactate levels show a strong correlation to both the magnitude of blood loss and the risk of death from hemorrhage in initial evaluation and through resuscitation. A lactate goal of 2 mmol/L can be used as a resuscitation goal. In cases of post-trauma sepsis, however, impaired tissue oxygenation is not the primary source of lactate accumulation and loses its value as a resuscitation surrogate. Use of all mentioned parameters rather than a single data point can best provide a comprehensive picture of resuscitation status in the trauma patient.

Inflammatory Response

As hypovolemic shock progresses, the body experiences a drop in temperature and gradually becomes coagulopathic. Hypovolemia and ischemia will also result in capillary permeability changes, which will continue to influence resuscitative efforts. These factors all contribute to systemic inflammation, described as systemic inflammatory response syndrome (SIRS). Following the initial cascade, there will be a period of recovery followed by a counter-regulatory anti-inflammatory response (CARS), which can progress to a temporary, immunosuppressed state. The positive feedback of fluid leak, hypovolemia, and systemic-inflammatory bursts followed by an immunosuppressed period place the trauma patient at great risk for sepsis, ARDS, and multi-organ system failure.[167]

Damage Conrol Orthopedics

Patients who sustain polytraumatic patterns of injury frequently require orthopedic care during their hospital stay. Appropriate timing of fracture fixation and soft tissue repair is critical for surgical success; patients must be assessed in light of the collective severity of their injuries and their clinical condition. The timing of fracture care remains controversial. Pape et al[165] recommend assessing patients on multiple parameters, including hemodynamics, coagulatory lab values, temperature, lung function, and chest/abdomen/pelvis injury scores. These parameters are used to separate patients into one of four categories as detailed in Table 49-1.

In summary, stable patients have no physiologic abnormalities; these patients should receive classically timed fixation. Borderline patients experience a delayed response to resuscitation; hemodynamic stabilization may allow for early fixation,[168] yet some authors advocate for rapid procedures such as unreamed, unlocked nails to be used with delayed locking to minimize the initial physiological insult to the patient. Unstable patients remain hemodynamically unstable; lifesaving procedures are performed, and orthopedic operations are limited to temporizing measures to minimize further insults to the initial systemic inflammatory response. Patients in extremis, if there is continued uncontrolled bleeding, are limited to life-saving measures. Roberts et al demonstrated significantly reduced sepsis rates in multiply injured patients using damage-control orthopedics in Hannover, Germany, compared with performance using previous protocols at the same institution.[167] Extensive operative intervention has been shown by Harwood et al to increase the systemic inflammatory response (not a good thing!).[169]

Plans for fixation of pelvic ring fractures can be made based on the patient's condition. Patients with unstable and displaced pelvic fractures are associated with up to a 20% incidence of hemodynamic instability. Bleeding cancellous bone and disrupted venous plexus flow can tamponade in the closed peritoneal space. However, the retroperitoneal space is not a confined space and injuries involving this region can result in exsanguination. Stable patients can receive ORIF of their fractures without delay. Borderline patients must first be stabilized with resuscitation. If successful, they may also receive definitive fixation in the acute setting. Patients that are unstable or in extremis may require temporary fixation with an external fixator or pelvic c-clamp to aid in rapid tamponade; these patients may also require pelvic packing or angiographic embolization of pelvic vessels to control hemorrhage. Prolonged operations in these patients risk additional complications from the traumatic inflammatory cascade, and definitive fixation should be delayed in an effort to reduce complications.

Why Might This Be Tested? While orthopedic surgeons logically focus on the extent of musculoskeletal injury, any plans formulated for a patient must consider the context of the patient's condition and other injuries. Additionally, rural orthopedic surgeons may need to take part in the care of acutely injured patients.

Here's the Point!

Trauma patients must be first managed according to the ABCs of the ATLS protocol. APC pelvic fractures are associated with higher transfusion requirements and mortality than LC fractures. Patients may benefit from the delay of definitive orthopedic procedures and other physiologic insults in the acute setting of severe traumatic injury.

Vignette 50: My Arm Won't Stop Hurting After I Fell Off My Bicycle

A 23-year-old male has had an increase in left arm pain after falling off of his bicycle 1 month ago. The pain has improved steadily with rest, and he had no symptoms prior to this incident. A recent left arm x-ray is shown in Figure 50-1. Hematoxylin-eosin slides of a biopsy specimen are shown in Figures 50-2 and 50-3.

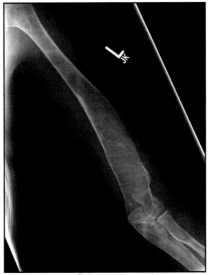

Figure 50-1. AP x-ray of the left humerus.

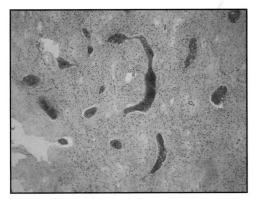

Figure 50-2. Hematoxylin-eosin stain (100× magnification) of the biopsy specimen.

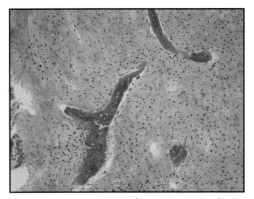

Figure 50-3. Hematoxylin-eosin stain (200× magnification) of the biopsy specimen.

▶ *What is the diagnosis?*

▶ *What additional findings would you look for on physical examination?*

▶ *What are management options for this patient?*

Vignette 50: Answer

This is a case of fibrous dysplasia, a benign fibro-osseous lesion representing an abnormality in normal bone maturation and stress remodeling. Most lesions are discovered in childhood and adolescence, but they may present at any age. Fibrous dysplasia has a predilection for the long bones (femur is most common), ribs, craniofacial bones, and pelvis. It is one of the few tumors that commonly affects the diaphysis of long bones. On radiographic analysis, the lesions characteristically involve the IM canal with well-defined borders and a "ground glass" appearance, although cystic areas may be present (see Figure 50-1). Severe shepherd's crook deformities of the proximal femur can develop in polyostotic disease. The differential diagnosis includes unicameral bone cysts, aneurysmal bone cysts (ABCs), osteofibrous dysplasia, nonossifying fibroma, adamantinoma, low-grade IM osteosarcoma, and Paget's disease.

The lesions can be monostotic (affect a single bone), often asymptomatic and discovered incidentally, or polyostotic (affects multiple bones). Polyostotic disease can also be associated with syndromes, and key elements should be looked for on physical exam (question writers love these syndromes!). McCune-Albright syndrome presents with endocrine abnormalities (precocious puberty) and café-au-lait macules. The café-au-lait spots have sharp, irregular borders (coast of Maine) distinguishing them from smoother lesions found in neurofibromatosis type 1 (coast of California). Mazabraud syndrome is polyostotic fibrous dysplasia in concordance with intramuscular myxomas and may present with multiple soft tissue masses (there's no easy way to remember these, so commit them to memory). Polyostotic disease is much more likely to be painful and progress compared with monostotic involvement, which tends to become quiescent at skeletal maturity.

In this patient, there is an abnormal appearance to the humerus, ulna, and radius. The bones have undergone expansile remodeling and have "ground-glass mineralization." The cortex appears thinned, and there is a bowing deformity of the humerus (see Figure 50-1). The deformity is a result of biomechanically insufficient bone. Upon closer inspection, there is a subtle oblique, subacute pathologic fracture of the distal humerus.

Histologically, characteristic features include a haphazard arrangement of immature bone that are often compared with "Chinese letters" or "alphabet soup." The lesion is generally well circumscribed and is composed of fibrous and osseous elements present in varying degrees. The curvilinear bony trabeculae are composed of metaplastic woven bone distributed in a hypocellular spindle cell stroma without atypia.

An abnormality in the $G_s\alpha$ gene is correlated to fibrous dysplasia and is thought to represent a spontaneous mutation. This gene codes for a guanine-nucleotide binding protein. The net result of the mutation is an inhibition of GTPase activity and increased cAMP formation.

Many lesions that are found incidentally may be observed with serial x-rays. Bone scans may be performed at presentation to search for polyostotic disease. Surgical indications include progressive deformity, impending or present pathologic fracture, and unclear diagnosis. Impending pathologic fractures, particularly in the proximal femur, may be treated with curettage and bone grafting, internal fixation, or a combination. Cancellous allograft and autograft notoriously form back into fibrous dysplasia when used as a surgical adjunct. Therefore, the best biological augmentation is cortical allograft because it is absorbed the slowest.

Why Might This Be Tested? Fibrous dysplasia is a common tumor with distinct radiographic and histologic findings. Furthermore, the gene abnormality is a commonly tested item; the $G_s\alpha$ gene mutates in its coding for a guanine-nucleotide binding protein (increased cAMP and decreased GTPase activities). There are several associated syndromes (McCune-Albright and Mazabraud). Just know them!

Here's the Point!

Fibrous dysplasia is a developmental abnormality of bone that is mono- or polyostotic in nature and often found incidentally on plain x-rays. Remember the histology buzzwords "Chinese letters" and "alphabet soup." Treat progressive deformities or impending fracture cases with curettage and bone grafting ± internal fixation.

Vignette 51: Coach, My Shoulder's Catching

A 26-year-old, right-hand-dominant minor league baseball pitcher has had persistent, vague right shoulder pain for the past 12 months. He reports deep shoulder pain with lifting weights and throwing, most notable during the late cocking phase, with an associated painful catching of the shoulder with rotational movements. Rest, physical therapy, and NSAIDs have failed to provide relief. Examination reveals pain with O'Brien's test but no signs of instability. A coronal MRI is shown in Figure 51-1.

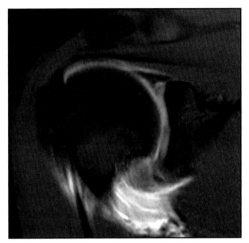

Figure 51-1. Coronal T2-weighted MRI.

▶ *What is the patient's most likely diagnosis?*

▶ *What is the pathophysiology of this disease process?*

▶ *What diagnostic tests should be ordered?*

▶ *What is the classification of these lesions?*

▶ *What are other commonly associated pathologies with this disease process? What is a Buford complex?*

▶ *What is the appropriate treatment?*

Vignette 51: Answer

The underlying diagnosis is a superior labral anterior to posterior (SLAP) tear, or injury to the superior labrum extending from anterior to posterior along the biceps root. SLAP tears may occur as isolated lesions or may be associated with internal impingement, rotator cuff tears (usually articular sided), or instability.[170-174]

The labrum is a fibrocartilaginous ring of tissue that surrounds and attaches to the glenoid, serving to deepen the glenoid and provide enhanced stability for the shoulder joint. The superior labrum is triangular in shape and typically attaches to the superior glenoid rim but more commonly attaches medial to the articular margin. At the 12-o'clock position, the supraglenoid tubercle, the attachment site for the long head of the biceps, is approximately 5 mm medial to the superior rim of the glenoid, and there is a synovial reflection between the long head of the biceps tendon and the superior aspect of the labrum connecting the 2 structures. The SLAP lesions typically occur in this area, affecting the SLAP to the insertion site of the long head of the biceps tendon.

The function of the superior labrum/biceps complex is not fully understood; however, several studies have demonstrated a joint-stabilizing role via enhancement of concavity compression and increasing the effective diameter of the glenoid. In an abducted and externally rotated position, the long head of the biceps is thought to depress the humeral head into the glenoid and limit external rotation of the shoulder. The presence of a SLAP lesion decreases this restraint, contributing to the potential for instability and decreasing the torsional rigidity of the shoulder (shoulder feels sloppy with throwing-type motion).

The most common mechanisms of injury in patients with SLAP lesions are traction injuries (eg, water skiing or sudden attempt to reach overhead), compression injuries (eg, fall onto an outstretched arm that is positioned in slight forward flexion and abduction), and overuse injuries (overhead throwers; most common mechanism, like our case). The existence of a cascade in overhead athletes resulting in an increased propensity for a peel-back SLAP tear has been proposed. Throwers have increased shoulder external rotation and decreased internal rotation (glenohumeral internal rotation deficit = GIRD, not GERD!) with subsequent posteroinferior capsular contracture, anterior capsular laxity, and increased proximal humeral retroversion. The essential lesion is the posterior capsular contracture of the posterior aspect of the inferior glenohumeral ligament, leading to increased posterosuperior migration of the humeral head in the late cocking phase, displacing the labrum/biceps complex medially (ie, peel back) over the glenoid rim and creating attritional SLAP lesions over time.

A careful history will provide clues as to the mechanism of injury. Although many cases are traumatic in nature, up to one-third of patients with SLAP lesions will report an insidious onset of shoulder pain. Symptoms may vary from a sharp pain anterosuperiorly to a sensation of a "dead arm" with activity, with or without complaints of mechanical symptoms, such as catching or locking with rotational movements of the abducted shoulder due to interposition of the labrum between the humeral head and glenoid.

Although physical examination findings may be suggestive of a SLAP tear (positive O'Brien's, anterior slide, or crank tests), it is rarely conclusive. Throwers often present with GIRD during ROM testing (must stabilize the scapula for accurate assessment). Complicating the examination is that partial and complete rotator cuff tears, in addition to instability and internal impingement, are often associated with SLAP injuries. There are several provocative tests with relatively high sensitivity but low specificity for detecting SLAP lesions, including O'Brien's test (pain with resisted forward flexion of the slightly adducted and pronated arm; most reliable for SLAP lesions) and Speed's test (biceps or biceps labral complex pathology). Eighty-five percent of patients with SLAP tears will have a positive apprehension test, and 86% will have a positive relocation test.

Plain x-rays are typically ordered but usually normal. The best imaging modality for diagnosis of SLAP lesions is MRI. Although CT arthrography is better for detecting bony abnormalities, MRI with fine cuts in the oblique coronal, oblique sagittal, and axial planes is superior for diagnosing labral lesions and rotator cuff pathology. To improve the accuracy of MRI, MRA has recently gained in popularity. However, the routine use of MRI vs MRA is a matter of debate despite findings that MRA offers significantly improved sensitivity, specificity, and accuracy compared with MRI for diagnosis of SLAP lesions.

MRI/MRA findings indicative of a SLAP lesion include high signal intensity in the labrum-biceps anchor (see Figure 51-1), high signal between the superior glenoid labrum and the superior glenoid fossa, displacement of the labrum, and the presence of a paralabral cyst. Importantly, if a spinoglenoid or paralabral cyst is located on MRI/MRA, there should be a high index of suspicion for an underlying labral lesion and shoulder instability, and assessment for suprascapular neuropathy should be pursued because this nerve may be compressed by the cyst within the spinoglenoid notch. Despite advances in MRI technique, the accuracy of detecting SLAP tears on MRI/MRA remains variable and definitive diagnosis is usually made with arthroscopy.

Diagnostic arthroscopy may be necessary if the physical examination is suggestive of a SLAP lesion and the MRI is nondiagnostic (Figure 51-2). It is important to recognize variations in normal glenohumeral anatomy to appropriately diagnose SLAP lesions. These include appreciation of the frequently normal sublabral foramen at the 2-o'clock position with a cordlike middle glenohumeral ligament (most common), a meniscoid appearance of the superior labrum, or the Buford complex (Figure 51-3), a cordlike middle glenohumeral ligament that attaches to the base of the biceps anchor with complete absence of labral tissue on the anterosuperior glenoid. Reattaching a Buford complex can result in marked restriction of external rotation.

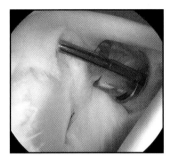 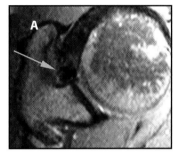 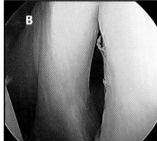

Figure 51-2. Intraoperative image of a SLAP tear.

Figure 51-3. (A) Axial MRI showing the rounded appearance of the cordlike middle glenohumeral ligament, or Buford complex. (B) Arthroscopic image from the same patient showing a nonpathologic sublabral foramen.

There are 4 types of SLAP lesions as defined by Snyder, but other subtypes have also been described. Type I involves fraying and degeneration of the edge of the superior labrum with a firmly attached labrum and biceps anchor. In a type II SLAP tear, the labrum and biceps anchor are detached from the insertion on the superior glenoid. In type III, there is a bucket-handle tear of the superior labrum, but the remaining portions of the labrum and biceps anchor are still well attached to their insertion. In type IV, there is a bucket-handle type tear of the superior labrum with extension of the tear into the biceps tendon. Complex lesions involve a combination of 2 types of lesions, typically types II and IV.

First-line treatment involves nonoperative management, such as NSAIDs and physical therapy to strengthen the rotator cuff muscles and improve posterior capsular flexibility. If symptoms persist despite an adequate trial (>3 months) of nonoperative management, surgery is indicated. Early intervention should be considered for patients with evidence of suprascapular nerve compression secondary to spinoglenoid notch cysts (look for this—they love to test this point). Careful consideration should be given to the older athletes (40- to 60-year-old weekend warriors) with a SLAP tear and multiple concomitant pathologies because the SLAP lesion is often not the primary cause of shoulder pain, and surgical intervention with SLAP repair may have little to no benefit and may even worsen shoulder stiffness.

Surgical treatment depends on the type of SLAP lesion. Type I and III lesions can frequently be treated with simple debridement while addressing any potential instability. The management of type II lesions is controversial but should include stabilization of the detached biceps tendon-superior labrum complex (if unstable and no other pathology) using a suture anchor. Treatment of type IV lesions depends on the extent of tearing of the biceps tendon. If the segment of biceps tendon is less than 30% of the substance of the tendon, the detached fragment of labrum and biceps tendon can simply be resected. If it is greater than 30%, the decision is more complex, ranging from labral debridement and biceps tenodesis or tenotomy in older patients to arthroscopic anchor fixation of the labrum with biceps tenodesis in younger patients. Associated lesions should be appropriately addressed. For example, in patients with GIRD, correction should be attempted with a posterior capsular release.

Rehabilitation involves a short period of immobilization followed by progressive ROM and strengthening exercises. Typically, the patient can return to sports or labor 6 to 9 months following surgery.

Why Might This Be Tested? SLAP tears are a well-recognized cause of shoulder pain. Recent examination questions have focused on normal vs abnormal labral anatomy (ie, Buford complex), as well as associated pathology (spinoglenoid or glenoid labral cysts leading to suprascapular neuropathy).

Here's the Point!

SLAP tears are common in the overhead throwing athlete, present with variable signs and symptoms, and are diagnosed with advanced imaging such as MRI/MRA or, more definitively, arthroscopy. Treatment is dependent on the classification type, with management of SLAP II tears remaining controversial. Do not repair a Buford complex, treat associated pathology, and decompress all paralabral cysts!

Vignette 52: Case of the Costly Rebound

A 35-year-old male returns to your office with difficulty bearing weight and an inability to actively extend his knee. He says that he was trying to "bring down" a rebound during a weekend basketball game when he felt a tearing pain in his knee. He collapsed and has had difficulty walking on his leg since the injury. He had been recently seen in your office for jumper's knee that was worsened after strenuous/sporting activities.

▶ *What is the most likely diagnosis?*

▶ *What are the most common mechanisms of injury?*

▶ *What is the relevant pathoanatomy?*

▶ *What clinical and radiographic findings are necessary to diagnose this condition?*

▶ *When is surgery indicated?*

Vignette 52: Answer

The patient has suffered an acute patellar tendon rupture (aka, jumper's knee, based on extensor lag and prior patellar tendinitis). Although this injury is uncommon, the consequences of improper diagnosis and failure of treatment can be devastating if delayed or missed. Usually, the patient is an active individual younger than 40 years. Although this vignette may apply to a patient with acute quadriceps rupture, and quadriceps rupture is more commonplace, the patient is usually older than 40 years.[175]

The extensor mechanism of the knee includes the patella, the patellar tendon, the quadriceps muscle group (rectus femoris, vastus medialis, vastus lateralis, vastus intermedialis), the quadriceps tendon, and the tibial tubercle. The lateral retinaculum is composed of the tendinous expansion of the vastus lateralis connecting the lateral patella to the tibia; and the medial retinaculum is formed by the vastus medialis tendinous expansion.

The patellar tendon receives its blood supply from the retinaculum and the infrapatellar fat pad. The distal and proximal attachments of the patellar tendon, composed mainly of fibrocartilage, are vascular watershed areas and are frequently the site of rupture.

Biomechanically, the patellar tendon experiences its greatest force with the knee at 60 degrees of flexion. Most ruptures happen with the knee in a flexed position, usually against a fixed surface. In addition, the tensile strain seen by the tendon is at the insertion sites of the tendon (patella and tibial tubercle). Although the force seen by the patellar tendon climbing stairs is about 3.2 times body weight, studies estimate that the force required to cause a patellar tendon rupture is 17.5 times body weight.[176]

The important considerations in this patient's history are an injury related to forceful quadriceps contraction against a fixed surface, previous history of patellar tendonitis, age younger than 40 years, feeling a tearing or popping sensation in his knee, and the inability to bear weight after the injury. Other predisposing factors to patellar tendon ruptures include TKA, use of the middle third of patellar tendon for ACL repair, long-term systemic steroid therapy, lupus, RA, diabetes mellitus, and renal failure.

Patients usually have difficulty bearing weight on the affected leg and have a significant hemarthrosis. One must also rule out an ACL tear, fracture (patella, tibial tubercle, or tibial plateau), or meniscal injury. One may also feel a palpable defect along the patellar tendon along with localized tenderness at this site. The most significant physical exam finding is the lack of active knee extension or the inability to maintain extension against gravity. Incomplete ruptures or tendon ruptures with an intact medial and/or lateral retinaculum will experience an extensor lag.

Orthogonal x-rays (Figures 52-1 and 52-2) of the knee may demonstrate patella alta (often this is all that is needed). The plain x-rays may also reveal an area of calcification along the patellar tendon, indicating chronic patellar tendinitis. Views of the patellofemoral compartment may help rule out osteochondral injury, patella fracture, or patellar dislocation.

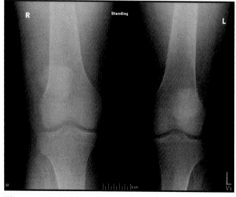

Figure 52-1. AP radiograph of the knees showing asymmetry of the patella.

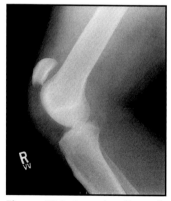

Figure 52-2. Lateral radiograph of the knee with patella alta, indicative of a patellar tendon rupture.

Another useful modality, in less obvious cases, is high-resolution ultrasonography in acute and chronic settings. Acute patellar disruptions are identified with an area of hypoechogenicity spanning across the entire tendon. Chronic ruptures show disruption of the normally hyperechoic tendon pattern along with thickening at the site of rupture.

Although not recommended for evaluation of acute tendon ruptures, MRI can be useful in determining if the tear is partial or full thickness. MRI (Figure 52-3) shows an increase in signal intensity on the sagittal T2-weighted image along the tendon, as well as fiber discontinuity.

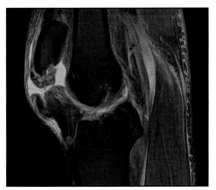

Figure 52-3. Sagittal MRI section showing an acute patellar tendon rupture..

Only with early diagnosis and prompt treatment can one expect the best results. Nonoperative management is indicated with partial tendon ruptures without an extensor lag. Surgery is indicated with a complete tendon rupture or evidence of an incompetent extensor mechanism. Siwek and Rao[177] showed that surgery is best performed within the first 2 weeks of injury so that the tissues are not retracted and scarred down. Surgical management includes a suture repair of the tendon through the patella with or without cerclage of the patella to the tibial tubercle. Postoperative management consists of toe-touch weight bearing for the 6 weeks. The patient should perform isometric quadriceps and hamstrings exercises immediately with gentle active ROM at the knee by 2 weeks (avoid passive ROM). Active extension should be encouraged 3 weeks after surgery.[178]

Why Might This Be Tested? An acute knee injury affecting active knee extension can be patella tendon tear, patella fracture, or quadriceps tendon tear. Plain x-rays can provide diagnostic evidence to determine where the injury has occurred along the extensor mechanism—the patella alta in a patella tendon tear, a patella fracture, or the patella baja in a quadriceps tendon tear.

Here's the Point!

Acute patella tendon tears occur in young patients and require primary repair to restore the extensor mechanism. Quadriceps tendon rupture occurs in older patients.

Vignette 53: That First Step Is a Doozie!

A 30-year-old female presents to the emergency room after a fall down a full flight of stairs. There was no loss of consciousness in the field. She complains of isolated neck pain. On careful neurological exam, the patient is intact to motor and sensory function, except for pain radiating down her arm. She has no evidence of objective weakness in her arms. She has no other confounding injuries, and she is cooperative with the history and physical exam. She has no prior history of neck pain or radicular symptoms. Cervical MRIs and a CT scan section are shown (Figures 53-1 to 53-3).

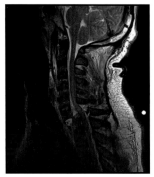

Figure 53-1. Sagittal T2-weighted MRI of the cervical spine.

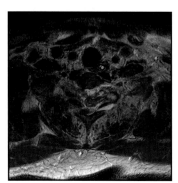

Figure 53-2. Axial T2-weighted MRI of the cervical spine.

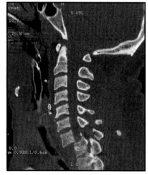

Figure 53-3. Sagittal section of a cervical spine CT scan.

▶ *What type of injury is this?*

▶ *What should the treatment algorithm be?*

Vignette 53: Answer

This patient had a facet dislocation from a flexion-distraction injury. For this injury, one should attempt closed reduction; if the deficit is progressive or pain increases, then perform an open procedure.

Facet dislocation is caused by a flexion-distraction injury. Allen and Ferguson mechanistically categorized these injuries into 4 stages: stage 1 (facet subluxation), stage 2 (unilateral facet dislocation), stage 3 (bilateral facet dislocation with 50% displacement), and stage 4 (complete dislocation).[179]

As for management, the use of cervical traction to reduce facet dislocations has been studied extensively due to the potential risk of iatrogenic injury during reduction from a concomitant disk herniation. This risk has caused some clinicians to advocate MRI prior to any reduction; however, there has been no documentation of permanent spinal cord injury in an awake, cooperative, neurologically intact patient. Nevertheless, because of this potential risk, an MRI should be obtained before any surgical procedure (even after successful closed reduction) to help guide treatment. An immediate closed reduction should also be performed before the MRI in the awake and alert patient with a complete or high-grade partial injury because the patients may be considered to have little to lose, even in the presence of herniation.[180]

Definitive management of cervical spine facet dislocation can be accomplished with several techniques. Traditionally, these injuries have been treated with closed reduction techniques and external orthotic immobilization or dorsal arthrodesis. With modern technology, performing an anterior arthrodesis is rapidly gaining favor. However, if a large disk herniation is present, an anterior diskectomy will be necessary with or without posterior fusion. Unfortunately, closed reduction techniques do not always work. Neurological deterioration can occur during or after attempted closed reduction procedures. Therefore, open reduction techniques have become more popular in recent years. Open reduction procedures can be performed via the ventral or dorsal approach. Dorsal open reduction is performed most frequently, and the technique consists of a partial or complete facetectomy, reduction of deformity and dorsal fixation, and fusion. Fusion and instrumentation techniques include facet wiring, interspinous wiring, and placement of a lateral mass fixation (plate or screw/rod). Any method will suffice; however, if a decompression or facetectomy is required, interspinous and facet wiring are not possible. Furthermore, lateral mass plating is biomechanically superior to laminar wiring or clamps. Facet wiring requires the use of an external orthosis for immediate stability. Alternatively, interspinous wiring does not provide as much rotational control. In general, most surgeons today rely on lateral mass fixation, albeit with rod/screw constructs because plating is hard to contour and the screw positions are dictated by the holes in the plate. Posterior plating or screw/rod construct provides immediate fixation.

Why Might This Be Tested? Although cervical spine trauma occurs in only 2% to 3% of patients who sustain blunt trauma, the potential for instability and devastating injuries is high. This requires prompt identification and proper management of these patients. A commonly tested and perhaps controversial topic that is tested on the Boards is facet dislocation.

Here's the Point!

If the patient is obtunded or noncooperative or has distracting injuries, a prereduction MRI is warranted to rule out a large disk herniation. In an awake, cooperative patient without deficits, closed reduction should be attempted with close monitoring of the physical exam.

Vignette 54: Doc, I Can't Wash My Hair Anymore!

A 55-year-old, right-hand-dominant female with type 2 diabetes mellitus presents to your office with worsening right shoulder pain over the past 8 months. She reports that she is now unable to wash her hair. She denies any previous trauma, surgery, or similar problems in the past with her shoulder. On examination, she demonstrates painful active abduction to 100 degrees, forward elevation to 110 degrees, external rotation to 20 degrees, and internal rotation to her gluteus. Passive ROM is limited to the same numbers for all directions of motion. She has pain with resisted forward elevation. Plain x-rays show a well-preserved joint space in the setting of osteopenia.

▶ *What is the most likely diagnosis?*

▶ *What other tests should be ordered?*

▶ *What are the treatment options?*

Vignette 54: Answer

In this case, the history and physical are screaming for the diagnosis of adhesive capsulitis. The combination of insidious onset of pain and stiffness with no inciting event or previous surgery is characteristic of this condition; in addition, diabetes mellitus is a significant predisposing factor. Concurrent limitation in active and passive ROM is critical to confirming this diagnosis. Pain patterns reproducing impingement or rotator cuff pathology may also be seen.[181] X-ray findings are usually unremarkable except for osteopenia. No further imaging is needed at this point based on the history and physical exam. If other pathology is suspected, MRI may be indicated.

Adhesive capsulitis is also known as frozen shoulder; however, this term is general and can also indicate posttraumatic or postsurgical stiffness. Adhesive capsulitis is more accurately thought of as the idiopathic loss of shoulder motion. Although the exact pathogenesis remains unclear, thickening and contracture of the joint capsule is characteristic. It is most closely associated with diabetes mellitus, but it also correlates with other systemic conditions, such as thyroid disease, endocrine disorders, or renal disease. Similarly, posttraumatic causes are possible, including immobilization from chest wall or breast surgery. Patients with diabetes mellitus have a greater risk of developing adhesive capsulitis than the general population. In case you missed it before, on physical examination, pain and global loss of active and passive ROM are diagnostic. If focal loss of motion is present, an alternative diagnosis should be considered. Close attention must be paid because patients may compensate for glenohumeral motion loss with increased scapulothoracic motion.[181] Loss of external rotation may be particularly noticeable. Imaging may show evidence of osteopenia but typically reveals no other source of stiffness. On advanced imaging, loss of the axillary recess indicates the characteristic decrease in glenohumeral joint volume.

The natural history of adhesive capsulitis is that it tends to resolve within 1 to 3 years.[181] It progresses through 3 stages, beginning with a freezing (painful) stage characterized by gradually increasing pain, followed by a frozen (stiff) stage in which decreased ROM affects activities of daily living, and a thawing stage in which motion gradually returns.[182] In this case, the adhesive capsulitis appears to be in the frozen stage (stage 2).

Physical therapy is the mainstay of treatment and is effective in improving pain and restoring motion. If physical therapy fails, manipulation under anesthesia should be considered. Corticosteroids can provide short-term relief to allow therapy to be tolerable. Arthroscopic capsular release should be performed only in severe refractory cases that have failed therapy. (Arthroscopically, there are 4 phases: 1, patchy fibrinous synovitis; 2, capsular contraction and synovitis; 3, increased contraction with improving synovitis; and 4, severe contraction.) The capsule acts as a tether, limiting humeral head rotation. Therefore, anterior capsular release of the rotator interval would increase external rotation, and posterior capsular release increases internal rotation. Any residual motion defects that persist after successful nonoperative intervention or arthroscopic capsular release do not appear to affect long-term outcomes.[182]

Why Might This Be Tested? Adhesive capsulitis can present with pain patterns and limitation of shoulder function similar to other shoulder pathologies. However, it responds favorably to nonoperative interventions in most cases. Questions will most likely be based on associated risk factors for adhesive capsulitis, as well as diagnosis and exam findings.

Here's the Point!

Adhesive capsulitis is associated with diabetes mellitus and presents with limitation of active and passive ROM. It usually responds to nonoperative interventions.

Vignette 55: Knock Knees

A 9-year-old male presents with a several-month history of knock knees and left-sided hip pain. The child always had a valgus alignment to his lower extremities, but his parents report that it appears to be accentuated over the past year. He was the result of a full-term delivery and has met all childhood milestones in an age-appropriate manner. Leg-length and AP pelvis x-rays are shown in Figure 55-1.

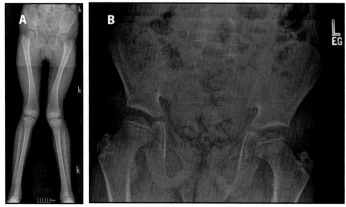

Figure 55-1. (A) Leg-length and (B) AP pelvis x-rays.

▶ *What is the diagnosis?*

▶ *What is the inheritance pattern?*

Vignette 55: Answer

The patient has multiple epiphyseal dysplasia (MED). Skeletal dysplasias occur in 1/5000 live births, and more than 450 are described in the literature.[183] Multiple epiphyseal dysplasia is a disproportionate dwarfism that results in shortened limbs. Our 9-year-old patient falls right into the classic time for presentation (5 to 14 years old) with bilateral symmetric involvement of his extremities. It is transmitted via autosomal-dominant inheritance. It is mapped on chromosome 10, and its gene product is the cartilage oligomeric matrix protein. Initial presentation is usually joint stiffness, pain, and/or limping, and it is often genu valgum or varus. The diagnosis is often made during early adolescence because the patients may be slightly shorter than their peers and are viewed as being shorter but not pathologically shorter. Other features include small metacarpals and metatarsals and multiple abnormal ossification centers. A detailed family history should be assessed to delineate any patterns of inheritance of skeletal dysplasias. In addition, the upper and lower trunk segments should be measured to determine a ratio. Typically, this ratio is 1.7 as a newborn, approximately 1 between ages 2 and 8 years, and 0.95 as an adult.[183]

X-rays of the long bones will reveal an abnormal epiphysis, but it may be subtle. When pelvis x-rays are taken and it appears as though the patient has bilateral Perthes' disease in the exact same stage, the suspicion for MED should be high. Bilateral Perthes' is rare. Let's restate that: bilateral Perthes' is extraordinarily rare. If both hips are involved in a Legg-Calvé-Perthes disease case, the x-rays will almost always show different stages (ie, one hip will be in the fragmentation stage and the other hip will be in the reossification phase). Knee x-rays may reveal a double patella (in older children), a shallow intercondylar notch, and an abnormal epiphysis. Metacarpal and phalange x-rays may also show shortened metacarpals and phalanges. A skeletal survey may be warranted when disproportionate body segments are noted, significantly short height prediction for the family, unexplained short stature, family history, and short child or an absent puberty growth spurt.[184]

Differentiating MED from spondyloepiphyseal dysplasia (SED) can be done by obtaining spine x-rays. In MED, the spine is unaffected, whereas in SED, the spine will have abnormalities identified. Table 55-1 shows some of the common dwarfisms and distinguishing features found with each condition.

For a full lecture on molecular genetics, review the references for this vignette; however, it is important to understand some of the basics. Type II collagen is expressed in early chondrogenesis and is an important constituent of the growth plate. Qualitative and quantitative defects will lead to varying degrees of skeletal dysplasias (SED, Kneist dysplasia, Stickler's syndrome, and achondrogenesis type II). However, COMP is a noncollagenous extracellular matrix protein that binds collagen types I, II, and X. Defects in COMP can lead to decreased chondrocyte viability and are likely responsible for the cell death of growth-plate chondrocytes. They are often found in MED and pseudoachondroplasia. In addition, a complex pathway involving a transcription factor Twist-1 and Runx2 can positively regulate FGF18, which activates FGFR3. Activating mutations of FGFR3 cause achondroplasia, hypochondroplasia, and thanatophoric dysplasia.[183,185] And that's all I have to say about that!

Why Might This Be Tested? MED has numerous presentation scenarios (knee pain, hip pain, genu valgum, genu varum, etc). It is important to be aware of this when a patient presents with these common complaints. Question writers love dwarfism questions, including inheritance patterns, molecular genetics, and the key distinguishing features of each condition.

Here's the Point!

Know your dwarfisms, particularly the AR and X-linked patterns of inheritance. MED is symmetric, whereas Perthes' may be found in bilateral cases but typically at different stages of the disease.

Table 55-1.

DWARFISMS AND COMMON ASSOCIATED FINDINGS

Dwarfism	Inheritance	Common Features	Genetic Defect	Locus
Achondroplasia	AD	Short limbs, prominent forehead, presents at birth	FGFR3 (98% with glycine arginine substitution)	4p16.3
Pseudoachondroplasia	AD/AR	Short limbs, lax joints, normal face, presents at birth/childhood	COMP (defects cause 40% of cases)	19p12-13.1
Thanatophoric dysplasia	AD	Short limbs, trident hands, narrow chest, presents at birth, can be lethal	FGFR3 (multiple mutations noted)	4p16.3
Spondyloepiphyseal dysplasia congenita	AD	Lordosis, myopia, presents at birth, retinal detachment later	COL2A1/type II collagen	12q13.1
Spondyloepiphyseal dysplasia tarda	X-linked recessive	Spine involvement, spares hands and feet, mild to moderate epiphyseal dysplasia in extremities	SEDL	Xp22
Kniest dysplasia	AD	Joint stiffness, flat facsies, myopia, cleft palate, presents at birth	COL2A1/type II collagen	12q13.1
Stickler's syndrome (hereditary arthro-opthalmopathy)	AD	Flat face, Pierre-Robin (micrognathia, glossoptosis, cleft palate)	COL2A1/type II collagen and/or COL2A2	12q13.1
Metaphyseal chondro-dysplasia				
Jansen	AD	Bowed limbs, presents at birth/infancy	PTH-PTHrP	3p22-21.1
Schmid	AD	Lumbar lordosis, bowed limbs, presents at childhood	COL10A1	6q21-22.3
McKusick	AR	Cartilage hair hypoplasia, flared fragmentation at knees, hips often spared	RMRP	9p13
Diastrophic dysplasia	AR	Rhizomelic shortening, hitchhiker thumbs	DTDST/SLC26A2 Sulfate transporter	5q32-33
Multiple epiphyseal dysplasia	AD	Short statue, waddling gait, presents at childhood	COL9A2, COMP, MATN3	1p32.2-33, 19p13.1, 2p23-24

AD = autosomal dominant; AR = autosomal recessive; COMP = cartilage oligomeric matrix protein; FGFR3 = fibroblast growth factor receptor 3; SEDL = spondyloepiphyseal dysplasia tarda.

Adapted from Alanay Y, Lachman RS. A review of the principles of radiological assessment of skeletal dysplasias. *J Clin Res Pediatr Endocrinol.* 2011;3(4):163-178; Brook CG, de Vries BB. Skeletal dysplasias. *Arch Dis Child.* 1998;79(3):285-289; and Phornphutkul C, Gruppuso PA. Disorders of the growth plate. *Curr Opin Endocrinol Diabetes Obes.* 2009;16(6):430-434.

Vignette 56: I Can't Go Up and Down Stairs With My Replaced Knee!

Approximately 1 year ago, a 57-year-old female underwent an uncomplicated primary CR TKA with excellent early clinical results. She notes a feeling of instability while ascending and descending stairs. Serum and synovial infection markers were negative on her preoperative workup. Her physical examination demonstrates an active ROM of 0 to 120 degrees and no varus/valgus laxity in extension but more than 10 mm of AP translation of the tibia on the femur at 90 degrees of flexion. Quadriceps strength is symmetrical, and she can straight leg raise without pain. Current x-rays demonstrate a well-fixed CR TKA with neutral mechanical alignment.

▶ *What is the most likely diagnosis?*

▶ *Name the possible etiologies of this problem.*

▶ *What clinical and radiographic findings may be associated with this condition?*

▶ *What is the best treatment option?*

▶ *How may this problem manifest in a posterior cruciate–substituting design?*

▶ *What are the causes and treatments of flexion instability?*

Vignette 56: Answer

This patient has the classic clinical complaints of flexion instability in the setting of a CR prosthesis.[186,187] One possible etiology is incompetence of the PCL from an iatrogenic injury during surgery or attenuation or traumatic rupture postoperatively. Incompetence of the PCL may be accompanied by a posterior sag sign and/or the ability to subluxate the tibia posteriorly on the femur during the physical examination. Other causes of flexion instability derive from a flexion/extension mismatch created when the femoral component is too small or excessive posterior slope has been cut into the tibia (both of which may be appreciable on the lateral x-ray). In addition, a weight-bearing lateral x-ray with the knee in flexion may display paradoxical role forward of the femur on the tibia. Revision surgery for flexion instability must address not only an incompetent PCL but also any flexion/extension mismatch (with component revision, cutting less slope in the tibia, and/or upsizing to a larger femoral component with posterior augments). Optimizing component placement is favored over settling for a greater level of constraint as such components place added stress on the revision TKA construct (hinge > semi-constrained > PS).

Flexion instability in posterior cruciate–substituting designs may present with an acute knee dislocation ("jumping the post").[188] This often occurs when the patient places the leg in a figure-4 position to put on a shoe in the setting of flexion instability. Patients with a large preoperative valgus deformity requiring extensive lateral release to balance the knee are at an increased risk for this complication. This problem can often be solved by increasing the size of the post (semiconstrained) on the polyethylene at the added expense of potential post wear and early tibial component loosening.

Extension instability results from imbalance of the collateral ligaments. Iatrogenic injury during surgery, as well as inadequate release, have been implicated as potential causes.[189] Further recurvatum and hyperextension instability of the knee can lead to anterior tibial post wear and possibly even catastrophic failure. Such deformity is often difficult to treat and may require the use of a hinged component.

Why Might This Be Tested? Flexion instability is not an uncommon cause for revision TKA. Furthermore, CR and PS designs have different manifestations of flexion laxity and are fair game to be quizzed. Flexion and extension gap balancing is a critical part of primary and revision TKR.

Here's the Point!

You have to know the table for balancing flexion and extension gaps. The posterior femur affects knee flexion, the distal femur affects extension, and the tibia impacts both gaps in general. Appropriate gap balancing is the key to minimizing component constraint, which is the crucial element for revision TKA success and longevity.

Vignette 57: I Have a Few Questions About My New Hip

A healthy 40-year-old male presents to your office with a 5-year history of right hip pain. He was diagnosed with ON of the femoral head in his 30s and has subsequently gone onto collapse and secondary DJD. He has discussed surgery with several other physicians and has many questions for you regarding the procedure. He is particularly interested in the type of replacement you would perform for him. After confirming that his x-rays show severe DJD secondary to ON, a discussion on THA ensues. His x-rays show normal-appearing metaphyseal and diaphyseal bone with no specific abnormal findings outside of the ON. He has no past surgical history.

▶ *The patient asks you to discuss cementless fixation in primary THA. Describe the material properties and necessary microenvironment for osseointegration.*

▶ *The patient is an engineer by trade and would like to better understand the concept and outcomes of the various bearing options in THA.*

▶ *In addition, he has heard a lot on television regarding problems with the metals involved in THA and would like you to explain some of these modern issues.*

Vignette 57: Answer

Cementless THA requires early stability for osseointegration, and recent bearing concerns have centered on ceramic component fractures and failed metal-on-metal bearings.

Cementless fixation in THA relies on early stability because micromotion must be kept to a minimum (< 150 µm, best between 50 and 100 µm). The optimal pore size is 50 to 300 µm, and the optimal porosity is at least 40% to 50% (newer coatings maintain 60% to 80% porosity); greater percentiles of porosity were thought to increase the risk of shearing off the coating from the implant. In addition, intimate contact is required between the host bone and the implant, with gaps being kept to less than 50 µm. Early fixation can be achieved with various techniques and material properties. Initial stability is reliant on a press-fit (1 to 2 mm is best) or adjunct fixation (screws, pegs, or surface modifications). Surface roughness and coefficient of friction (impacted by the nanotexture of the implant) are properties of the coating or finish of the implant and are important for early stability. It is important to explain that implants must be placed in the bone tightly to avoid aseptic loosening but that this can lead to fracture intraoperatively (1% to 4% of the time). Technique is important because proper preparation of the acetabulum (eccentric or aggressive reaming) and the femur (avoid varus reaming/broaching) is necessary to obtain a good fit and maximize host-bone contact.

These 5 bearing options are discussed with the patient in full detail:

- Metal-on-standard polyethylene: Polyethylene is a polymer of ethylene molecules organized into chains and connected by tie molecules. Most components are composed of GUR 1020 or 1050 polyethylene resins and treated by direct compression molding or ram extrusion (machining from bars).[190] Traditional polyethylene has been reported to have wear rates of 0.18 mm/year for the initial 5 years and then 0.1 mm/year at longer-term follow-up.[191] With modern sterilization techniques (avoiding irradiation in air, which typically led to polyethylene oxidation 0.5 to 2 mm below the implant surface and early wear), standard polyethylene is a good bearing surface (and cheaper) but will likely wear out over time for this 40-year-old patient.

- Metal-on-cross-linked polyethylene: To improve upon traditional polyethylene, components can be irradiated with 5, 7.5, or 10 Mrad to induce cross-linking of the polymer chains. Greater cross-linking leads to a harder surface with reduced articular wear rates (40% to 80% less wear) and greater resistance to surface damage.[192] After cross-linking, the polyethylene is then remelted (decreases component strength) or annealed (may lead to increased oxidation). Despite excellent early reported wear rate reduction, concerns for material fracture have been reported with malpositioned components and thin polyethylene liners. Component fracture risk has to be weighed against the lower dislocation with larger-diameter femoral heads with thinner cross-linked polyethylene liners.

- Ceramic-on-ceramic: Ceramic is an inorganic material noted for its high modulus of elasticity, wettability, biocompatibility, and corrosion resistance. Ceramic bearings maintain enhanced lubrication and lower susceptibility to third-body wear. Extremely low wear rates and osteolysis are found with alumina-on-alumina ceramic bearing surfaces. Despite these positives, the concern is for component fracture risk, which has been reported to be 1/2000 to 3000 for femoral heads and 1/6000 to 8000 for liners.[193] Revision is difficult in such a setting because the ceramic component shatters into many pieces that are difficult to retrieve. Furthermore, squeaking has been another concern, with up to 7% of ceramic-on-ceramic cases presenting with squeaking (often associated with malpositioning, failure to restore hip biomechanics, and component impingement), thought to be due to microseparation of the head and liner resulting in stripe wear.[193]

- Ceramic-on-polyethylene: Due to concerns with fracture, there has been a recent trend toward pairing ceramic femoral heads with polyethylene liners. In addition, ceramic femoral heads have been strengthened (150% fracture toughness and 160% burst strength) by adding zirconia to the prior alumina construct.[193] Favorable wear characteristics have been reported with this articulation because the resistance to third-body wear is improved with ceramic femoral heads.

- Metal-on-metal (MOM): This articulation involves a cobalt-chromium femoral head articulating with a like acetabular component/liner. The cobalt-chromium alloys typically consist of cobalt, chromium (provides corrosion resistance), molybdenum (increases strength and decreases grain size), and carbon (aids in strength and wear resistance). A resurgence occurred 5 years ago with large-diameter MOM implants coming back with improved manufacturing (decreasing grain size and improved carbide distribution). The early benefits were improved dislocation rates and lower wear with a fluid-film mode of lubrication (better than the boundary lubrication typically found with polyethylene articulations). However, the resurgence has essentially been derailed with the significant number of early failures and associated adverse local tissue reactions.

A detailed discussion with the patient ensues, and the concept of adverse local tissue reactions are reviewed. These reactions occur from abnormal host responses to excessive or rapid development of MOM, polyethylene, and foreign debris. This can occur from component malposition, poor implant design, increased frictional torque, aseptic loosening, or insertional deformation of the components. Adverse reactions can range from minor fluid collections to massive pseudotumors that cause soft tissue damage or local neurovascular compression. Recent warnings have led to decreased use of these components and widespread recalls. Based upon these discussions, he elects to undergo a ceramic-on-polythene THA.

Why Might This Be Tested? The concept of osseointegration is frequently tested, and you must know the ideal parameters. Similarly, the pros and cons of the various bearing options are fair game and are frequently tested.

Here's the Point!

Early fixation is important for cementless implants and can be obtained with a press-fit and or adjunct fixation. Minimizing micromotion and host bone-implant gaps are important for osseointegration. As for bearing surfaces, MOM and ceramic-on-ceramic bearings have the lowest wear rates but are associated with adverse local tissue reactions and squeaking/fracture, respectively.

Vignette 58: Careful on the Fire Escape Route

A 28-year-old, healthy, nonsmoking, male medical student was climbing out of a second story window to escape a fire when he fell and landed on his right foot. He noticed immediate pain and inability to bear weight and went to the emergency room for evaluation. Physical exam at that time demonstrated that his skin was intact without tenting or concern for compartment syndrome and that he had no associated injuries. A lateral x-ray is shown in Figure 58-1.

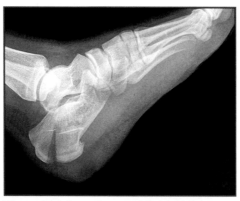

Figure 58-1. Lateral x-ray of the right foot.

▶ *What is the most likely diagnosis?*

▶ *What other tests should be ordered?*

▶ *What is the classification of this injury and the treatment options?*

▶ *What are key factors in determining operative vs conservative management?*

Vignette 58: Answer

The patient's history, physical exam, and x-rays are consistent with a calcaneus fracture. These account for about 2% of all fractures, and more than 75% of them have an intra-articular component. The patient's history, as in this case, usually involves an axial loading mechanism (fall from height or high-speed motor vehicle accident). Exam should include a careful exam of skin integrity because up to 10% of these are open injuries (typically a transverse medial wound at the level of the sustentaculum). Open fractures have a high likelihood of having complications related to infection, nonunion, and wound breakdown.[194] Key factors in the history and exam that are indications for nonoperative management are smoking, diabetes mellitus, vascular disease, workers' compensation,[195] and age older than 50 years. The lumbar spine and pelvis should also be examined secondary to the axial load mechanism.

Imaging should begin with x-rays of the foot, including AP, lateral, and oblique views. Specifically, Böhler's angle (20 to 40 degrees) is assessed on the lateral view (Figure 58-2), along with a double crescent sign from the depressed superolateral fragment. Other specific views are the Harris axial view (lateral wall blow-out, shortening, widening, and varus angulation of the tuberosity) and Broden's view (intra-articular step-off of depressed superolateral fragment). The Harris view is obtained by angling the beam 10 to 45 degrees in the sagittal plane from behind the leg, centered on the posterior portion of the subtalar joint. CT is obtained to help differentiate fracture characteristics; the coronal projection can be specifically used for the Sanders classification.

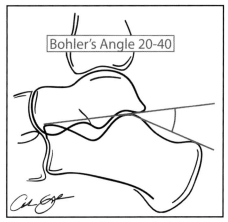

Figure 58-2. Simplification of a lateral foot x-ray showing a normal Böhler's angle of 20 to 40 degrees. (Reprinted with permission from Adam B. Yanke, MD.)

Classification and treatment should begin with separating intra- from extra-articular injuries. The latter are often avulsion fractures of the anterior process, sustentaculum, or tuberosity. These can be treated with restricted weight bearing and cast application. One specific entity in this group to be aware of is an Achilles avulsion because it is at increased risk of skin breakdown and may require ORIF. Intra-articular fractures include the tongue-type in which the posterior articular facet remains in continuity with the tuberosity. This is in contrast to the joint depression type in which the tuberosity is separate from the posterior articular facet. The typical pattern is a line crossing the posterior facet from anterolateral to posteromedial.[196] This can be accompanied by other fragments as follows: sustentacular (constant), superolateral depressed, tuberosity, and anteromedial. Sanders classification on coronal CT is based on the number and location of posterior facet articular fragments (I, nondisplaced; II, 2 fragments; III, 3 fragments; IV, 4 or more fragments).

Treatment options can be conservative (extra-articular fractures and smokers) and operative. The latter should include closed reduction and percutaneous fixation for tongue-type and Sanders types I and II. Displaced Sanders II through IV should be treated with ORIF. One should consider subtalar arthrodesis along with ORIF in patients with severe type IV injuries. All operative patients should be nonweight bearing for 8 to 12 weeks.

Pain and functional outcome are similar in conservative and operative management, with improved operative results seen in women, young men, high Böhler's angle, simple intra-articular involvement, nonworkers' compensation cases, and more sedentary jobs.[197] Patients older than 50 years, especially men, should be treated conservatively. Outcomes in patients for whom the inciting injury involved a motor vehicle accident tend to have worse outcomes than those with axial loading mechanisms.[198]

Given the presentation of this patient, he is well suited for closed reduction and percutaneous fixation. Again, this it because he is young and healthy, doesn't smoke, sustained a closed tongue-type injury, and does not perform heavy labor.

Why Might This Be Tested? Calcaneal fractures are relatively common, and the treatment algorithm can be simplified greatly with a basic understanding.

Here's the Point!

First, determine if the injury should be treated operatively or conservatively based on patient factors (smoking = conservative management) and fracture characteristics. This is the most important factor, followed by the different surgical options based on the level of comminution, which is one of the greatest predictors of outcome.

Vignette 59: What's Holding My Replacement in My Bones?

A 67-year-old male with a history of a cemented right TKA presents to the office with endstage degenerative changes to his left hip. After a discussion in the office, he is surprised to hear that his THA will be placed without the use of cement and inquires how the hip will be held in place without the "glue." The patient and his wife have multiple questions they would like you to answer prior to surgery.

▶ *What are the mechanisms of cementless fixation?*

▶ *What are the components coated with to facilitate this fixation?*

▶ *What are the characteristics of these coatings that facilitate optimal fixation?*

Vignette 59: Answer

Prosthetic components can be held in place with the use of biocompatible cement or with cementless techniques. Cementless techniques allow for a secure interface between the implant and surrounding bone. This interface is not static and can remodel according to the forces placed on the bone surrounding the implant. Implants are specially coated to allow for ingrowth, in which bone grows into a porous coating, or ongrowth, in which bone grows onto a roughened surface. This requires relatively intimate (< 50-μm gaps) and firm contact at the bone-prosthesis interface; by limiting micromotion to less than 150 μm, the formation of interposing fibrous tissue can be avoided.[199] Porous coatings are typically attached to a substrate material (hence, failure can occur from shedding of the coating), whereas roughened implants are surface treated (ie, plasma sprayed) and are not truly a porous coating.

Although polymethylmethacrylate use has dramatically declined in THA, it is an acceptable form of fixation, particularly in elderly patients. The major concern is that bone cement serves as a grout and cannot remodel with the femoral canal as it expands with age. Cementing techniques have improved over time to include canal preparation, vacuum mixing, use of a cement restrictor, pressurization, and heating of the femoral component. If a complete 2-mm cement mantle is achieved, long-term success with cemented stems is very good. If there are voids and/or the implant is in contact with bone, the success rate plummets drastically. On test questions, look for cracks in the cement mantle, varus alignment, or component contact with the cortex to signify that the implant is loose.

Implants that rely on bone ingrowth for fixation via a porous coating typically have pore sizes ranging from 100 to 400 μm.[200] Deeper pores are correlated with stronger fixation, as are more open cell structured materials with excellent pore interconnectivity. Ingrowth materials include porous metals, sintered beads, or fiber mesh. Most recently, these coatings have been updated to include greater porosity (60% to 80%), higher surface coefficient of friction (closer to 1), greater strength, and favorable implant characteristics. Despite these improved characteristics, it is important to remember that only 10% to 30% of ingrowth into the surface of the component will provide stable long-term fixation.

Implants that rely on bone ongrowth are roughened using various techniques. Grit blasting involves spraying a large number of small abrasive particles at the implant surface. Plasma spraying involves mixing metal with inert gas, pressurizing it, and spraying molten metal at the component surface. Surface roughness, which is proportional to the strength of the implant fixation, is defined as the average peak-to-valley distance.

Hydroxyapatite coating may also be used with ongrowth or ingrowth stems to supplement fixation due to its osteoconductive properties. Osteoblasts can adhere to the hydroxyapatite, which may shorten the time to biologic fixation. The addition of hydroxyapatite requires a thickness less than 70 μm because a coating that is too thick has the potential to delaminate. In addition, the hydroxyapatite must have high crystalline content because areas with low crystallinity will dissolve and be nonfunctional. However, although animal studies have been promising, long-term outcomes have not definitively demonstrated clinical superiority with hydroxyapatite coating.[201]

Why Might This Be Tested? The majority of THA implants used in this country use cementless, press-fit fixation and are coated with materials that facilitate this process. It is important to understand the characteristics of these coatings, the mechanisms of fixation, and the reasons for failure.

Here's the Point!

Components are coated with materials that facilitate bone ongrowth or ingrowth. Fixation for ingrowth components is optimized with deep pores sized 100 to 400 μm, within 50 μm of bone surface, and with less than 40 m of micromotion. Ongrowth fixation is optimized with increased surface roughness and, similarly, minimal micromotion and minimal bone-prosthesis distance. Hydroxyapatite may shorten time to biologic fixation.

Vignette 60: Flexor Tendon Injury

A 21-year-old male was playing intramural football 6 weeks prior to presentation. Shortly after making a tackle, he was unable to fully flex the DIP joint of the ring finger. He thought it would get better on its own, but it has failed to improve since the injury. On physical exam, he has an absence of flexor digitorum profundus (FDP) function and tenderness with a nodule in the distal palm but not in the digit. He has full flexor digitorum sublimis function, active PIP flexion, and full DIP passive flexion. His x-rays show no fracture and a congruently reduced DIP joint.

▶ *What is the patient's underlying diagnosis?*

▶ *What is the classification of this injury and time factors in treatment?*

▶ *How is treatment different in the chronic setting as in this case?*

Vignette 60: Answer

The underlying diagnosis in this case is a traumatic rupture of the insertion of the FDP on the distal phalanx of the ring finger, or Jersey finger, and represents a zone 1 flexor tendon injury.[202] This injury typically occurs in young, active males and not infrequently presents in a delayed fashion because it appears innocuous at the time of injury. The injury occurs almost pathognomonically in the ring finger. Zones of tendon injury include the following: zone 1 (distal to flexor digitorum sublimis insertion), zone 2 (between the distal palmar crease and the flexor digitorum sublimis insertion), zone 3 (the palm), zone 4 (carpal tunnel), and zone 5 (wrist and forearm).

Leddy[203] classified these injuries into 3 types based on the presence or absence of fracture and to where the proximal stump is retracted, which has a direct implication on the timing of treatment. Type I ruptures occur without fracture and retract into the palm with no intact vincula. Patients will often be tender in the palm at the area of tendon retraction. The combination of muscle contracture and noncompliance of the empty sheath make primary repair difficult or impossible after just a few days. Type II ruptures have intact vincula on the proximal stump and retract to approximately the PIP joint, where patients will often be tender. The relatively maintained sheath compliance and muscle length in contrast to type I will allow primary repair for 6 weeks or more after injury. Type III injuries include a bony avulsion of the tendon insertion on the volar base of the distal phalanx and retract only as far as the distal edge of the A4 pulley. These injuries are amenable to treatment with screw or wire fixation or fragment excision and tendon advancement even if the fragment is small and presents several months after the injury. Uncommonly, a type III injury can convert to a type IV injury in which the tendon is separate from the bony fragment and requires separate repair to bone after fixation of the bone fragment.

This patient has evidence of a type I injury; given the time course, this is an injury not amenable to primary repair. If this had been diagnosed early, treatment would have consisted of repair using a pullout suture over a button for 6 weeks or repair to the bone with a suture anchor.[204,205] The most widely accepted treatment options for this patient now are 2-stage flexor tendon reconstruction or nonoperative treatment for the FDP itself and DIP arthrodesis if the patient has symptomatic joint hyperextensibility in the future. The former includes a first stage that comprises resection of the FDP, typically from 1 cm proximal to its insertion then back proximally just distal to the takeoff of the lumbrical. A silicon rod is sutured to the distal stump and routed under the pulley system into the palm or as far as the wrist at the surgeon's discretion. The second stage is performed 2 to 3 months after the first stage once a new flexor sheath has formed and consists of placement of a tendon graft, most often palmaris longus, toe extensor, or plantaris depending on the length required.[206,207] Although good results have been obtained with this treatment, caution must be exercised because chronic Jersey fingers usually have full active PIP flexion from a functioning flexor digitorum sublimis and there is a risk of worsening PIP motion with flexor tendon reconstruction. This risk and the lengthy rehabilitation inherent in 2-stage reconstruction must be weighed with the importance of regaining active DIP flexion for the patient.

Why Might This Be Tested? It is a common injury with a well-defined anatomic basis and a classification with implications on treatment and outcome.

Here's the Point!

Jersey finger is an FDP avulsion typically found in young, active patients. The farther a purely tendinous injury retracts, the less time you have to treat with primary repair. Treatment in chronic cases requires careful consideration of the risks and benefits of 2-stage reconstruction in the setting of an intact flexor digitorum sublimis.

Vignette 61: Case of the Persistently Draining TKA

A 58-year-old female is 2 weeks status post left TKA. She initially did well following the procedure but has developed increased pain, swelling, erythema, warmth, and drainage from the knee over the past 24 to 48 hours. Inflammatory markers are elevated, and aspiration reveals a WBC count of around 50,000 with 91% PMNs. Cultures are sent to the microbiology laboratory.

▶ *What are common bacteria that cause this patient's current condition?*

▶ *What are some of the more common bacteria encountered by orthopedic surgeons?*

Vignette 61: Answer

This patient has an acute periprosthetic joint infection (PJI). *Stapholococcus aureus* and *Stapholococcus epidermidis* are frequent pathogens in PJI.[208] Cell count in the early postoperative time frame is more variable than with chronic aspiration (a WBC cutoff of 27,800 cells/μL gives a 94% positive predictive value and a 98% negative predictive value; in addition, optimal levels of CRP and polymorphonuclear cells were 95 mg/nL and 89%[209]), laboratory tests may be falsely elevated from recent surgery, and Gram stain is a relatively poor test in diagnosing periprosthetic infection. It is also important to make sure antibiotics are held for 2 weeks prior to aspiration; however, prophylactic antibiotics do not have to be withheld prior to obtaining cultures intraoperatively at the time of revision surgery. Clinical suspicion, persistent draining, warmth, erythema, and nonhealing wounds are signs of infection. The Musculoskeletal Infection Society definition of PJI should be well known as the following:

1. An open sinus tract to the prosthesis is present.
2. Positive cultures from 2 different samples obtained from the affected joint.
3. Four of the 6 following criteria exist:
   a. Increased ESR or CRP (> 30 mm/hr and > 10 mg/L, respectively)
   b. Elevated synovial WBC (chronic 1100 to 4000 cells/uL)
   c. Elevated PMN percentage (chronic 64% to 69%)
   d. Presence of purulent fluid
   e. Isolation of a pathogen on culture about a prosthetic joint
   f. Frozen section consistent with more than 5 WBC per high-power field in 5 high-power fields on histological exam

Table 61-1 contains an overview of commonly encountered bacteria in orthopedic surgery.

Why Might This Be Tested? Infections of native tissues and postoperative infections will be diagnosed and treated by orthopedic surgeons in all fields. It is important have a basic understanding of the most common causative organisms.

Here's the Point!

Table 61-1 outlines many of the basic facts about bacteria that are tested on orthopedic standardized exams (sorry, they have to be memorized).

	Table 61-1.	
	COMMON BACTERIA ASSOCIATED WITH ORTHOPEDIC CONDITIONS AND PERTINENT FACTS	
Group	*Bacteria*	*High-Yield Facts*
Gm pos cocci	Stapholococcus aureus	Most common cause of septic arthritis, abscess formation; MecA gene production by methicillin-resistant *S aureus* resist beta lactam antibiotics
Gm pos cocci	Stapholococcus epidermidis	Normal skin flora; forms biofilm to resist immune system and attach to implants
Gm pos bacilli	Bacillus anthracis	Spore forming; cause of anthrax; cutaneous, pulmonary, and gastrointestinal forms of disease
Gm pos bacilli	Clostridium tetani	Cause of tetanus; update vaccine with open wounds
Gm pos bacilli	Clostridium botulinum	Neurotoxin causes flaccid muscle paralysis; injections used for muscle spasm
Gm pos bacilli	Clostridium difficile	Antibiotic associated diarrhea or more severe pseudomembranous colitis; treat with flagyl or oral vancomycin; commonly associated with clindamycin use
Gm pos bacilli	Listeria monocytogenes	Found in soil, unpasteurized dairy; more often causes diarrhea, bacteremia, central nervous system infection, septic arthritis, periprosthetic joint infection, listeriosis in pregnancy
Gm neg cocci	Neisseria gonorrhoeae	Migratory polyarthritis, tenosynovitis, dermatitis is classic triad; also monoarticular septic arthritis in sexually active young adults
Gm neg bacilli	Escherichia coli	Common cause of urinary tract infection, normal gut flora, postoperative infections
Gm neg bacilli	Salmonella	Common cause of osteomyelitis in sickle cell patients
Gm neg bacilli	Vibrio species	Undercooked seafood and marine infections
Gm neg bacilli	Pseudomonas aeruginosa	Common after foot puncture wounds (through the sole of the shoe), septic arthritis in IV drug users; can cause fatal bacteremia after spread from local infection
Gm neg bacilli	Pasteurella multocida	Infection due to domesticated animal bites
Gm neg bacilli	Bartonella henselae	Causative bacteria for cat scratch disease; more common in immunocompromised patients
Mycobacteria	Mycobacterium tuberculosis	Pott's disease in spine, hips, and knees also can be affected; acid-fast bacilli testing
Mycobacteria	Mycobacterium leprae	Causes Hansen's disease (leprosy); most commonly found in tropical climates
Spirochete	Borrelia burgdorferi	Cause of Lyme disease; vector is the Ixodes tick
Spirochete	Treponema pallidum	Sexually transmitted; causes syphilis, congenital infection, monoarticular arthritis, Charcot knee
Gm pos rod	Propionibacterium acnes	Slow growing in cultures; may colonize axilla and cause infection after shoulder surgery
Gm neg bacilli	Eikenella corrodens	Consider in human bite infections, diabetics/IV drug users who lick needles
Gm neg=gram-negative; Gm pos=gram-positive; IV=intravenous.		

Vignette 62: Doc, Why Does My Elbow Clunk?

A 58-year-old male sheet metal worker has noticed gradually worsening pain and mild stiffness of the dominant right elbow over 7 months. There was no trauma or specific inciting event. He denies any locking or clunks with elbow ROM. He has pain with holding heavy things at his side and full flexion of the elbow. He gets occasional swelling and denies numbness and tingling. He has tried a compressive elbow sleeve with only partial relief. Physical examination shows a muscular well-developed male with ROM of 30 to 125 degrees on the right compared with 5 to 145 degrees on the left. Pain is reproduced by maximal passive flexion and extension but there is no pain in the mid-arc of motion. He has good varus and valgus stability, and forearm rotation is full and causes no pain. He is tender at the medial and lateral ulnohumeral joints but not at the radiocapitellar joint. His neurologic exam is intact. A lateral x-ray is shown in Figure 62-1.

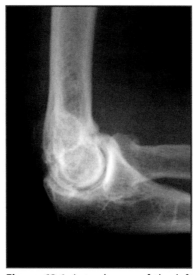

Figure 62-1. Lateral x-ray of the left elbow.

▶ *What is the patient's underlying diagnosis?*

▶ *How does this disease typically progress?*

▶ *How does it differ from inflammatory arthritis of the elbow?*

▶ *What are the surgical treatment options depending on stage?*

Vignette 62: Answer

The underlying diagnosis in this case is idiopathic OA of the elbow, which usually arises in middle-aged men who use their hands heavily for work or recreational activities (eg, football lineman, racquet sport players, and throwers). It usually presents with a combination of motion loss and pain of varying degrees. It classically starts with impinging osteophytes at the coronoid and olecranon fossae/processes that limit flexion and extension, respectively. It is this impingement that leads to pain at the extremes of motion in flexion and extension. Due to the high articular congruity of the ulnohumeral joint, the majority of the ulnohumeral joint in mid-arc is typically spared until later in the disease process.[210,211] In addition to bony impingement, capsular thickening and contracture often contribute to loss of motion. In the setting of OA, the radiocapitellar joint often has a degenerated appearance but rarely is the primary pain generator. In the absence of substantial pain with forearm rotation or radiocapitellar tenderness, treatment can usually focus on the ulnohumeral joint without addressing the radiocapitellar joint. Inflammatory elbow arthritis, most commonly RA, typically presents with more evenly distributed joint space narrowing with erosive changes and minimal osteophyte formation (typically managed with injections, synovectomy interposition arthroplasty, or semi-constrained total elbow arthroplasty [TEA]). Ulnar neuropathy at the cubital tunnel is common with elbow arthritis and must be evaluated for on physical exam.

Treatment is initially similar to OA elsewhere, starting with activity modification, NSAIDs, and corticosteroid injections. The surgical options vary depending on the stage. If a patient has pain limited to the extremes of motion with impinging osteophytes but an otherwise well-preserved joint space, open or arthroscopic surgical debridement can be offered. The procedure includes bony debridement of the olecranon and coronoid tips and re-establishing their respective fossae, as well as anterior and posterior capsulectomy.[210,211]

Most series report between a 20- and 30-degree improvement in ROM arc, and 80% to 90% good to excellent results for pain relief. The procedure also tends to have good longevity, but long-term results are only available for open techniques. At 10 plus years, patients may lose approximately 10 degrees of their motion gained, and osteophytes will typically recur in 50% or more of patients, but the great majority (85%) will have no or minimal pain.[210,211] Although there are no long-term results for arthroscopic debridement, early results appear similar to open techniques in experienced hands.[212] Arthroscopy portals and potential risks include the following: anterolateral (1 cm distal and anterior to the lateral epicondyle; beware the lateral antebrachial cutaneous and radial nerves), anteromedial (2 cm distal and anterior to the medial epicondyle; beware the medial antebrachial cutaneous and median nerves), and posterolateral (2 cm proximal to the olecranon).

Once the arthritis has progressed to involve the entirety of the ulnohumeral joint, debridement is not reliably successful. This scenario can be treated with TEA in the older low-demand patient who is willing to accept a permanent 5- to 10-pound lifting restriction or with fascial resurfacing arthroplasty, such as Achilles allograft resurfacing in the higher-demand patient. The latter is a technically demanding procedure with less predictable results that should only be reserved for the most refractory cases. Elbow arthrodesis is an option for very young patients but carries great functional impairment.

Why Might This Be Tested? Elbow OA isn't common, but it presents in specific patient demographics and progresses in a classic pattern. The treatment is well described and varies depending on stage and patient demand.

Here's the Point!

Elbow OA is typically found in middle-aged men with heavy use of the arms. It begins with impinging osteophytes anteriorly and posteriorly with associated capsular contracture, for which open or arthroscopic debridement yield similar results for pain and motion. Progressive degenerative disease will require more formal arthroplasty procedures depending on each patient's demand level. Radiocapitellar disease is often present but is rarely the pain generator and does not usually need to be addressed.

Vignette 63: My Child's Foot Looks Like a Slipper!

A 3-month-old male is brought to the office for evaluation of his feet. He was the born via a normal vaginal delivery and has no associated medical problems. His mother is concerned about the rounded nature of his feet. A clinical photograph and lateral x-ray are shown in Figure 63-1.

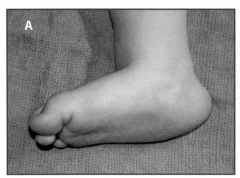 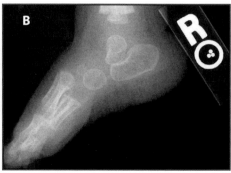

Figure 63-1. (A) Clinical photograph and (B) lateral x-ray of the child's foot.

▶ *What is the diagnosis?*

▶ *What else is it associated with?*

▶ *What type of radiographic study is necessary to make the diagnosis?*

▶ *What is the initial treatment?*

▶ *What is the definitive treatment?*

Vignette 63: Answer

The patient has a congenital vertical talus (CVT) as depicted on the lateral x-ray. Foot deformities are relatively common, with an incidence of up to 4.2% in newborns. Although metatarsus adductus accounts for 75% of these cases, the others that should immediately come to mind for pediatric/newborn foot abnormalities are talipes equinovarus, calcaneovalgus foot (aka clubfoot), and vertical talus.[146] A neurologic issue (tethered cord, sacral agenesis, syrix, intraspinal pathology, etc) needs to be ruled out and a genetic evaluation contemplated because up to 60% of cases may be associated with arthrogryposis or myelomeningocele.[146] File it away; it is a rare finding to see CVT in a child with no neurologic issue.

The diagnosis is made clinically and on plain x-rays. Clinically, the foot will have a Persian slipper appearance. The plantar surface is convex with the apex, and convexity is located at the talar head. The calcaneus is in equinus and the foot is everted. In addition, the Achilles tendon will be tight, resulting in a dorsiflexed forefoot with a midfoot dislocation through the talonavicular joint.[146] The clinical appearance can also be present with an oblique talus. CVT can occasionally be confused with a clubfoot deformity; however, the lack of flexibility and rigid deformity differentiate the 2 conditions. The diagnosis is confirmed with a forced plantarflexion lateral view x-ray. The parent holds the forefoot in plantarflexion while a lateral x-ray is obtained. No further fancy imaging studies are required! A CVT or an oblique talus will reveal the talus pointing downward on the lateral x-ray. In the case of an oblique talus, the forced plantarflexion view will demonstrate the talus aligned in a normal position in relation to the navicular. With a true CVT, the navicular will remain dorsally displaced on the talus and the talus will remain vertical.

Initial treatment may include manipulation and serial casting, particularly in the neonatal period. However, the definitive treatment is a full release, usually reserved until the child is 6 to 12 months old. Even with reduction, the incidence of recurrence is high (best results occur with surgery before 2 years old) due to the underlying neurologic condition. Some recent success has been found with serial casting followed by a percutaneous tendo-Achilles lengthening and pin fixation of the talonavicular joint.[146]

Why Might This Be Tested? This foot deformity is associated with numerous other neurologic conditions that are important to identify. CVT is different from a clubfoot deformity in that is not flexible and often has underlying associated neurologic abnormalities. Neurologic deformities tend to be rigid and recur despite casting or surgical management.

Here's the Point!

Persian slipper foot is likely CVT; however, check the lateral x-ray and forced plantarflexed lateral x-ray to make sure the talus stays vertical. When you see CVT, look for an associated neurological condition, such as arthrogryposis or myelomeningocele.

Vignette 64: Doc, What's Wrong With My Prosthetic Leg?

A 37-year-old male with a history of a right below-knee amputation presents to your office with pain in his residual limb and progressive walking difficulties. He reports his pain is localized to his anterolateral residual limb with prolonged periods of walking and that he has recently noticed some mild redness in the same area when he doffs his prosthesis. His amputation occurred years ago after a traumatic injury to his leg in a motorcycle accident. Since then, he has had minimal problems and has gotten back into running and even recently skiing. He denies any recent trauma or other skin issues. His exam reveals increased knee flexion at initial contact on his right leg.

▶ *What type of socket does this patient likely have? What are the pressure-tolerant areas?*

▶ *Besides a poor-fitting socket, what other gait abnormalities may cause his excessive knee flexion?*

▶ *What type of foot is recommended for this patient?*

Vignette 64: Answer

The standard socket used for most transtibial amputees is a patellar tendon–bearing socket. This is a custom-molded plastic socket that distributes weight over certain pressure-tolerant areas, including the patellar tendon, pretibial muscles, popliteal fossa, lateral shaft of the fibula, and the medial tibial flare. Reduced weight bearing over the bony prominences, including the tibial crest, fibular head, and distal tibia and fibula, minimizes any associated pain and skin breakdown.

This socket is characterized by a bar incorporated into the anterior wall of the socket that applies additional pressure on the patellar tendon. For various reasons, a poor-fitting socket can lead to pain, gait abnormalities, prosthesis failure or abnormal wear, and skin issues.[213]

Due to the kinetic chain, excessive knee flexion at initial contact can be caused by a variety of biomechanical problems throughout the lower limb. At the ankle and foot, increased ankle dorsiflexion or a heel cushion (or foot) that is too firm can both cause this pattern. A knee flexion contracture, excessive anterior displacement of the socket over the foot, or moving the socket anteriorly in relation to the foot can also present similarly.[213] If this patient had instead presented with excessive knee extension at initial contact, the opposite could be possible etiologies, along with quadriceps weakness or habit.

Other common prosthetic problems for transtibial amputations include the following:

- Pistoning: This can be related to poor suspension of the prosthesis if this occurs through the swing phase or poor socket fit if during the stance phase of walking.

- Foot alignment problems: If the foot is dorsiflexed, the gait is impacted by increased patellar pressure and the opposite for a plantarflexed position. If the foot is placed too far forward, there tends to be increased knee extension and patella pain; when it is too far posterior, there is an increased knee flexion moment and instability.

For transfemoral amputations, gait abnormalities are associated with prosthetic problems, including the following:

- Vaulted gait: prosthetic is too long or suspension is ineffective, allowing the leg to feel longer

- Knee instability: foot is too hard or knee is too anterior (increased flexion moment)

- Lateral trunk bending: prosthetic is too short or fits poorly

- Terminal snap: inadequate prosthetic knee flexion secondary to quadriceps weakness or insecure patient

- Excessive lumbar lordosis: flexion contracture of the hips, similar to native hip pathology

Given the active lifestyle of this patient, an energy-storing/dynamic-response prosthetic foot would be most appropriate. This type of foot, such as the Springlite foot (Ottobock), Endolite foot (Endolite), or Seattle foot (M+IND), is made of flexible, energy-storing material that absorbs energy at heel strike when the foot is compressed and is then transferred back to the person at the time of push-off. They are also more lightweight, they conserve energy, and they allow for a smoother roll-over. Another option for this active patient may be a multiaxis prosthetic foot, which permits some controlled movement in the normal anatomic planes, allowing for ambulation on uneven surfaces and absorbing some of the torsional forces associated with ambulation. However, these feet can be relatively bulky and heavy, making them less ideal for those interested in jogging and vigorous sports.[213,214]

Why Might This Be Tested? Prosthetic options and their associated medical issues have significant functional implications for amputees. Residual limb care is a significant part of postamputation medical care, and understanding the biomechanical and practical use of lower extremity prostheses is also pertinent.

Here's the Point!

Appropriate load transfer for socket fit minimizes the risk of common complications, including dermatologic conditions and gait abnormalities. Heel strike with the knee abnormally flexed or extended can represent a poorly aligned lower extremity axis, joint contracture, or conditions related to the foot components themselves. A dynamic-response foot optimizes energy conservation for athletic use in active amputees.

Vignette 65: This Back Pain Is Limiting My Soccer Game

A 20-year-old male presents with severe low back pain and occasional bilateral leg pain in the antero-lateral aspect of his legs. In the past, he has tried a corset brace, muscle strengthening in a formal physical therapy program, and NSAIDs when he had bouts of low back pain. Now, the pain is affecting his ability to walk to class. He also maintains a very active lifestyle, playing soccer at the collegiate level. He has been unable to play the last semester because of his back and leg pain. He has no ambitions to play professional soccer and just wants to be pain free and live a normal life. A full set of lumbar spine films are obtained, with the lateral x-ray shown in Figure 65-1.

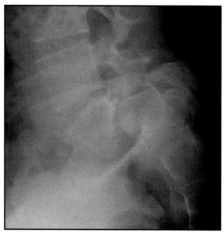

Figure 65-1. Lateral x-ray of the lumbar spine.

▶ *What is his diagnosis?*

▶ *What is the treatment algorithm for this patient now?*

Vignette 65: Answer

Spondylolisthesis, or the forward slippage of a cephalad vertebrae on the caudad vertebra, can be categorized by etiology (Table 65-1). Isthmic spondylolisthesis is caused by a defect in the pars interarticularis. This is typically a pediatric condition, but it is more commonly symptomatic in adults (presents as back pain, abnormal gait, and hamstring tightness). Furthermore, isthmic spondylolisthesis can be divided into low grade (less than 50% slip) and high grade (greater risk of progression).[215] In general, the grading is I (5% to 25%), II (25% to 50%), III (50% to 75%), IV (75% to 100%), and V (> 100%). It is very common in Eskimos and those who perform activities with an emphasis on repetitive hyperextension of the lower back (football lineman).

Table 65-1. CLASSIFICATION, TYPE, AND DEMOGRAPHICS ASSOCIATED WITH VARIOUS DEGREES OF SPONDYLOLISTHESIS		
Class	Type	Demographics
I	Dysplastic	Childhood
II (most common)	Isthmic	Ages 5 to 50 years, more common in younger age group, related to repetitive hyperextension
III	Degenerative	Older patients, more common in Blacks, diabetics, and women older than 40 years
IV	Traumatic	Young, acute fracture
V	Pathologic	Any age, related to tumor
VI	Postsurgical	Typically in adults

Pediatric and adolescent patients with asymptomatic low-grade slip only need observation. Patients with such grade I slips may return to normal activities, including contact sports, when they are asymptomatic. It may be advisable for the patients to avoid contact sports and sports that require lumbar hyperextension if they have a grade II slip. If symptomatic, conservative treatment is usually successful. Indications for surgery include slip progression, high-grade slip with significant lumbosacral kyphosis, neurological deficit (most cases in isthmic is the L5 nerve root), low back pain unresponsive to a prolonged course of nonoperative measures, and radicular pain.[216]

In low-grade slips, 1-level fusion usually suffices. In high-grade slips, 2-level fusion is usually the minimum, with complete reduction of the slip remaining unnecessary. Most surgeons attempt to attain partial reduction if lumbosacral kyphosis exists in a high-grade slip. Reduction increases the risk of nerve damage, particularly the L5 nerve root.[217] A reasonable goal is to improve the slip angle by 30 to 40 degrees and achieve a grade 2 slip on a lateral fluoroscopic view. Slip angle is defined as the angle formed by lines parallel to the inferior end plate of L5 and a line perpendicular with the posterior aspect of S1 (> 10 degrees is indicator for possible progression). If reduction takes place, a circumferential fusion is usually needed. If no lumbosacral deformity or sagittal imbalance is present with the high-grade slip, the literature does not support reduction as routine. Decompression is also indicated to relieve nerve root compression in many adult patients. In young adolescents, nerve root compression is usually due to dynamic instability rather than degenerative changes, so decompression is not as critical and fusion alone is often adequate.

In pediatric patients with low-grade slips, a direct pars repair may be an option instead of a fusion. The ideal patient is one who has a positive single-photon emission CT scan, has failed nonoperative treatment, has a normal intervertebral disk on MRI, has no radiculopathy and no or minimal spondylolisthesis, and has only axial back pain. However, long-term studies demonstrate that the theoretical benefits of direct repair cannot be proven.[218]

Why Might This Be Tested? Although spondylolisthesis is not very common (approximately 5% of the population), a lot has been published in the literature in regard to this condition. The severity of the slip determines the treatment and surgical techniques used in treating this condition.

Here's the Point!

Isthmic spondylolisthesis needs to be distinguished from degenerative spondylolisthesis, which results from arthritis of the functional spinal unit rather than from a defect in the pars. Degenerative spondylolisthesis most commonly occurs at L4-L5 and isthmic spondylolisthesis occurs at L5-S1. Both conditions tend to affect the L5 nerve roots (L4-L5 because of lateral recess stenosis and L5-S1 because of foraminal stenosis). Isthmic spondylolisthesis is a condition of the young but usually becomes symptomatic when the patients age.

Vignette 66: My Pitching Arm Takes Forever to Warm Up

A 24-year-old, right-hand-dominant baseball pitcher has had right shoulder pain during pitching for the past 6 months. He reports pain in the posterosuperior aspect of his shoulder, most notably during the late cocking phase, and often requires more time to loosen up than his other teammates. He denies any mechanical symptoms, such as locking or catching. A standard radiographic series reveals an exostosis off the posterior aspect of his glenoid, and an MRI shows increased signal along the undersurface of the supraspinatus tendon.

▶ *What is the patient's most likely diagnosis?*

▶ *What is the pathophysiology of this disease process?*

▶ *What other shoulder conditions are associated with this condition?*

▶ *What is a Bennett lesion? What specific radiographic view best evaluates for the presence of this lesion?*

The patient undergoes an extensive course of therapy, and nonoperative management ultimately fails. Arthroscopic surgery is indicated, and he is found to have a partial articular-sided rotator cuff tear of approximately 40% of the width of the tendon.

▶ *What is the appropriate treatment?*

Vignette 66: Answer

The underlying diagnosis is internal impingement, characterized by pathologic contact between the articular side of the posterior rotator cuff and the posterior margin of the glenoid, resulting in tearing or fraying of the undersurface of the rotator cuff or labrum. With shoulder abduction, external rotation, and extension, the greater tuberosity with its attached supraspinatus impinges on the posterosuperior aspect of the glenoid rim. While similar impingement occurs in asymptomatic, nonthrowing shoulders, repetitive activity in the shoulders of overhead athletes predisposes these athletes to pathologic changes, resulting in the clinical diagnosis of internal impingement. This diagnosis is different than subacromial (outlet) impingement, which describes pain associated with entrapment of the bursal-sided rotator cuff (supraspinatus) between the anteroinferior corner of the acromion (and coracoacromial ligament) and the greater tuberosity with humeral elevation or internal rotation.[158,170,219]

The specific etiology of internal impingement is controversial. The most accepted theory suggests that impingement results from a combination of anterior microinstability and excessive tightness of the posteroinferior capsule, driving the humeral head superiorly during overhead activities, such as throwing. This ultimately leads to impingement and related pathology, such as SLAP tears. Others suggest that impingement results primarily from posterosuperior instability, with an intricate association between partial rotator cuff tears and the posterior subtype of type II SLAP lesions. Finally, some argue that natural physiological adaptations to throwing, such as increased humeral external rotation, increased humeral and glenoid retroversion, and anterior laxity, may predispose the thrower to a continuum of pathology, including internal impingement.

Impingement results in a wide spectrum of pathology, including fraying, partial articular-sided tendon avulsions (PASTA), full-thickness tears of the articular-sided rotator cuff, hypertrophy and/or scarring of the posterior capsule at the margin of the glenoid, cartilage wear in the posterior glenoid or posterosuperior humeral head, biceps lesions, and anteroinferior (Bankart) or posterosuperior (SLAP) labral lesions. A Bennett lesion is a common finding in patients with internal impingement and is defined as an extra-articular posterior glenoid ossification associated with a posterior labral injury and a posterior undersurface rotator cuff injury (kissing lesion).

Patients are predominantly overhead athletes who report posterior shoulder pain while throwing or performing other repetitive overhead motions. Similar to SLAP lesions, pain is usually elicited during the late cocking or early acceleration phase of throwing with the arm in abduction and external rotation. Shoulder stiffness requiring a prolonged warm-up period is commonly found in throwing athletes. On physical examination, the patient will usually demonstrate an internal rotation deficit (GIRD), indicating excessive tightness of the posterior capsule. The patient will have the same total arc of motion but will sacrifice internal rotation for external rotation. Loss of more than 20 degrees of internal rotation with the shoulder abducted at 90 degrees indicates excessive tightness of the posterior band of the inferior glenohumeral ligament (IGHL). The examiner must stabilize the scapula to get a true measure of rotation. Specific exam findings, such as the Jobe relocation test (instability) and Hawkins and Neer's signs (subacromial, not internal, impingement), may be elicited on exam, but are neither sensitive nor specific.

Standard x-rays are usually normal, but a posterior capsule exostosis (Bennett lesion) may be present and is best appreciated on axillary (Figure 66-1) or West Point views. MRI is the most useful imaging modality, with a 95% sensitivity and specificity for detection of labral tears and rotator cuff disease. MRAs improve the diagnostic potential of this modality. MRI/MRA findings in internal impingement are subtle (Figure 66-2), usually with increased signal on the undersurface of the supraspinatus or infraspinatus tendon or cystic changes in the posterior aspect of the humeral head associated with posterosuperior labral pathology. The classic Bennett lesion may also be visible on MRI. Often, a distinct diagnosis is not obtained until the time of arthroscopy (Figure 66-3).

Most cases of internal impingement can be treated nonsurgically with NSAIDs, rest, and physical therapy (rotator cuff and serratus strengthening). Posterior capsular stretching (ie, sleeper stretch) regimens in overhead athletes may be therapeutic and protective against further injury. Injections are not recommended.

Surgical therapy is indicated for those who fail nonsurgical management and is largely dependent on the specific pathology and addressing comorbidities. For PASTA lesions that are less than 50% of the thickness of the tendon, debridement of the rotator cuff is recommended. For PASTA lesions involving more than 50% of the tendon thickness, a transtendon repair should be performed by repairing the tendon to the insertional footprint without taking down the intact tendon. If a Bennett lesion is suspected, debridement or excision is indicated. For associated GIRD or anterior microinstability, surgical treatment remains controversial. Some surgeons will perform a posterior capsular release, but others will perform anterior stabilization. During

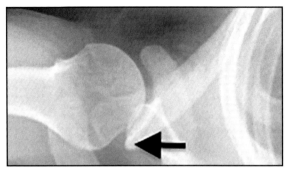

Figure 66-1. Axillary view of the beginning stages of a Bennett lesion.

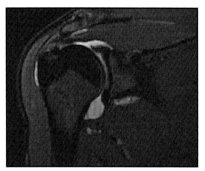

Figure 66-2. T2-weighted fat-suppressed MRA showing mildly enhanced signal intensity on the undersurface of the supraspinatus, suggestive of a partial-thickness cuff tear.

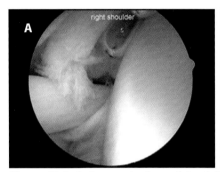
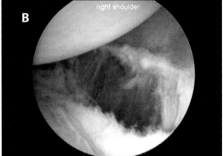

Figure 66-3. Arthroscopic views of the right shoulder showing (A) a partial undersurface rotator cuff tear and (B) the posterior rotator cuff following debridement and posterior capsular release secondary to posterior capsular contracture (GIRD).

posterior capsular release, the inferior suprascapular nerve (to infraspinatus) is at the greatest risk. For gross instability with a labral tear, labral repair and/or capsulorrhaphy are indicated. Typically, after rehabilitation, the patient can return to sports or labor 4 to 6 months after surgery.

Why Might This Be Tested? The concept of internal impingement has continued to evolve, and the frequency of diagnosis is increasing. Most commonly, questions will focus on the definition of internal impingement, possible etiology (GIRD/posteroinferior capsular tightness leading to superior migration of humeral head with subsequent rotator cuff tendinopathy and SLAP tears), classic radiographic findings (Bennett lesion), and treatment (usually nonoperative with posterior capsular stretching).

Here's the Point!

Internal impingement of the shoulder is one of several diagnoses to consider in the overhead throwing athlete. GIRD is common, and treatment is usually nonsurgical with posterior capsular stretching, but surgical repair should address all associated pathologic lesions and include labral repair and/or capsulorrhaphy if instability is present. Debridement of the rotator cuff is typically performed for PASTA lesions that are less than 50% of the thickness of the tendon, whereas substantial lesions (> 50%) require repair.

Vignette 67: This Mass Is Beginning to Be a Pain in the Butt

A 64-year-old male has a mass over his right buttock that has been slowly enlarging over the past year. The mass itself is not tender to palpation. He has a history of low back pain, which is being treated with physical therapy. He feels there has been partial relief with this treatment. A CT scan and histology slide are shown in Figures 67-1 and 67-2.

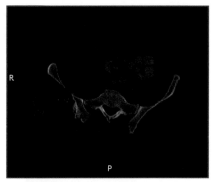

Figure 67-1. Axial CT scan of the pelvis showing the mass in the right buttock.

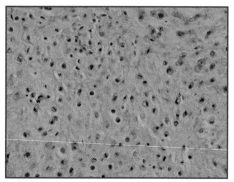

Figure 67-2. Histology of the tumor (400× magnification).

▶ *What is the diagnosis?*

▶ *What is the most appropriate treatment?*

Vignette 67: Answer

CHS is the second most common primary sarcoma of bone after osteosarcoma. It has a predilection for older adults, with the majority of cases in patients older than 50 years (in this case, the patient is older than 50 years and male [there is a slight male predilection] and has a pelvic mass→CHS has to pop into your head). The most common sites of involvement are the pelvis, proximal femur, proximal humerus, distal femur, and ribs. Around 90% of CHS arise in a previously normal bone, but benign cartilaginous lesions (osteochondroma, enchondroma) may also dedifferentiate into CHS.

Most patients present with pain, although this is not a universal finding. Clinical suspicion should be heightened when the pain is at rest or at night, not associated with activity, not related to previous trauma, and worsens over time. Three to 8 percent of patients present with a pathological fracture, and the presence of prodromal symptoms should be elicited. In this age group, metastatic disease to the bones is more common than a primary sarcoma. However, a diagnosis of sarcoma must be investigated and eliminated prior to skeletal fixation with a plate or IM device.

Radiographically, CHS usually appears as a partially radiolucent lesion in the pelvis and metaphysis or diaphysis of long bones. The characteristic finding is stippled ("popcorn") calcifications—mineralization that is punctate and very dense (bright white on x-ray or CT). When you see popcorn-like calcifications, you must think cartilaginous tumor and, in the right age range, CHS. The bone can show expansion or cortical thickening; cortical erosions and perforations are often visible as well. When a chondroid matrix is suggested radiographically, the differential includes CHS, enchondroma, chondroblastoma, and chondromyxoid fibroma.

The most common subtype is conventional CHS. Others include mesenchymal CHS, which shows a greater predilection for the spine and younger patients. Analogous to small cell osteosarcoma, histologically this looks like a mixture of CHS and Ewing's sarcoma. Clear cell CHS is an epiphyseal lesion that should be considered when diagnosing giant cell tumor (GCT) or chondroblastoma. The affected age range is younger than conventional CHS (25 to 50 years old). When an area of low-grade conventional CHS is adjacent to a high-grade spindle cell neoplasm, the tumor is called dedifferentiated CHS and carries an ominous prognosis (< 20% two-year survival).

Secondary CHS is suspected when a previously benign enchondroma or osteochondroma becomes symptomatic or increases in size. For osteochondromas, enlargement is concerning after skeletal maturity. An MRI or CT scan is used to look at the size of the cartilage cap. Although there is some debate on the exact size of the cartilage cap that indicates malignant transformation, a thickness greater than 2 cm is worrisome and should be excised. Enchondromatosis (Ollier's disease and Maffucci's syndrome) have an increased risk of malignant degeneration compared to solitary enchondromas, osteochondromas, or multiple exostoses.

Histologically, low-grade CHS (most often found as stage 1 or 2 disease) is relatively acellular with a bluish matrix, indicative of a chondroid background, with irregularly shaped lobules of cartilage. The lobules vary in size and are separated by fibrous bands. Mitoses are rare, and bilobed nuclei may be present. The grading of CHS is based on the cellularity of the tumor as well as nuclear pleomorphism. It is histologically challenging to differentiate an enchondroma from a grade 1 CHS, and the diagnosis must be made in the context of the patient's history and radiographic findings (such as a permeative lesion with cortical breach). The exception is the small bones of the hands and feet, in which benign enchondromas can appear radiographically and histologically aggressive. At higher grades, the nuclei become more atypical, the cellularity increases, and mitotic figures are visible.

CHS is primarily a surgical disease, and adjuvant treatments, such as radiation and chemotherapy, are fairly ineffective and reserved for recurrent or metastatic disease. The accepted treatment is wide resection with reconstruction when possible. Some (but not the question writers!) advocate for intralesional curettage of contained low-grade lesions, although this is controversial. Survival is excellent in low-grade tumors and is 90% and 65% for grade I and II tumors, respectively.

Why Might This Be Tested? There are several types of CHS, so review the subtle differences. The fact that x-rays and histology can easily be confused with other tumors and that CHS is associated with other syndromes (Ollier's and Maffucci's) make this subject a common one for question writers.

Here's the Point!

In general, a man in his mid-60s with a growing, painful pelvic mass must have CHS on the differential. Treatment is typically wide resection without chemotherapy or irradiation. Remember, popcorn calcification equals a cartilage tumor until proven otherwise.

Vignette 68: Shoulder Injury During a Scrum

A 19-year-old male collegiate rugby player presents to the emergency department after being tackled during a match. He states that his arm was "bent back" when he was midway through a throw and had immediate onset pain to his shoulder. He has never had pain in this shoulder before. On examination, his shoulders have a slight difference in the contour, with a more "squared off" look to the painful shoulder. He has significant pain with any attempt at ROM and holds his arm at his side. His distal neurovascular exam is symmetric to the contralateral limb. A complete series of plain x-rays is shown in Figure 68-1.

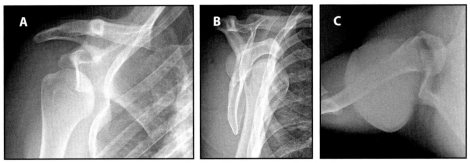

Figure 68-1. (A) AP, (B) scapular Y, and (C) axillary x-rays of the shoulder.

▶ *What is the most likely diagnosis?*

▶ *What, if any, immediate treatment should the patient receive?*

▶ *After initial management in the emergency room, what further evaluation and treatments, if any, are necessary?*

▶ *Under what circumstances would operative treatment be considered?*

Vignette 68: Answer

The history and imaging are consistent with an anteroinferior glenohumeral dislocation. The shoulder is the most frequently dislocated joint in the body,[220] and 95% of these dislocations are anterior.[221] Usually, these injuries occur after a traumatic incident in young males when the arm is abducted and externally rotated (throwing or tackling position). The main restraints to anterior dislocation are the anterior labrum, the anterior band of the inferior glenohumeral ligament, and the osseous glenoid rim.[222] These structures are damaged in 97% of cases and are often described in the classic Bankart lesion.[223] Often, the humeral head recoils and collides at its posterosuperior aspect against the anterior glenoid, leading to a characteristic impaction fracture called the Hill-Sachs lesion.[223] Recurrence is common, occurring in 57% of cases.[224]

Initial diagnosis can be made on physical examination and radiographic imaging. Physical examination will commonly demonstrate a loss of the normal shoulder contour, occasionally with the humeral head palpable anteriorly. ROM will typically be severely limited, and patients will often use their contralateral limb to support the dislocated arm. Initial evaluation should include a complete neurovascular assessment, including axillary nerve function, by assessing motor function in the deltoid muscle and sensation over the lateral deltoid in Sergeant's patch. In the office setting, the patient with concern for recurrent anterior subluxation can be tested for apprehension with the arm in the abducted and external rotation position with an anterior force upon the proximal humerus (patient will guard and not be happy). In the relocation sign, this apprehension will resolve with a posterior force.

Initial x-rays commonly show loss of congruency between the humeral head and the glenoid fossa, with the humeral head lying anterior and inferior to the glenoid fossa. The best view to confirm concentric reduction of the joint is the axillary view, which can also show the anterior glenoid to evaluate for fracture or bone loss. These x-rays should also be inspected for fracture, osseous Bankart lesions (Figure 68-2), Hill-Sachs lesions (Figure 68-3), and other abnormalities of the glenoid and proximal humerus. CT and MRI can provide a more detailed view of the osseous pathology and soft tissues, respectively, but should not delay a reduction attempt.

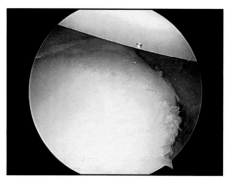

Figure 68-2. Intraoperative image of a Bankart lesion.

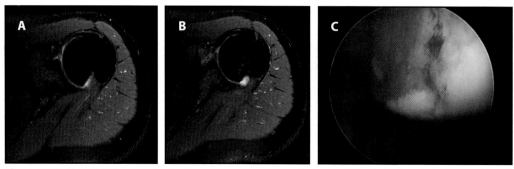

Figure 68-3. (A, B) MRI views and (C) arthroscopic appearance of a large Hill-Sachs lesion of the humeral head.

Initial treatment should focus on reduction of the joint. The least painful and most effective maneuver for reduction is the Fast, Reliable, Safe technique.[225] In this technique, the patient lies supine with the arm adducted and with no sedation or analgesia. While applying gentle traction and making vertical short-arc oscillating movements a rate of 2 to 3 Hz, the arm is slowly abducted. Once 90 degrees of abduction is reached, external rotation is added until reduction is achieved. The Hippocratic method is performed with simultaneous downward traction on a slightly abducted arm and countertraction via a circumferential sheet at the level of the axilla by an assistant. Reduction is commonly associated with a palpable "clunk" but should be radiographically confirmed with an axillary view. Ideally, some muscle relaxation/sedation should be maintained to make the reduction attempt easier and less painful for the patient.

After reduction, the patient should be treated with a brief period of immobilization followed by physical therapy. Therapy is directed to focus on strengthening of the rotator cuff and periscapular musculature. Surgical stabilization should be reserved for patients who suffer a recurrence.[226] Operative interventions are tailored based on intraoperative findings.

Why Might This Be Tested? Anterior shoulder instability is a common problem in young patients and often requires surgical management. In cases of subtle subluxation, instability can also be easily missed, which makes this an important diagnosis to keep in mind.

Here's the Point!

In the patient with a traumatic injury to the shoulder, always evaluate for concentric reduction of the joint with an axillary view. Acute dislocation should be reduced immediately and treated with immobilization followed by therapy. Patients with recurrent instability often require open vs arthroscopic capsulolabral stabilization.

Vignette 69: Congenital Limb-Length Discrepancy

A 4-year-old female presents with a limb-length inequality (right shorter than left). When she was born, the limb-length inequality was initially identified. Her right leg is now significantly shorter than the left side, with the shorter leg lying just below her contralateral knee. Her thigh appears short and bulky. The family has growing concerns and is in to discuss management of her congenital leg-length discrepancy. A leg-length view plain x-ray is shown in Figure 69-1.

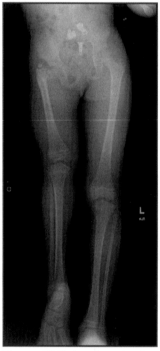

Figure 69-1. Leg-length view plain x-ray.

▶ *What is the diagnosis?*

▶ *Is the limb-length inequality stagnant (always remaining the same difference) or progressive?*

▶ *When lengthening the femur, what needs to be considered with the knee?*

▶ *When lengthening the femur, what needs to be considered with the hip?*

Vignette 69: Answer

The patient has proximal femoral focal deficiency (PFFD), which is a congenital defect leading to abnormal growth of the proximal femur during embryological growth.[227] The disorder can include proximal femoral dysplasia (coxa vara), limb-length inequality, an ACL-deficient knee (as well as other ligamentous deficiencies), lateral femoral condyle deficiency, ulna hypoplasia, fibula hemimelia (50%), clubfoot, unusual fascies, and Pierre Robin syndrome (micrognathia and glossoptosis). PFFD is a rare disorder found in less than 0.2/10,000 births and is noted to involve both extremities in 10% to 15% of cases.[228] The hip is usually flexed, abducted, and externally rotated, and the thigh is short and bulky. The limb-length inequality is different than limb-length inequalities from a femur fracture in that it is not a stagnant discrepancy but is progressive. As the children grow, the difference increases proportionally, which is what prompted the family to bring the child in with our case.

Treatment is based on the quantitative leg-length discrepancy, associated anomalies, and muscle strength/function. The Aiken classification is used to describe the disorder, with types A and B maintaining a femoral head and C and D not having a femoral head. Reconstructive options are possible when a femoral head remains. Typical surgical options include Brown's procedure (femoral-pelvic arthrodesis), limb lengthening (using a fixator), Van Ness' rotationalplasty, and amputation.

Other causes of a leg-length discrepancy that must be considered include hemihypertrophy, dysplasias, DDH, polio, infection, tumors, and trauma. In general, projected limb-length discrepancies less than 2 cm are observed; 2 to 5 cm are treated with contralateral epiphysiodesis or shortening or limb lengthening; and greater than 5 cm are treated with limb lengthening. The following assumptions are important to calculate the limb-length discrepancy anticipated at maturity:

- Males mature at the following rates up to 16 years old and females up to 14 years old:

    o   Distal femur: 3/8 inch/year (9 mm)
    o   Proximal tibia: 1/4 inch/year (6 mm)
    o   Proximal femur: 1/8 inch/year (3 mm)

When lengthening the femur following Ilizarov principles, the fixator needs to span the knee. Because knees in patients with PFFD are ACL deficient, if the knee is not spanned then as the femur is lengthened, tibial subluxation may occur. In addition, because of the presence of hip dysplasia, the hip can also subluxate or dislocate with lengthening, so this needs to be observed closely.

Why Might This Be Tested? Proximal femoral focal deficiency is easy to identify on x-rays, especially in the more severe form. However, milder forms can be subtler and present as a congenitally short femur. It is important to be aware what other anomalies are associated with PFFD when it comes time to pick a treatment option. Also, it is important to be aware that the limb-length discrepancy is progressive in order to give the parents a better understanding of what to expect. For example, if the difference is 50%, as the child gets older and the legs grow, the difference becomes even larger!

Here's the Point!

PFFD is a progressive limb-length discrepancy disorder. Look for associated conditions, such as ligamentous deficiencies of the knee, fibular hemimelia, and foot disorders, as these affect treatment options. Beware hip and knee subluxation as the femur is lengthened. Remember, 9:6:3 = growth at distal femur:proximal tibia:proximal femur in mm.

Vignette 70: Case of the Disappearing Femoral Condyle

A 40-year-old female presents with a 2-year history of left knee pain, predominantly on the medial side of her knee. She has a history of renal and hepatic failure with transplantation of both solid organs. She has a long history of using immunosuppressant agents and oral corticosteroids. The patient had a limited course of NSAIDs due to her renal disease and a corticosteroid injection, which provided minimal relief. Her plain x-ray and representative cuts of her CT scan are shown in Figure 70-1.

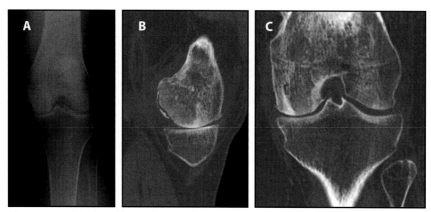

Figure 70-1. (A) Flexed knee x-ray and (B, C) representative CT cuts of the left knee.

▶ *What is her diagnosis?*

▶ *What is the proposed pathogenesis of this disease process?*

▶ *What are appropriate treatment options?*

Vignette 70: Answer

The patient's diagnosis is secondary ON of the left distal femur due to chronic use of corticosteroids and solid organ transplant. Osteonecrosis of the knee is less commonly seen than in the hip but is a debilitating disease process nevertheless. It is composed of 3 distinct conditions: spontaneous ON of the knee (SPONK), secondary ON, and postarthroscopic ON of the knee (Table 70-1).[229]

In this patient, the etiology is hypothesized to be related to a relative intraosseous hypertension secondary to an increase in adipocyte size and deposition within the bone. Subsequent vascular collapse and ischemia occurs, leading to ON. A modified version of the Ficat and Arlet classification for ON of the femoral head can be used to stage these lesions.

- Stage 1: Normal joint space, patchy lucencies noted on x-rays
- Stage 2: Normal joint space, wedge-shaped areas of sclerosis mixed with stage 1 lucencies
- Stage 3: Subchondral collapse, irregular joint space, significant sclerosis, and lucencies on plain x-rays
- Stage 4: Advanced DJD in joint, significant collapse, and extensive condylar destruction

Similar to the hip scenario, the stages are basically broken down into precollapse (1 and 2) and postcollapse (3 and 4). Joint-sparing techniques[230] are more appropriate for precollapse lesions and arthroscopy with grafting techniques, HTO, and arthroplasty (uni- and tricompartmental) reserved for postcollapse cases. Due to the large area of ON and the patient's medical history, she underwent a TKA.

Why Might This Be Tested? Osteonecrosis is a commonly tested subject on standardized tests, typically focusing on how to treat these lesions. However, knowing the potential etiologies of ON may make the diagnosis more apparent to you. Spontaneous ON of the knee and postarthroscopy ON are becoming more popular diagnoses and will likely show up on these tests for the next several years.

Here's the Point!

Recognize ON of the knee and determine the stage of the disease; this will direct your treatment. Precollapse=nonoperative treatment and joint-sparing techniques. Postcollapse=joint reconstruction techniques (typically uni- or tricompartmental arthroplasty).

Table 70-1.

GENERAL CHARACTERISTICS OF THE FORMS OF OSTEONECROSIS OF THE KNEE

	SPONK	*Secondary ON*	*Postarthroscopic ON*
Demographics	>55 years old, female:male=3:1	<45 years old, more common in females with autoimmune disorders and males with alcohol use	No age or demographic bias after a knee arthroscopy (thermal or RF use increases risk)
Findings	Sudden onset of pain worse at night and with WB, rarely bilateral, typically one lesion	Gradual onset of pain, often history of increased risk factors, >80% bilateral, multiple lesions	Sudden onset of pain, never bilateral, one lesion, often mistaken for a failed arthroscopy
Areas affected	One condyle (most often femur vs tibia), no other bones involved	Multiple condyles (most often femur vs tibia); hip, shoulder, ankles often involved	One condyle (almost exclusively in the femur), no other bones involved
Etiology	Unknown, thought to be subchondral fractures with subsequent increased intraosseous pressures	Typically related to corticosteroids, alcohol, SLE, sickle cell, thrombophilia, etc	Related to subchondral fractures (similar to SPONK), often occurs within 6 mo of scope
Diagnostic exams	Plain x-rays, often in medial femoral condyle; MRI is very sensitive test, will see high signal on T2-weighted and low signal on T1-weighted	Plain x-rays, often more diffuse lesions; consider x-rays of contralateral side MRI is a very sensitive test (100%)	Plain x-rays, look for patchy areas of sclerosis and lucency as well as collapse; MRI is obtained for early diagnosis
Treatment: Noncollapse	Protected WB and NSAIDs; successful in up to 89% of early lesions (small>medium>large lesions), with recovery expected to take 3 mo	Protected WB and NSAIDs; successful in ~20% of cases, bisphosphonates and various medicines now being tried, most lesions progress	Protected WB and NSAIDs; successful in early-stage lesions, core decompression and HTO remain viable options in early stages
Treatment: Post-collapse	Arthroscopy: can debride or use OATS to treat lesions <20 to 30 mm Core decompression: extra-articular procedure, successful in early lesions UKA: successful with small, unicondylar lesions TKA: successful with modern-day implants	Core decompression: improved outcomes with percutaneous drilling Bone grafting: small series report good results with osteochondral grafts UKA: contraindicated due to multicondylar disease TKA: improved results with augmented fixation	UKA: remains a good procedure for small unicondylar disease TKA: good results with more extensive ON or preexisting DJD

DJD=degenerative disk disease; HTO=high tibial osteotomy; MRI=magnetic resonance imaging; NSAIDs=nonsteroidal anti-inflammatory drugs; OATS=osteochondral autograft transplantation; ON=osteonecrosis; RF=radiofrequency; SLE=systemic lupus erythematosus; SPONK=spontaneous osteonecrosis of the knee; TKA=total knee arthroplasty; UKA=unicompartmental knee arthroplasty; WB=weight bearing.

Vignette 71: Flag Football Gone Awry!

A 20-year-old male is playing flag football when he sustains a fall on top of his nondominant left arm, with immediate pain and deformity of the elbow. He is evaluated in the emergency department, where he has an intact neurovascular exam, and symptoms are isolated to the elbow, including deformity and pain with any attempted ROM. His x-rays show a posterolateral elbow dislocation. No fracture is seen. Under conscious sedation, a closed reduction is successfully performed with correction of coronal translation, followed by traction coupled with direct distally directed pressure on the olecranon.

▶ *How should the reduced elbow be tested for stability?*

▶ *What findings in this patient would lead you to recommend surgery?*

▶ *If a fracture was present in the setting of this dislocation, how may it change your recommendation?*

▶ *If this elbow dislocation is amenable to nonoperative treatment, how would you immobilize and rehabilitate it, and what results could be expected?*

Vignette 71: Answer

Elbow dislocation is one of the most common elbow injuries and is second only to the shoulder in frequency of dislocation in the upper extremity. It is an injury primarily seen in patients in their 20s and 30s and usually results from a fall on an extended and abducted arm. This patient's posterolateral direction of the forearm in relation to the humerus is the most common, with posterior directed dislocations comprising 90% of all dislocations.[231] The most common mechanism of injury has been shown to be a combination of a direct posterior force coupled with forearm supination. This allows the radial head to spin posteriorly as it clears the capitellum and translates posteriorly out of the socket.

In addition to inspecting static postreduction x-rays for an uneven joint space, which may represent an intra-articular osteochondral fragment, the elbow should be taken through a ROM under lateral fluoroscopic imaging, and an attempt should be made to reach maximal allowable extension. The simple elbow dislocation will usually be stable throughout the arc. If the elbow demonstrates widening of the ulnohumeral joint or posterior translation of the radial head with respect to the capitellum, it should be documented how much flexion is required to keep the elbow reduced. If greater than 50 to 60 degrees of flexion is required, this increased instability probably represents not only collateral ligament insufficiency but also a partial or complete rupture of the flexor pronator and common extensor masses. Surgical treatment with LCL repair or reconstruction is indicated. The medial side typically does not require surgical attention unless instability remains after repair of the lateral side, which is uncommon.[232]

Redislocation after a stable simple (no fracture associated with dislocation) elbow dislocation is rare, occurring in only 1% to 2% of cases. This low recurrence rate is due largely to the high articular congruity and bony support, especially anteriorly from the coronoid process and radial head that prevent posterior displacement of the forearm. For that reason, clinically significant fractures to the anterior structures of the elbow render the reduced elbow unstable and require surgical attention. These include partial articular radial head fractures greater than 30% to 40% of its width, which are sufficient to affect lateral support, as well as any comminuted complete radial head fracture. Partial articular fractures and noncomminuted complete fracture patterns are amenable to ORIF, but complex and comminuted patterns require radial head arthroplasty to restore stability and allow early ROM. Radial head excision is not a viable option in the setting of elbow instability. Coronoid fractures are uncommon with elbow dislocation. When present, the most common is a tip fracture that represents a shearing of the trochlea rather than an avulsion. Larger coronoid fragments (>50%) and anteromedial facet fragments contribute to stability and should be considered for ORIF.[231,232]

If our patient demonstrates a stable elbow on postreduction imaging, he should be immobilized full-time for a 7- to 10-day period to rest the elbow and then start early ROM with the arm adducted. Supination and pronation should be performed with the elbow flexed 90 degrees, with simultaneous elbow extension and supination avoided in the first 6 weeks. Strengthening and static progressive splinting can be added at 6 to 8 weeks. While patients commonly end up with small (< 10 degree) flexion contractures after simple elbow dislocations, this is usually of no functional consequence. Patients should be warned of the risk, albeit low, of recurrent instability and motion-limiting HO. Although evidence of chondral injury is seen arthroscopically in nearly all simple elbow dislocations, there seems to be no risk of clinically significant early onset OA. Transient nerve palsy of the median or ulnar nerves may occur in up to 20% of cases.

Why Might This Be Tested? Elbow dislocation is common, and the well-known factors of postreduction instability in extension and clinically significant fractures change management from nonoperative to operative.

Here's the Point!

Simple elbow dislocation is usually stable after reduction and should be treated with early mobilization to prevent stiffness after a brief period of rest. Operative treatment is indicated in the setting of clinically significant fracture and instability in extension to achieve an elbow that is stable for early ROM and prevent recurrent instability.

Vignette 72: Basketball Player With High Arches

A 37-year-old male presents to the office with an inversion injury ("Doc, I twisted my ankle!") to his foot while playing basketball. He gives a history of multiple ankle sprains as he was growing up, particularly in the past decade. He has previously been treated for bilateral stress fractures of the fourth and fifth metatarsal shafts and states that he has "always had a high-arched foot." When questioned, the patient also states, "I frequently get calluses underneath my big toe."

▶ *What is the patient's most likely underlying diagnosis?*

▶ *What deformities and foot conditions are typically seen with this condition?*

Vignette 72: Answer

Pes cavus describes a foot with a high arch that fails to flatten out upon weight bearing. It describes a spectrum of deformities, from mild to severe, brought on by an elevated longitudinal arch. This condition can run the gamut from mild cavus, with only flexible clawing of the toes being the predominant issue, to severe cavovarus, in which ankle instability, rigid deformity, callus formation, and recurrent stress fractures dominate the clinical picture.

The common thread in all cavus feet is an imbalance of the musculature leading to weakness and stiffness of the ankle and foot. Although the etiology of this foot disorder is idiopathic, most have some subtle, underlying neurogenic cause. Charcot-Marie-Tooth (CMT) disease is by far the most common of these neurological diagnoses, and a thorough neurological exam (and punt to your local neurologist for a consultation) is part of the initial workup of a high-arched foot. Now, a little bit more on CMT: this range of conditions refers to a series of 7 hereditary motor sensory neuropathies (HMSN-I through VII). Remember the following: CMT-1 is the most common form, accounting for more than 50% of cases, and it is transmitted by autosomal-dominant penetrance. Other less common causes of cavovarus include poliomyelitis, syringomyelia, spinal cord tumors, cerebral palsy, arthrogryposis, and residual deformities associated with clubfeet or compartment syndrome.

The key to understanding the deformity in CMT is in recognizing 3 components of the muscle imbalance present:

1. Weakness of the tibialis anterior allows for unopposed pull of the peroneus longus, creating marked plantarflexion of the first ray.
2. Loss of the peroneus brevis muscle strength allows the posterior tibialis to markedly adduct the forefoot and pull the heel into varus. Progression of the deformity occurs as the intrinsic muscles and plantar fascia contract.
3. As the intrinsics weaken, clawing of the toes occurs as overpowering of the extensors prevents the MTP joints from maintaining a neutral position.

Long-standing cavovarus frequently leads to lateral foot and ankle pathology. Laxity of the lateral ankle ligaments is frequently seen in athletes as a consequence of varus positioning of the heel. Furthermore, peroneal tendon pathology (tenosynovitis, tear, subluxation) is extremely common in this situation. Preferential weight bearing on the lateral column of the foot often leads to recurrent stress injuries to the fourth and fifth metatarsal bones (sounds familiar!).

On physical examination of the cavovarus foot, the aforementioned ankle and foot deformities are assessed. As the disease progresses, the deformity becomes more rigid. With the patient standing, the Coleman block test is performed, which helps to determine how supple the deformity is and is therefore critical to guiding treatment. While observing the patient from behind, the lateral side of the foot is placed on a block (0.5 to 1 inch in size), while allowing the medial column to fall off the side and contact the ground. In a flexible deformity, the heel varus will correct to neutral or to a valgus position. In a rigid foot, the heel will remain in varus. Did we mention that the Coleman block test is a critical guide to the treatment algorithm? A flexible deformity can be addressed through nonoperative measures or by means of surgical reconstruction, whereas a fixed deformity is typically corrected with fusion.

Depending on the degree of deformity and amount of muscle weakness exhibited, nonoperative treatment can often be entertained. This typically involves stretching of the plantar fascia to help maintain suppleness of the foot, custom orthotics with lateral posting of the heel, and/or a molded AFO device (in the case of significant motor weakness).

With significant deformity, failure of nonoperative treatment, and in the setting of recurrent lateral foot and ankle pathology (ankle instability, peroneal tears, fifth metatarsal fractures), surgery is indicated. The goal of surgery is to provide a stable, plantigrade foot in a way that preserves the motion of the joints. In a flexible foot, this is accomplished through a series of soft tissue and bony procedures that are addressed through a laundry-list type of approach. Typically, a combination of these is used to address forefoot overload, varus of the heel, ankle equinus, and clawing of the toes. As a general rule, the more flexible the deformity, the less need to use bony procedures.

First, the soft tissue procedures:

- Plantar fascia release (Steindler stripping): The contracted plantar fascia becomes secondarily tight and contributes to the cavus deformity. Release of the fascia helps to reduce the height of the longitudinal arch and retain some element of flexibility.

- Achilles tendon lengthening: Relative overpull of the gastrocnemius-soleus complex typically leads to an equinus contracture.
- Extensor hallus longus tendon transfer to first metatarsal neck (Jones' procedure): Extensor hallus longus tendon overpull leads to clawing of the hallux with subluxation of the MTP joint and callus formation over the interphalangeal (IP) joint. Moving the insertion of the extensor hallus longus tendon to the neck of the first metatarsal alongside a fusion of the IP joint relieves the cockup deformity of the hallux.
- Peroneus longus to peroneus brevis tendon transfer: This procedure acts to weaken the plantar pull of the longus on the first ray while simultaneously augmenting the strength of the failing brevis. This short procedure often has a profound effect on a supple cavus deformity.
- Claw-toe correction: In a fixed clawing of the MTP joints, extensor tendon tenotomies and joint capsulotomies are done, with flexor to extensor tendon transfers performed to maintain a neutral position.
- Lateral ankle ligament reconstruction (Broström-Gould): Repair of the anterior talofibular ligament and calcaneofibular ligaments with incorporation of the extensor retinaculum is advisable in cases of chronic ankle instability.

Now for the bony procedures:

- Dorsiflexion osteotomy of the first metatarsal: In advanced cases of cavovarus, the plantarflexion deformity of the first ray is rigid. In such instances, a closing-wedge dorsal osteotomy of the first metatarsal is performed to elevate the first ray.
- Dwyer calcaneal osteotomy: When fusion can be avoided, a lateral closing-wedge osteotomy of the heel is very effective in correcting the heel varus seen in CMT.
- Midfoot osteotomies: A variety of procedures are available to address fixed forefoot equinus. Closing-wedge osteotomies (Cole, Japas, Jahss) have been described through the metatarsals and cuneiforms to elevate the forefoot.
- Triple arthrodesis: Most surgeons reserve this for severe, rigid cavovarus.

Why Might This Be Tested? Pes cavus is often a subtle, but recognizable, cause of lateral ankle and foot pathology. The etiology of the cavovarus foot is often attributable to CMT disease, and a neurological evaluation is a standard component of the diagnostic algorithm.

Here's the Point!

In a high-arched foot with varus of the heel and callus formation under the first metatarsal head, think CMT and neurology consult! When diagnosed early on, cavovarus can usually be adequately addressed through nonoperative or reconstructive means to preserve flexibility within the foot. Failure to recognize and intervene at an early point in the pathologic development of cavovarus often leads to a rigid deformity, and a triple arthrodesis may then be in the patient's future.

Vignette 73: Neuropathic Arthropathy

A 62-year-old male with mild hypertension who has not seen his primary care physician in 7 years presents with a 6-month history of increasing left knee pain. He has a history of mild to moderate OA of the left knee, which is being treated conservatively. Corticosteroids, bracing, and injections have not provided significant relief of his symptoms. On physical examination, his ROM is 0 to 130 degrees, with significant crepitus. The left knee is unstable to varus/valgus stress testing without defined endpoints, and there is a gross deformity of the knee that is new in the past 6 weeks. The patient has a moderate effusion and calor to the knee in the absence of erythema. There is some subjective numbness to his left foot and ankle, with normal motor function throughout. The patient has been running a low-grade fever of 99.8°F. Initial and follow-up x-rays are shown in Figure 73-1.

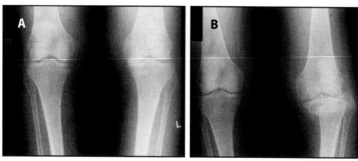

Figure 73-1. (A) AP x-ray of the left knee. (B) AP x-ray of the left knee 6 months later, just prior to surgery.

▶ *What is the underlying etiology of the degenerative changes in the pictured x-rays?*

▶ *What is the differential diagnosis?*

▶ *List appropriate treatment options.*

Vignette 73: Answer

There are several key phrases to decipher from the history and physical exam described in this vignette, including calor, rapid development of structural deformity, vague lower extremity dysesthesias, knee instability, and good ROM. The question writers will often try to trick you into reading this as a septic joint by throwing in distractors, like low-grade fever, mild erythema, and painful ROM. The key is to look at the details closely; this is a rapidly destructive process that has far worse radiographic findings than clinical examination leads you to believe, and it presents similar to septic arthritis but with less pain and a near-full ROM. At this point, you should be settling in on the diagnosis of some form of neuropathic arthritis. In this case, this was his first presentation of Charcot arthropathy.

The differential diagnosis in this case would include DJD, septic arthritis, neuropathic arthritis, crystalline arthropathy, fracture, internal derangement, and tumor.[233] With the correlation of x-rays that are well advanced of the noted clinical examination, the diagnosis is Charcot arthropathy, which holds its own differential diagnosis for determining its pathogenesis as well. The most commonly associated disorders include diabetes mellitus (most common), tabes dorsalis (related to syphilis infection), syringomyelia, and a variety of other peripheral nerve disorders. The common pathway for these conditions that leads to a Charcot joint is centered around the development of a neuropathic situation in which the patient has a relative insensitivity to pain and loss of proprioception. The loss of neuromuscular reflexes in the knee leads to injury from repetitive stresses with progression to cartilage damage, bone fragmentation, and joint subluxation. Clinically, this translates into a rapid destruction (can be as little as weeks to a couple of months) of the affected joint with gross deformity, swelling, and calor in the setting of a near-normal ROM and much less pain than one would anticipate. Charcot arthropathy most commonly affects the foot and ankle, has an onset usually between 40 and 59 years old, and affects men more commonly than women. Despite the relatively common diagnosis of diabetes mellitus in the United States, there is only approximately a 0.5% prevalence of Charcot arthropathy in this population.[234,235]

The knee is not commonly affected by Charcot arthropathy, and few data exist in the literature to support an evidenced-based review of treatment options. The most important aspect is making the correct diagnosis and making sure one is prepared for the rapid progression of this process and severe destruction that might be encountered at the time of surgery. Traditionally, arthrodesis (optimal position: slight valgus, 10 degrees of external rotation, 0 to 20 degrees of flexion depending on degree of bone loss) was the treatment of choice; however, with modern-day implants, an enhanced awareness of bone loss and improved options for constraint, TKA is now a viable option to consider. Typically, supplemental fixation of implants will be required to maintain stability, including stemmed tibial and femoral implants, augments, metaphyseal sleeves/cones, and possibly structural bone graft. Good outcomes can now be anticipated if the standard principles of restoring the joint line and mechanical axis using the least possible constraint with well-supported implants are followed.[233]

Why Might This Be Tested? Charcot arthropathy is a great imitator and can be difficult to diagnosis and manage. It is a good topic for questioning due to the difficulty in making the diagnosis and ultimately how much the disease affects the outcomes of the various treatment options.

Here's the Point!

Do not confuse charcot arthropathy for an infected joint. Remember that joint destruction is typically out of proportion to the level of pain (patients often do not complain of pain). Look for associated comorbidities, including diabetes mellitus, tabes dorsalis, syringomyelia, and peripheral nerve disorders. Err on the side of greater constraint when replacing a knee for Charcot joint destruction.

Vignette 74: Weekend Warrior With a Basketball Injury

A 32-year-old healthy male presents to the clinic complaining of knee pain after sustaining a twisting injury 3 months prior. He reports being a former collegiate lacrosse player and being able to run more than 5 miles per day without limitations prior to this injury. He states that 3 months ago, he twisted his right knee while playing recreational basketball, felt a pop, and had immediate pain and swelling. He was able to bear weight, but the swelling and pain have persisted. In addition, he reports night pain and a sensation of clicking/catching along the medial aspect of his right knee. He denies current fevers, chills, or weight loss. He also denies previous episodes of similar pain or trauma. He has been managing his pain with NSAIDs and ice packs but has been unable to return to impact- or pivoting-based activities. Physical examination is notable for a mild effusion and medial joint line tenderness to palpation. He is ligamentously stable with firm endpoints to varus and valgus stress testing, as well as to anterior drawer, posterior drawer, and Lachman's testing. He has normal patellofemoral motion. X-rays are unremarkable, and a subsequent MRI study is performed.

▶ *What is the presumed diagnosis?*

▶ *What tests are required to confirm the diagnosis?*

▶ *What are the treatment options?*

Vignette 74: Answer

The presumed diagnosis in this case is either an articular cartilage (hyaline cartilage) defect or meniscus (fibrocartilage) lesion. The clues in this vignette are the isolated traumatic injury, continued effusion, night pain, isolated medial compartment pain, and sensation of clicking/catching. These key words indicate a unilateral, intra-articular source of knee pain. A distractor placed to confuse the reader is the history of a pop, which may lead toward the diagnosis of an ACL injury or patella dislocation. The stable ligamentous and patellofemoral physical examination findings should help guide toward the correct diagnosis. In order to understand the diagnosis and treatment of cartilage/meniscus pathology, it is critical to understand the basic science of cartilage, including its structure and function.

There are several forms of cartilage, including hyaline or articular cartilage, fibrocartilage (meniscus, intervertebral disk, pubic symphysis), and elastic cartilage (trachea).

Articular cartilage essentially comprises 2 components, including extracellular matrix and cells (chondrocytes).[236-238] The extracellular matrix is composed of water, collagen, PGs, and noncollagenous proteins. Water makes up approximately 65% to 80% of the total mass of cartilage. The water content normally decreases with aging and increases in certain pathologic conditions, such as OA. Increases in the water content of articular cartilage lead to decreased strength and increased permeability, which may possibly lead to more wear and tear with aging. Collagen makes up approximately 10% to 20% of the total mass of cartilage. Type II collagen accounts for 90% to 95% of the collagen in articular cartilage and functions to provide a framework and tensile strength. Other less common types of collagen found in articular cartilage are highlighted in Table 74-1. Finally, PGs comprise approximately 10% to 15% of total articular cartilage mass. These function to provide compressive strength and also to attract water molecules. Proteoglycans are produced by chondrocytes and are composed of GAG subunits, including chondroitin sulfate and keratin sulfate. The cells of articular cartilage—chondrocytes—produce collagen, PGs, and various enzymes. Chondrocyte metabolism is known to respond to mechanical and chemical stimuli; however, only immature articular cartilage has these capabilities because mature articular cartilage does not have stem cells.

Table 74-1.

TYPES OF COLLAGEN IN ARTICULAR CARTILAGE

| Type II: 90% to 95% total collagen composition |
| Type V: small amounts |
| Type VI: small amounts, anchors chondrocyte to matrix |
| Type IX: small amounts |
| Type X: often found in hypertrophic cartilage and matrix mineralization areas |
| Type XI: small amounts acting as an adhesive |

There are 4 layers of articular cartilage, including 3 zones and the tidemark. The zones are based on their location (superficial to deep) and, more importantly, on the shape of the chondrocytes and the orientation of the type II collagen. The superficial zone, also referred to as the tangential zone, contains flattened chondrocytes, type II collagen oriented parallel to the joint, and rare PGs. It is in this zone where articular cartilage progenitor cells have been identified. The intermediate zone is the thickest layer and contains round chondrocytes, type II collagen in an oblique or random orientation, and substantial PGs. The deep zone, or basal layer, contains round chondrocytes arranged in columns and type II collagen that is orientated perpendicular to the joint. Finally, the tidemark, found only in joints, is beneath the deep layer and separates the true articular cartilage from deeper calcified cartilage. This layer also represents division between nutritional sources for the chondrocytes. Type II collagen from the deep layer crosses the tidemark.

Articular cartilage functions to decrease friction and distribute load within the joint. With its high water content and its structural organization of PGs and collagen molecules, articular cartilage exhibits stress-shielding of the solid matrix components. As cartilage ages, several changes in its composition occur. Notably, there is an increase in chondrocyte size, protein content, and overall stiffness. Furthermore, there is an increase in the ratio of keratin sulfate to chondroitin sulfate with regard to the PGs. However, as articular cartilage ages, there is a decrease in the absolute number of chondrocytes, water content, PG size, elasticity, and overall solubility.

Articular cartilage injuries, including full-thickness injuries, such as the one described in this vignette, are difficult to treat. This is because of the relatively avascular nature of articular cartilage. Superficial articular cartilage injuries that do not extend to the tidemark rely on chondrocyte proliferation, but no true healing occurs. Deeper articular cartilage lacerations that extend through the tidemark lead to fibrocartilaginous healing. This only occurs when the injury penetrates the subchondral bone and undifferentiated MSCs initiate a healing response. For reasons that are still not well understood, type I collagen is produced, resulting in fibrocartilage as opposed to hyaline cartilage. Unfortunately, this healed cartilage is less impressive with reported wear characteristics.

The menisci are composed of fibrocartilage, which differs from hyaline cartilage in both its composition and function.[239,240] Fibrocartilage is composed of collagen, PG, glycoproteins, cells, and water. Similar to articular cartilage, water accounts for most of the mass of fibrocartilage, comprising approximately 65% to 75%. The collagen component is predominately type I collagen, which accounts for approximately 90% of all collagen found in fibrocartilage. The meniscus, specifically, functions to optimize force transmission across the knee and to deepen the tibial service and act as a secondary stabilizer. In the ACL-deficient knee, the fibrocartilage of the menisci becomes the primary stabilizers to tibiofemoral translation. There are 2 types of fibrocartilaginous fibers in the meniscus that permit expansion under compressive forces, increasing the overall contact area of the joint. These fibers are radial and longitudinal/circumferential (which help to dissipate hoop stresses). Because the menisci are more elastic than articular/hyaline cartilage, they are better able to absorb shock on impact. Similar to articular cartilage, the menisci are relatively avascular. Only tears in the peripheral third of the meniscus (red zone) have the potential for healing with blood supply from the medial (medial meniscus) or lateral (lateral meniscus) inferior geniculate artery. Following appropriate repair of a meniscus tear in the peripheral zone, there is a potential for healing via fibrocartilaginous scar formation with type I collagen. Tears in the central portion of the meniscus, however, have essentially no potential for healing.

In this clinical vignette, the next most appropriate step in the evaluation of this patient's knee pain is obtaining an MRI. The findings from an MRI, which are likely to include a full-thickness articular cartilage defect of the medial femoral condyle and also possibly a medial meniscus tear, may need to be verified with diagnostic arthroscopy. Depending on the depth/thickness of the articular cartilage defect and the location (peripheral vs central) of the meniscus tear, treatment strategies can then be determined. A thorough appreciation of the anatomy, structure, and function of the various types of cartilage is necessary in order to determine the treatment strategy most likely to be effective.

Why Might This Be Tested? Articular cartilage injuries and meniscal pathology remain some of the most commonly treated and most often tested diagnoses in sports medicine. Understanding the structure and function of cartilage, including the blood supply and changes in composition as aging occurs, is critical to getting these questions correct.

Here's the Point!

Articular cartilage is composed of type II collagen, and fibrocartilage is composed of type I collagen. As articular cartilage ages, chondrocytes increase in size, protein content increases, stiffness increases, and the ratio of PG keratin sulfate to chondroitin sulfate increases. Deep defects in articular cartilage across the tidemark have the potential to heal with fibrocartilage and type I collagen. The fibrocartilage of meniscal tissue will only heal with repair of tears in the peripheral zone of the meniscus.

Vignette 75: Did I Wear My Hip Out Already?!

A 68-year-old male presents 12 years after a left THA for a routine follow-up. He has no pain and ambulates without assistive devices with a minimal limp. He is concerned that things could wear out because he was told this hip would only last 10 years. In addition, he is worried that he may not be able to tolerate a large procedure at his age and wants to know if there are nonoperative options if his implants are worn out. His x-rays and a CT cross-section are shown in Figure 75-1.

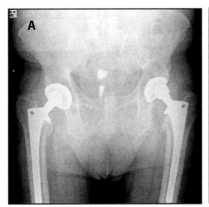 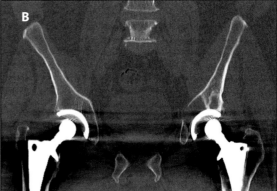

Figure 75-1. (A) AP pelvis x-ray of eccentric polyethylene wear and peri-implant osteolysis. (B) Coronal cross-section CT scan showing extensive retroacetabular osteolysis.

▶ *What is the diagnosis?*

▶ *What are the pathogenesis and biologic pathways that led to his condition?*

▶ *What are his potential treatment options?*

Vignette 75: Answer

The etiology of this patient's symptoms and radiographic findings is likely reactive synovitis due to osteolysis with possible component loosening. Osteolysis is a reactive process initiated by wear debris, propagated by macrophages, with a resultant increase in osteoclast activity. This process may range from an asymptomatic random finding on routine x-rays to gross loosening and migration of affected components.

The process begins with creation of wear particles that are debris from the components. Wear can occur at any place where there is motion between 2 surfaces, such as the polyethylene-metal junction of an acetabular component or at taper junctions where modular components attach (don't forget about screw fretting in the cup as well). However, the most common area is at the interface of the bearing surfaces where motion purposefully occurs with joint motion. One of the goals of THA is to recreate the process of elastohydrodynamic lubrication (where there is a constant film separating the surfaces at all times and the lubricant properties determine the coefficient of friction) while minimizing the direct contact of the bearing surface elements. Historically, we have only been able to recreate a boundary lubrication scenario in which the synovial fluid does not fully separate the bearing surfaces.

The process of articular wear follows several well-described mechanisms, including the following:

- Adhesion: bonding of the surfaces when they are loaded, with material removed from the weaker material (ie, polyethylene wear against the femoral head)

- Abrasion: deviations on the surface of one material (femoral head) cut through the surface of the weaker material (polyethylene)

- Transfer: film from the softer material is transferred to the harder material (like markings on a ceramic head after scraping against metal)

- Fatigue: local strain may lead to subsurface stresses that can cause fatigue after repetitive cycling

- Third-body involvement: trapping of particulate debris (bone, cement, etc) leads to increased local stress concentrations (most common form).

The most common material to undergo this type of wear is ultra-high-molecular-weight polyethylene (UHMWPE) at the bearing surface, which can be highly cross-linked or nonhighly cross-linked. The wear rates of UHMWPE have been reported to be approximately 0.18 mm/year for the first 5 years and then 0.1 mm/year thereafter.[241] Typically, wear rates will change based on patient age, activity level, condition of adjacent joints, sterilization techniques (gamma sterilization in air leads to oxidation, increased density and crystallinity, and reduced mechanical properties, with a subsurface band located 1 to 2 mm beneath the surface), and component alignment and design (compression molded more favorable than machined from bar stock).[242] Standard UHMWPE has been associated with greater wear and larger particles compared with its highly cross-linked counterpart. Highly cross-linked UHMWPE is irradiated to induce a more wear-resistant surface. However, this creates free radicals in the material that can oxidize and weaken the component. To combat this concern, components are treated by remelting (weakens final materials) or annealing (may leave residual free radicals) processes. For highly cross-linked UHMWPE, there has been a reported 40% to 80% decrease in wear rates. The reduction in wear rate has been hypothesized to offset the potential increased biological activity of highly cross-linked particles, possibly explaining the lack of associated osteolysis seen with this bearing surface. One thing to keep in mind is that recent use of antioxidants (ie, vitamin E) has helped quench free radicals and improve the strength of UHMWPE.

There are 7 classic patterns of wear damage reported for UHMWPE surfaces, including embedded debris, scratching, pitting, burnishing, surface deformation, abrasion, and delamination.[243] Wear rates greater than 0.1 mm/year may be associated with more significant osteolysis. Metal-on-metal bearing surfaces produce low wear rates with relatively smaller particles, often an order of magnitude smaller than UHMWPE wear debris. Although the particles are smaller, there is a greater number and surface area that is in contact with host tissue, possibly explaining the increased propensity for metal wear products to be associated with adverse local tissue reactions, such as pseudotumor, aseptic lymphocytic vasculitis-associated lesions, or a lymphocyte-dominated immunological answer. Adverse local tissue reactions can present as massive muscular destruction, fluid collections, bony erosion, and periprosthetic osteolysis (cytokine response is similar to UHMWPE-triggered pathways). Ceramic has the lowest wear rates and is the least likely to be associated with osteolysis. Furthermore, there is some evidence that alumina particles elicit a decreased response compared with UHMWPE particles of the same size on volume in regard to stimulating the enzymatic process of osteolysis.

On a molecular level, osteolysis begins with phagocytosis of wear particles, which causes macrophage activation and further recruitment to the site of the wear debris. Much of this biologic response is related to the particulate characteristics, such as size, shape, and chemical composition. The next step is a cellular cascade (Figure 75-2),[244] which results in the release of signaling factors that activate osteoclasts and lead to bone resorption. Some of these factors include platelet-derived growth factor, prostaglandin E2, TNF-α, IL-1, and IL-6.[244] The bone resorption leads to loosening, micromotion, and increased subsequent wear that propagate this process. The bone resorption is primarily a result of osteoclasts (this is the basis of bisphosphonate medications slowing the rate of osteolysis) and fibroblasts. The areas of bone that undergo osteolysis are influenced by the effective joint space, which is essentially the area surrounding the prosthesis that is accessible to synovial fluid and wear debris. Therefore, femoral stems with contiguous circumferential coating may reduce femoral osteolysis because it prevents wear particles from accessing the femoral canal (if you see distal femoral osteolysis, you must think the component was patch coated, allowing transport of particles below the stem).

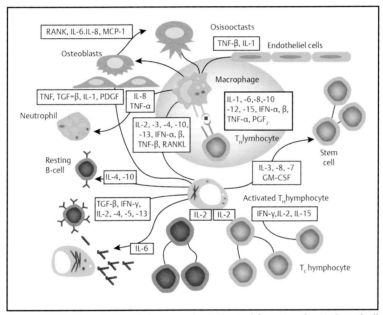

Figure 75-2. Osteolysis cellular cascade. (Adapted from Jacobs JJ, Campbell PA, T Konttinen Y; Implant Wear Symposium 2007 Biologic Work Group. How has the biologic reaction to wear particles changed with newer bearing surfaces? *J Am Acad Orthop Surg.* 2008;16 suppl 1:S49-S55.)

Why Might This Be Tested? Osteolysis and articular surface wear are common problems associated with THA. It is also an avenue to bring in molecular biology mechanisms, material properties, tribology, and THA complications. Therefore, numerous questions can stem from such cases.

Here's the Point!

Osteolysis is due to small wear particles at sites of motion between materials (can occur with all bearings and all junctions in which components come into contact with one another, including tapers, screw holes, etc). This is an inflammatory process, primarily initiated by macrophages/osteoclasts, that results in bone resorption.

Vignette 76: Doc, Why Does This Simple Cut Hurt So Bad?

A 35-year-old male presents to the emergency room with increasing pain, swelling, and erythema to his right lower extremity over the past 18 hours. He has a history of laceration around his ankle while working in his wood shop the previous day. He is up to date on his tetanus shot and has no significant medical problems. In the emergency room, it is noted that the erythema is rapidly spreading up his leg, as is the pain and edema. Skin blisters are noticed to be forming, and the patient has a heart rate of 120 bpm. Antibiotic therapy is initiated without response. His pain continues to worsen with passive stretch of the toes, and there is palpable crepitation in the surrounding soft tissues. The patient continues to spike fevers to 103.5°F and is becoming hypotensive.

▶ *What is the diagnosis?*

▶ *What are the treatment options?*

▶ *What is the typical prognosis?*

Vignette 76: Answer

Necrotizing fasciitis is a rare, life-threatening infection that rapidly disseminates along the fascial planes of an extremity. There are approximately 500 to 1500 cases per year in the US, with mortality rates averaging approximately 22% (range, 8% to 65%). Classic risk factors for this often fatal and disabling condition include the following[245,246]:

- Trauma
- Diabetes mellitus
- IV drug abuse
- Immunodeficiency
- Lacerations, minor abrasion, chronic ulcers
- Surgical site infections

The differential diagnosis includes cellulitis, soft tissue abscess, and pyogenic arthritis. As in the case presented, the patient has a relatively benign early presentation with rapid progression, and the spreading erythema is often replaced by blistering of the skin and, ultimately, necrosis. There are 3 stages of progressive skin lesions, as follows:

1. Early: tenderness to palpation, erythema, calor, and edema
2. Intermediate: Serous-filled blisters or bullae form in conjunction with skin fluctuance
3. Late: Hemorrhagic bullae, decreased sensation, and skin necrosis develop

The pathogenesis is related to a bacterial inoculation at the level of the muscle fascia. The bacteria rapidly multiply, spreading through the superficial fascial planes, destroying the nutrient vessels, and creating a scenario of progressive skin ischemia and full-thickness loss. The 3 most common organisms responsible for this infection include *Staphylococcus aureus*, group A *Streptococcus*, and *Streptococcus viridans*. Typically, necrotizing fasciitis is characterized by a polymicrobial flora; however, group A *Streptococcus* is one of the most prevalent and commonly tested organisms. Type I infections are the most common type and are polymicrobial. Type II infections are monomicrobial, often with group A *Streptococcus* as previously described. Streptococcal surface proteins (M1 and M3) can protect the bacteria from being removed by the body's defenses. The bacteria release exotoxins that activate the immune system, which triggers a release of inflammatory markers (TNF-α, IL-1, and IL-6), giving the symptoms of toxic shock syndrome. Diagnostic tests are typically not warranted acutely and may only delay the diagnosis and surgical management.[245,246]

Treatment is emergent surgery. If you suspect necrotizing fasciitis, do not pass go or collect your $200; head straight to the operating room for surgical exploration and debridement. Hesitating may compromise the outcome because early surgical debridement has been shown to decrease the mortality of this condition. A 9-fold increase in mortality has been shown if debridement is delayed greater than 24 hours after admission. Intraoperative cultures are taken, and the skin down to the fascia is widely (5- to 10-mm margins recommended) debrided as needed. Nonadherent wound dressings or negative-pressure wound-vacuum devices are placed, and laboratory values are obtained to make sure the coagulation parameters are close to normal, kidney function is maintained, and creatine kinase levels stabilize (related to muscle destruction). Close monitoring of the wound needs to be followed; if infection appears to be recurring, multiple debridements may be necessary before wound coverage begins. If adequate debridement is not achieved, the risk for amputation increases; however, remember, "life over limb." This may be a necessary evil. Typically, skin grafts and wound flaps are needed to cover these wounds. It is important to assure appropriate nutrition, IV antibiotics (clindamycin should be used in conjunction with beta-lactam drugs to help sequester the toxins), and supportive care are available. Adjunct therapies, such as hyperbaric oxygen (increased partial pressure of oxygen may enhance WBC-killing activity, improve tissue repair, and provide a synergistic effect on the antibiotics), and IV IgMs (may bind taphylococcal superantigens) are controversial at this time.[245,246]

Why Might This Be Tested? Necrotizing fasciitis is a deadly condition, and there is little argument as to what the treatment involves, therefore making this a good testing point.

Here's the Point!

Make the diagnosis quickly and take the patient to the operating room emergently. Debride, debride, debride, and then debride some more. Treat with supportive care, antibiotics, and, ultimately, wound coverage by a plastic surgeon.

Vignette 77: My Child Has Flat Feet

A 9-year-old healthy female soccer player has been treated for recurrent ankle sprains over the past 2 years. She complains of worsening lateral ankle and hindfoot discomfort, which increases during the course of her soccer games. She has been fitted with custom orthotics in the past for flat feet. On physical examination, she is noted to have a rigid pes planus deformity. She is point tender over the sinus tarsi region. The tibiotalar joint is supple, but no active or passive inversion or eversion is elicited.

▶ *What is the diagnosis?*

▶ *What is the most common age of presentation of this condition?*

▶ *What are the most common presenting symptoms?*

▶ *Which joints are the most commonly affected?*

▶ *What is the natural history of this condition?*

The recommendation is made to proceed with surgical intervention.

▶ *What options are available for early surgical intervention when diagnosed in the pediatric population?*

▶ *What salvage options are available for late (adult) presentation?*

Vignette 77: Answer

Tarsal coalition is caused by a failure of mesenchymal cells to segment and produce normal peritalar joints. A hereditary tendency for this condition has been suggested. Tarsal coalition should be considered in the pediatric population in any patient who presents with flat feet, recurrent ankle instability, or a family history of problematic feet.

The triad of rigid pes planus, tarsal coalition, and peroneal spastic flatfoot is often lumped together in the same discussion. The truth is that peroneal muscle spasm occurs as a manifestation of the shortening of the muscle unit from fixed valgus of the subtalar joint, rather than from true spasm, detectable by EMG. Although many patients have little or no deformity, the vast majority of patients with a coalition present with a rigid flatfoot deformity.

Ninety-two percent of all tarsal coalitions are seen in the middle facet of the talocalcaneal joint and in the calcaneonavicular joint. The remaining 8% include the talonavicular and calcaneocuboid joints. This condition is present bilaterally in up to 50% of cases. Tarsal coalitions are broadly classified as ossified or nonossified (fibrous or fibrocartilaginous).

Radiographic evaluation of the foot with a suspected talocalcaneal coalition consists of plain x-rays of the foot, including oblique and axial calcaneal views. Although CT scan is the gold standard for diagnosing an osseous coalition, MRI is necessary in order to detect a fibrous coalition. Plain x-rays will often suffice; in a calcaneonavicular coalition, the lateral oblique view will usually detect a bony bridge linking the anterior process of the calcaneus to the lateral body of the navicular. In talocalcaneal coalition, which typically involves the middle facet of the subtalar joint, the axial calcaneal view will often reveal the bony bridge. Beaking of the dorsal articular margin of the talar head is often pronounced in cases of talocalcaneal coalition.

Generally speaking, patients with calcaneonavicular tarsal coalition present between the ages of 8 and 12 years, whereas talocalcaneal coalition presents between ages 12 and 16 years. Recurrent ankle instability and lateral hindfoot discomfort (secondary to peroneal spasm) are common presenting complaints. In the setting of a delayed (adult) presentation, pain is most often attributed to degenerative changes in the remaining portion of the noncoalesced segment of the affected joint.

Initial treatment consists of activity restriction and immobilization. As patients become older, and as deformity and limitation in activities become more pronounced, surgical treatment emerges as the preferred treatment. The 2 most commonly performed procedures for tarsal coalition are resection of the coalition with interposition of muscle (extensor digitorum brevis, usually) or fat and selected arthrodesis. Resection of the fibrous or osseous coalition is indicated in most cases, unless degenerative changes are noted. Although most authors report best results in cases of takedown of tarsal coalition in the pediatric coalition, good results have been published in adults as well in the absence of degenerative findings on radiographic studies. Although subtalar ROM seldom equals that of the uninvolved side, 50% of normal is considered an excellent result. In cases of severe, fixed hindfoot valgus or in cases with large, ossified bony bridges (>2.5 cm in a talocalcaneal coalition), it is recommended that one opts to punt and perform a fusion or triple arthrodesis.

Why Might This Be Tested? Tarsal coalition is a common cause of rigid pes planus and recurrent ankle instability in the pediatric population.

Here's the Point!

When detected early and in the absence of subtalar DJD, tarsal coalition should be treated with surgical resection, whereas in cases with DJD, joint fusion is the treatment of choice.

Vignette 78: I Am Too Young to Have Hip Pain

A 38-year-old female presents to your office with a 6-month history of increasing right hip pain. Her past medical history is only significant for severe asthma. Upon further questioning, her asthma has been poorly controlled over the past few years, and she has been on intermittent regimens of oral corticosteroids. Physical examination reveals pain with rotational ROM of the hip and weight bearing. Despite the pain, her overall ROM is not significantly limited. At this point, her activities of daily living are significantly compromised and she is looking for treatment options.

▶ *What is the most likely diagnosis?*

▶ *What are some of the other etiologic factors for this pathologic condition?*

▶ *What is the relevant pathoanatomy?*

▶ *What is the classification system used to help guide decision making?*

▶ *What are the surgical options?*

Vignette 78: Answer

The patient has ON of the femoral head due to chronic corticosteroid use. ON of the femoral head accounts for nearly 5% to 18% of all THAs (10,000 to 20,000 cases) performed each year.[247] Typically, patients are relatively young, depending on the etiology of the ON, with ages often ranging between the late 30s and early 50s.[248] The contralateral hip is affected in up to 75% of cases, with males being 3 times more likely to develop ON than females.[247]

The etiology of ON of the femoral head is multifactorial, spanning both traumatic and atraumatic causes, with a final common pathway of a decreased blood supply to the femoral head. The ischemic injury leads to upregulation of tartrate-resistant acid phosphatase–positive osteoclasts, which remove the dead subchondral trabeculae.[247] Ultimately, this leads to collapse of the femoral head under repetitive loading and destruction of the hip joint. This case screams ON with the chronic use of steroids, which is a common etiology, and, along with alcoholism, smoking, trauma, and prior hip surgery, constitutes up to 75% to 90% of the cases of ON each year.[247] Other common history nuggets that should conjure up thoughts of ON of the femoral head include slipped capital femoral epiphysis, deep sea diving, SLE, autoimmune diseases, sickle cell anima, coagulopathies, HIV, organ transplantation, chronic liver disease, storage disorders (Gaucher's disease), gout, and metabolic bone disease.[247]

In the setting of a traumatic event, there may be direct disruption of blood to the femoral head as in a femoral neck fracture or hip dislocation. The somewhat tenuous blood supply of the femoral head stems from a large contribution from the medial femoral circumflex artery (major contributor to the extracapsular vascular ring at the base of the femoral neck) and, to a lesser extent, the superior and inferior gluteal arteries and the artery of the ligamentum teres.[247] In trauma cases, direct injury to the blood vessels may occur, along with the formation of a compressive local hematoma.

In atraumatic causes, the exact pathogenesis is not as clearly defined and may involve a spectrum of intra- and/or extravascular disorders. Intravascular insults leading to ON may be associated with direct osteocyte toxicity and alterations in blood flow caused by coagulopathies, thrombophilia, or embolic debris (fat, clots, immune complexes, and sickle cells). The direct causes for ON include trauma, irradiation, blood cancers, caisson disease, cytotoxins, Gaucher's disease, and sickle cell disease/trait. The indirect causes include corticosteroid use, alcohol consumption, SLE, organ transplant, renal failure, thrombophilia, hemophilia, and idiopathic. Alcohol consumption and corticosteroid use have been implicated in 90% of newly diagnosed cases of ON.[249] The pathogenesis of ON in these cases has been postulated to be secondary to adipogenesis and subsequent compression of venous structures. This causes increased intraosseous pressure and limits arterial blood flow, with resultant ON.[247]

The clinical presentation and patient's symptoms are crucial in ultimately determining treatment options. Most importantly, one must evaluate the duration of symptoms and limitations of function. Physical examination is often remarkable for painful ROM and groin pain that is exacerbated by weight bearing. More limited abduction, internal rotation, and flexion indicate more extensive femoral head destruction. One must take a detailed history to discover if the patient has any risk factors for ON. However, other causes of groin pain must be assessed, particularly in the younger patient population, to include a sports hernia, genitourinary concerns, and intrapelvic sources of pain. AP and frog-lateral x-rays can show the extent of the femoral head collapse, the size of the head destruction, the remaining joint space, and osteophytes. Classically, alternating areas of lucency and sclerosis will be present on plain x-rays, with the crescent sign representing more advanced disease and subchondral collapse. MRI may show focal increases in signal on T2-weighted images (double-line sign) or presence of a low-intensity band on T1-weighted images.[247] Although much has been written on the prediction of disease progression, no hard, fast rules exist; remember, the bigger the lesion, the more likely collapse will occur, making head-preserving procedures less reliable.

The Ficat classification is useful for initially staging ON (Table 78-1).

Collapse of the femoral head is a negative prognostic factor for preserving the femoral head. Conservative measures (limited weight bearing, physical therapy, and activity modification) rarely provide prolonged relief or alter disease progression. Ideally, causative factors should be stopped if possible (ie, alcohol, steroid, and smoking cessation). Medical management options include lipid-lowering agents (may decrease the prevalence of steroid-induced ON, with and without a concomitant anticoagulant), bisphosphonates (may slow the progression of ON), and hyperbaric oxygen, all of which may be beneficial in early stages of the

Table 78-1. FICAT CLASSIFICATION	
Stage	Symptoms/Imaging
0	No pain; MRI normal; diagnosis based on histology
I	Pain present; decreased internal rotation and abduction; normal x-rays; abnormal MRI
II	Pain worsened; x-rays show sclerosis and lytic lesions
III	Worsening pain/limp; x-rays show crescent sign and flattening of head; joint space normal
IV	Progressive loss of joint space; osteophyte formation; hip arthritis with flattened femoral head
MRI = magnetic resonance imaging.	

disease process.[247] New research has focused on means to treat ON using cellular therapies with CD34+ cells, stem cell injections into the femoral head, and combinations using a drug-coated scaffolding (calcium phosphate).[247]

For earlier stages of ON, core decompression of the femoral head is an option. This includes drilling a single or multiple holes into the femoral head with or without insertion of an autogenous or allogenic bone graft filler. Other head-sparing procedures include proximal femoral osteotomy, arthroscopic debridement/ drilling, and nonvascularized/vascularized fibular graft. An additional concern with head-preserving procedures is related to the ability to modify the cause of the ON. If the underlying disease cannot be corrected in some way, drastic head-preserving techniques may be futile and possibly compromise a future THA.

Because ON is primarily a disease of the femoral head, a hemiresurfacing arthroplasty may be indicated if the acetabular cartilage is preserved. However, one must take into account both the cyst formation in the femoral head and the quality of bone in the femoral head. Hip resurfacing results are not consistent in the literature in treating ON, and while not a contraindication, is often a reason a surgeon will choose THA. Furthermore, the MOM nature of the articulation precludes its use in women of childbearing age because metal ions have been shown to cross the placenta in vivo. THA is a valuable option because it provides predicable pain relief and reasonable complication rates. However, patients must be counseled on the increased risk of dislocation, limb-length discrepancy, and likely need for a second surgery (particularly in very young patients).

Why Might This Be Tested? ON is a commonly managed disease process in young adults with multiple etiologies, making it an attractive topic for test questions. Disease-based diagnostic testing and treatment options are all fair game for questioning.

Here's the Point!

Young patients with groin pain require assessment for ON of the femoral head. A detailed history will often elucidate the pathogenesis, with alcohol and corticosteroid use being the most common culprits. Head-preserving management may be considered prior to collapse of the femoral head and arthroplasty may be used when sphericity of the head is lost and arthritic changes are present.

Vignette 79: Doc, This Hip Keeps Popping Out on Me

A 70-year-old male with a history of endstage OA of the right hip undergoes an uneventful right THA using cementless components and a metal-on-polyethylene bearing. The early postoperative recovery goes extremely well, and he is discharged on postoperative day 2 with home health. An initial postoperative x-ray is shown in Figure 79-1. Two weeks later, the patient suffers immediate pain and inability to bear weight while attempting to rise from the bedside commode. X-rays upon presentation to the emergency department are shown in Figure 79-2.

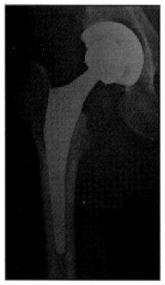

Figure 79-1. Postoperative x-ray showing what appears to be a well-functioning THA.

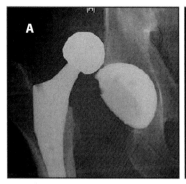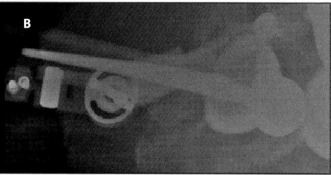

Figure 79-2. (A) AP and (B) shoot-through lateral x-rays of the right hip showing a posterior hip dislocation.

▶ *What patient factors are associated with instability after THA?*

▶ *What surgical techniques are associated with a decreased risk of instability?*

▶ *What is the treatment paradigm after a single episode of postoperative instability?*

▶ *What is the treatment paradigm for chronic, recurrent postoperative instability?*

Vignette 79: Answer

Instability after a THA occurs in 2% to 5% of cases and accounts for 23% of revisions as the single most common reason for revision. The majority (75% to 90%) of these dislocations are posterior, most (60%) occur as a single isolated event, and most (60% to 80%) can be treated successfully with conservative management. The remaining 20% to 40% require operative revision. Dislocations are typically classified as early (ie, within 6 to 12 weeks postoperatively) or late (ie, occurring later than 12 weeks postoperatively). Late dislocations are more likely to recur.[250-252]

A number of patient factors have been associated with instability. Females outnumber males 2 to 3:1 in the largest series. Developmental dysplasia of the hip, ON, and femoral neck fracture as indications for THA have all been associated with an increased risk of instability. Conditions that impair patient's neuromuscular status, such as Parkinson's disease, chronic alcohol abuse, and a decline in mental status, have also been associated with instability. A history of hip surgery or THA also increases the risk for instability. Factors that lead to the development of a loss of physiologic abductor tensioning, such as trochanteric malunion, marked weight loss, or extensive polyethylene wear, can also lead to instability.

A number of surgical factors have been associated with instability. Large retrospective trials have shown higher dislocation rates with the posterior approach than the anterior, anterolateral, and lateral approaches. However, other studies comparing the posterior approach with capsulorrhaphy and repair of the external rotator musculature to the lateral and anterolateral approaches have shown equivalent rates of dislocation. Component orientation, in particular acetabular orientation, has also been shown to play a role, with components ideally being placed in 40 degrees of abduction and 15 degrees of anteversion. Intraoperatively, poor exposure, poor patient positioning, extensive peripheral osteophytes, and anatomic variation can lead the surgeon to malposition the acetabular component. Revision surgery has also been associated with instability, particularly if the abductors or the proximal femoral bonestock is compromised. Instability after revision surgery is also a problem with factors such as female sex, increasing Paprosky grade of the cup, preoperative diagnosis of instability, and greater number of prior surgeries. Several factors in implant design have been associated with instability, in particular small femoral necks, low femoral head-to-neck ratio, a reduction in femoral offset, or an elevated liner (impingement).

Patients presenting with a first-time dislocation warrant radiographic evaluation to check for liner dissociation, implant neck failure, greater trochanter failure, and periprosthetic fracture prior to reduction. The surgeon may also wish to evaluate for infection with inflammatory serologies. An attempt should be made at closed reduction under conscious sedation or general anesthesia, which is successful in more than 90% of cases. Postreduction x-rays must then be scrutinized to examine for component malpositioning. If reduction is successful and the components are well positioned, then the surgeon can consider bracing with close clinical follow-up, although some evidence suggests bracing to be unnecessary.

Patients presenting with recurrent dislocation should be evaluated with x-rays and inflammatory laboratory tests. Before a treatment can be selected, the surgeon must determine the cause of instability. Patients with infection should undergo irrigation and debridement or 1- or 2-stage exchange depending on the chronicity of the infection. Patients with component malpositioning should undergo revision. Patients with impingement should undergo osteophyte resection and revision to improve component geometry by increasing head size, lateralizing the acetabular liner, or increasing the neck length or offset. Patients with inadequate soft tissue tension should be revised to increase offset by increasing head size, lateralizing the liner, or increasing neck length. In selected cases, this can be supplemented with capsulorrhaphy and/or trochanteric advancement. Cases that have failed other measures could be considered for a constrained liner, although this places significant stresses on the bone-implant interface of the acetabular component and may increase the risk of aseptic loosening of the cup (never place a constrained liner with malpositioned components or at the time of a tenuous acetabular reconstruction). The surgeon could also consider a dual-mobility component, although this remains controversial.

Why Might This Be Tested? Instability is a common complication after THA and is thus frequently tested. In addition, the evaluation and treatment requires a full understanding of the biomechanics that govern THA and allows question writers to access these basic principles through clinical scenarios.

Here's the Point!

Instability occurs after 2% to 5% of THAs. The posterior approach, loss of the abductor musculature, component malpositioning, and impingement are common causes. Acute isolated cases with well-positioned components are candidates for conservative treatment, whereas recurrent cases warrant revision once the etiology is determined.

Vignette 80: Doc, I Think I Tore Some Cartilage?!

A 16-year-old male begins to notice knee swelling after playing higher-level sports. Pain is difficult to reproduce on exam, but the patient notices that it is worse with stairs compared with level walking. X-rays show no evidence of arthritis or joint space narrowing. The patient's MRI can be seen in Figure 80-1.

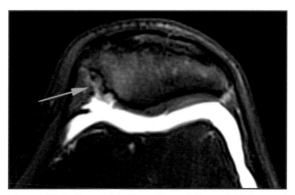

Figure 80-1. Coronal MRI section of the patellofemoral joint.

▶ *What is the healing potential for this lesion and why?*

▶ *What is the makeup of the tissue that would fill this void after treatment vs the original tissue?*

▶ *What biomechanical properties are inherent to the different layers of cartilage and why?*

▶ *What are the metabolic and histologic differences between what this lesion may lead to (arthritis) and normal cartilage aging?*

Vignette 80: Answer

Although specifics of articular cartilage defect treatment will likely not appear on the Boards, aspects related to its healing and pathology are more likely to be tested. Articular cartilage is avascular, aneural, and alymphatic. The only cellular component is the chondrocyte within cartilage; however, the synoviocyte also plays an important role. The type B synoviocyte helps blow up the joint balloon and produce lubricating proteins (described later). Because there are no direct channels of access to cartilage for nutrient delivery, all water content comes from diffusion from the synovial fluid.

Regarding this case, the MRI demonstrates that the calcified cartilage layer is intact; therefore, there is no inherent ability for healing secondary to a lack of MSC access.[253] Although "creeping substitution" can occur with cartilage, the body primarily repairs cartilage through production of fibrocartilage by MSCs. This brings us to the second portion of the case, in which healing cartilage is formed with a majority of type I collagen instead of type II. Therefore, many of the inherent properties of cartilage are devoid in this scar-like tissue.

Normal cartilage is 90% type II collagen, which is 60% of the dry weight, and type X collagen in the calcified zone. The other abundant molecules are PGs at 30%. PGs are composed of subunits (glycosaminoglycans [GAGs]), which are fabricated by cartilage cells and secreted into the surrounding matrix. The GAGs are either chondroitin sulfate or keratin sulfate. Cartilage exhibits viscoelastic properties, in which the amount of deformation relies on the amount of time the force is applied over or the pulse. Silly Putty acts in the same way, where slow gradual pressure causes deformation and quick impact results in fast reformation (or bouncing in the case of putty). The wet weight of cartilage is 74% water, which is a polar molecule. PGs have good compressive strength and attract water (negative charge attracts positive molecules, cations, which increase the ability of water to penetrate the tissue). A simple way to remember the organization of PGs is HULK: HyalUronic acid backbone with Link proteins that bind the protein core that contains Keratin sulfate and chondroitin sulfate (95% of the glycoproteins). The most active chondrocytes are in the deep layers, as is most of the PG production. In a similar manner, all water must come from diffusion from the joint fluid; therefore, most water content is in the superficial zones.

The following are the cartilage zones from superficial to deep, with the most important points of each one included:

- Superficial zone:
    - Lubricated by lubricin
    - Superficial zone protein
    - Resists shear force with tangential collagen fibrils
    - Mostly water because it comes from the joint fluid diffusion
- Middle or transitional zone:
    - Tangential collagen above and vertical below, so oblique collagen in transition
- Deep or radial zone:
    - Vertical collagen orientation with largest diameter
    - Resists compression and has the most PGs
- Calcified cartilage zone or tidemark:
    - Type X collagen
    - Requires injury for access to MSCs

Finally, it is important to understand the different characteristics of cartilage aging and arthritis, as these lead to 2 very different states.[254] An easy way to remember the 2 is that "arthritis is wet" and with "aging you dry up and get stiff." This covers one of the most important factors, which is that there is increased water content in arthritis, where it decreases in aging. Many other changes with aging can be remembered using the following: old people are not flexible and, therefore, are not responsive to change (growth factors); stiff and increased collagen cross-linking makes them less flexible. To make up for looking old, they decorate themselves (decorin) as you collect AGE (advanced glycosylation end products).

Why Might This Be Tested? Understanding cartilage biology/biochemistry/histology helps clinicians understand the current state of cartilage injury and repair as well as the pathogenesis of OA.

Here's the Point!

Normal cartilage is largely type II collagen and is replaced by fibrocartilage (type I collagen) if the calcified layer is violated. The other most abundant structures are PGs, which interact with water to give viscoelastic properties. Arthritis is wet, whereas aging is stiff (cross-linked collagen), stubborn (no growth factor response), and dried up (decreased water content).

Vignette 81: Monkey Bar Injury

A 5-year-old female fell off the monkey bars onto an outstretched right upper extremity. She complained of immediate pain, and her parents noted a deformity of her elbow. X-rays from the emergency room are shown in Figure 81-1.

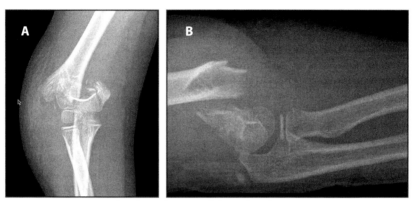

Figure 81-1. (A) AP and (B) lateral x-rays of the right elbow.

▶ *What is the diagnosis?*

Initial examination revealed a pulseless, pink hand. The emergency room physician stated that the patient was initially able to do an "OK" sign; however, when examined later by the orthopedic resident, it was noted that the patient could not flex the IP joint of the thumb nor the DIP joint of the index finger.

▶ *What nerve is most likely injured?*

▶ *What should the initial treatment be?*

After an uneventful period of healing, the patient achieved a full recovery. Three years after the injury, the patient returns for follow-up due to a deformity of the right elbow. On examination, the patient is noted to have an asymptomatic cubitus varus deformity of the elbow.

▶ *What is the appropriate treatment now?*

Vignette 81: Answer

Pediatric elbow injuries are extraordinarily common, and, as an orthopedist taking call, you will not be able to escape them. Supracondylar fracture of the humerus is the most common elbow fracture in children and accounts for 3% of all pediatric fractures.[255] These fractures occur most commonly in children between 5 and 7 years old, and 98% are extension-type injuries.[255] The mechanism of injury is typically a fall onto an outstretched hand with the elbow in full extension—one reason most orthopedists forbid monkey bars or a trampoline at home! A thorough physical exam is required to rule out an open fracture or an ipsilateral wrist or forearm fracture. The latter is more likely to develop a compartment syndrome.

The diagnosis is a Gartland type III supracondylar humerus fracture. These fractures are graded as 3 types: type I is nondisplaced with the anterior humeral line bisecting the middle one-third of the capitellum; in type II, the anterior humeral line does not transect the capitellum, but the posterior cortex is intact; and type III is displaced with no posterior cortical contact. In addition, a flexion-type supracondylar humerus fracture has been described and is much less common with the anterior displacement of the distal fragment.

The initial examination is extremely important and should be conducted despite pain and patient anxiety/ability to cooperate. The radial, median, and ulnar nerves should all be tested because nerve injuries are reported in up to 11.3% of cases.[255] In order of prevalence, the following nerve injuries can be found after supracondylar fractures: anterior interosseous nerve, median, radial, and ulnar (more commonly injured in flexion-type fractures) nerves. The anterior interosseous nerve can be tested by showing the "OK" sign, which is described as when the IP joint of the thumb and the DIP joint of the index finger are flexed. Most patients with focal neurologic deficits at the time of injury will experience resolution by 6 to 12 weeks after the injury. A change in the nerve function status is more concerning for incarceration of the nerve at the fracture site.

The next critical step is to determine the vascular status of the hand. Pulses should be palpated and/or evaluated with a Doppler. However, most important is the viability of the hand as judged by capillary refill, temperature, and color of the fingers. Perfusion of the hand can be adequate despite brachial artery spasm due to collateral circulation. A white dysvascular hand constitutes a surgical emergency.

Management of these fractures is based on the classification, described above. It is not common practice to reduce supracondylar humerus fractures and cast them. Type I fractures are managed with a long-arm cast for 3 to 4 weeks (elbow at 90 degrees and forearm neutral rotation). Type II and type III fractures are better treated with closed reduction and pinning; if reduction cannot be achieved, open reduction via an anterior approach is suggested.[256]

Timing of the surgery is a commonly tested topic, and it has been shown that there is no difference in complications if the surgery occurs less than or more than 8 hours after injury. In a well-perfused upper extremity, it is acceptable to delay surgery, even in a type III fracture, up to 12 to 18 hours from injury.[255] When there is a pulseless hand that is still pink, with a type III fracture, treatment should include closed reduction and percutaneous pinning (urgently/emergently) and assess whether the pulse returns. If the pulse returns, the elbow is pinned and splinted. If the pulse does not return and the hand remains pink, the patient can be closely monitored after the fracture is stabilized. If the pulse does not return and the hand is white, open exploration of the artery should be performed with possible fasciotomies to prevent reperfusion compartment syndrome. There are 8 factors that determine the urgency of fracture management: (1) open fracture, (2) dysvascular limb, (3) skin puckering (caused by the proximal fragment poking through the brachialis muscle), (4) floating elbow, (5) median nerve palsy, (6) evolving compartment syndrome, (7) young age, and (8) cognitive disability.[255]

Pin configuration has been classically described as one medial and one lateral K-wire; however, ulnar nerve injury can occur in up to 10% of patients.[255] Two lateral K-wires have been shown to have excellent strength and union rates. These pins must engage the medial and lateral columns of the elbow. After 2 pins are placed, the stability of the fracture is tested by stressing the elbow and, if unstable, another pin is placed (medially or laterally). The arm is splinted, and the K-wires are removed 3 to 4 weeks after surgery. Common complications (occur in ~4%) include pin migration (1.8%), pin site infection (1%), ulnar nerve injury, and malunion.[255] Common reasons for failure of fixation include the inability to obtain bicortical fixation with 2 pins, less than 2-mm pin spread at the fracture site, and inadequate purchase of both fragments with 2 pins. The important technical points for fixation with lateral-entry pins are to (1) maximize separation of the pins at the fracture site, (2) engage the medial and lateral columns proximal to the fracture, (3) engage sufficient bone in both the proximal segment and the distal fragment, and (4) maintain a low threshold for use of a third lateral-entry pin if there is concern about fracture stability or the location of the first 2 pins.[257]

Cubitus varus is a common complication of casting or pinning of supracondylar humerus fractures in children. Traditionally, this deformity is felt to be a cosmetic concern only because elbow ROM is typically unaffected. More recently, an entity known as *tardy posterolateral elbow instability* has been described; it is best treated by a valgus osteotomy and ligamentous reconstruction.[255] Based on the potential for developing this instability complex, it is suggested to treat significant cubitus varus early (> 1 year after surgery and when old enough to follow postoperative instructions) with a local osteotomy.

Why Might This Be Tested? It is important to know when a supracondylar humerus fracture requires surgery. These injuries will forever follow orthopedists on standardized tests and in the emergency room for those of us who take call.

Here's the Point!

Type II and III fractures can usually be treated with closed reduction and 2 lateral K-wires. Pulseless upper extremities require more urgent surgery and possible exploration of the neurovascular bundle via an anterior approach.

Vignette 82: Rotator Cuff Disease

A 65-year-old male presents with a 4-month history of insidiously worsening right shoulder pain. He denies any acute injury and reports that the pain is worse at night and when he combs his hair. On physical exam, he demonstrates full painless passive shoulder ROM bilaterally but actively abducts his right shoulder to only 85 degrees. He has weakness with resisted abduction and external rotation at 0 degrees of abduction. He has pain with passive forward elevation and an empty can sign. He demonstrates a negative belly-press test. An x-ray is shown in Figure 82-1.

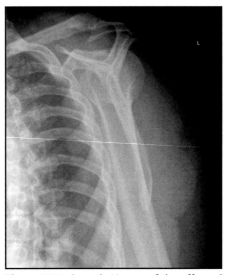

Figure 82-1. Scapula Y x-ray of the affected shoulder.

▶ *What is the most likely diagnosis?*

▶ *What other tests should be ordered?*

▶ *What are the treatment options for this condition?*

▶ *What are the benefits of arthroscopic vs open repair?*

Vignette 82: Answer

The obvious diagnosis is a rotator cuff tear. The age of the patient and the insidious nature of the pain suggest a chronic etiology. Often, these patients may report no history of trauma. In addition, night pain and pain with overhead activities are classic symptoms. On examination, weakness with resisted abduction is consistent with supraspinatus involvement. External rotation weakness at 0 degrees of abduction suggests that the infraspinatus may be involved as well. A negative belly-press test indicates that the subscapularis remains intact. The x-ray reveals no evidence of severe glenohumeral arthritis, a normal acromiohumeral interval, and a hooked (type III) acromion morphology (see Figure 82-1). MRI or ultrasound would be the next diagnostic study ordered. MRI is considered the gold standard and can clearly visualize tear patterns as well as associated shoulder pathology. Ultrasound is also used, but it is technician dependent and can be difficult to visualize glenohumeral joint changes. Arthrograms are of historical significance primarily but would demonstrate extravasation of fluid into the subacromial space in the setting of a rotator cuff tear.

Rotator cuff tears are common and increase with age. Screening of asymptomatic individuals has demonstrated partial or complete tears in 7% to 40% of the population.[153] Partial-thickness tears are more common. Rotator cuff tears can be thought of as a stage on a continuum of disease beginning with subacromial impingement and tendinopathy before progressing to rotator cuff tears and eventual rotator cuff arthropathy. Tears most commonly involve the supraspinatus, but they may extend to the infraspinatus and teres minor or, less commonly, the subscapularis. In younger patients (younger than 40 years), rotator cuff tears are typically the result of an acute traumatic event, such as a shoulder dislocation, and may be massive. In older patients (older than 60 years), the prevalence increases, and chronic, insidious presentation is more common. This may reflect a combination of intrinsic tendinous degeneration associated with aging, as well as extrinsic damage from the undersurface of the acromion and coracoacromial arch.

On physical examination, careful ROM testing is essential to rule out adhesive capsulitis, which would need to be addressed prior to any surgical intervention for the rotator cuff. Limitations of active ROM, or weakness associated with provocative testing of the rotator cuff, are characteristic of a rotator cuff tear.

Close radiographic review is also essential. Evidence of severe glenohumeral arthritis is a contraindication to surgical repair. In addition, fixed superior migration of the humeral head suggests chronic rotator cuff arthropathy. Acromial morphology, such as a type III (hooked) acromion, indicates that external subacromial impingement may be contributing to symptoms, and that if surgical intervention is undertaken, an associated acromioplasty may be performed. On MRI, it is important to note the characteristics of the tear, including size, shape, and amount of retraction. This is typically best visualized on T2 imaging. Tears can be classified as full or partial thickness, and partial-thickness tears can be determined to be articular or bursal sided. In addition, muscular atrophy or fatty infiltration can be seen, which suggests a more chronic etiology and portends a worse outcome. Associated glenohumeral pathology can also be visualized. The subscapularis should be carefully examined, and a medially subluxed biceps tendon may be a clue that a subscapularis tear has occurred.

Treatment options include nonoperative interventions, such as NSAIDs, physical therapy with scapular strengthening, and subacromial cortisone injections. These cortisone injections may diminish tendon quality, however. Older patients may do better with nonoperative intervention. Surgical intervention is indicated for patients with symptomatic rotator cuff tears that fail nonoperative intervention, younger patients with acute tears, acute loss of motion, patients with good-quality tendon and muscle on MRI, and those without significant glenohumeral arthritis or adhesive capsulitis. Contraindications include active infection, severe arthritis, severe chronic retracted tendons with muscle atrophy, fixed superior humeral head migration (indicative of chronic rotator cuff arthropathy), or deltoid dysfunction.[153] Moosmayer et al randomized patients with small- and medium-sized tears of the rotator cuff to nonoperative vs operative intervention and found improved pain and outcome scores in the operative group at 1 year.[258]

Operative intervention traditionally included open rotator cuff repair, but more surgeons are moving toward mini-open or all-arthroscopic repairs. Open rotator cuff repairs require deltoid detachment from the acromion, which requires careful repair and can produce subsequent deltoid detachment as a complication. In addition, protection of the deltoid repair limits postoperative rehabilitation. Mini-open repairs split the deltoid but must not extend more than 3 to 5 cm from the inferior edge of the acromion in order to avoid the axillary nerve. Arthroscopic repairs are more technically challenging, especially for large cuff tears (Figure 82-2). Careful application of concepts, such as margin convergence, interval slides, and anatomic footprint

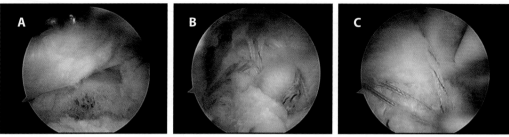

Figure 82-2. (A) Arthroscopic view of a massive rotator cuff tear. (B, C) Arthroscopic views of repair of a massive rotator cuff tear using double-row fixation.

restoration, are critical for repair of larger tears but are beyond the scope of this discussion. Mini-open and arthroscopic repairs have been shown to have similarly good results to open repairs, with less stiffness.[259] Postoperative rehabilitation begins with gentle passive ROM. Massive irreparable tears may be reconstructed with latissimus dorsi or teres major transfer, but latissimus dorsi transfer requires an intact subscapularis tendon.

Why Might This Be Tested? Rotator cuff tears are a common problem faced by orthopedic surgeons and, therefore, are frequently tested. Questions are common regarding cuff anatomy and physical examination. Asymptomatic cuff tears are common, and clinical indications for surgery are key, so careful attention must be paid to the entire case presentation and imaging to determine if surgical intervention is indicated. In general, older patients may do better with physical therapy, and younger patients with acute avulsion injuries may head straight to surgery. Differences between surgical techniques are also important.

Here's the Point!

Know rotator cuff anatomy, pathogenesis, and indications for surgical repair. Remember that screening of asymptomatic individuals has demonstrated partial or complete tears in 7% to 40% of the population.

Vignette 83: Gait and Upper Extremity Prostheses

A 45-year-old male construction worker was in a single-car accident and sustained an acute pelvic fracture and multiple open fractures to his forearm, wrist, and hand on his right upper extremity. The patient remained in a coma for several months and, secondary to infection, underwent a transradial amputation 2 weeks ago. His mental status has continued to improve over the past 2 weeks, and rehabilitation is set to begin. At this point, the patient is cleared to walk weight bearing as tolerated on his lower extremities, and the wound at the end of his amputated forearm is well healed.

▶ *Review the gait cycle and rehabilitation for this patient.*

▶ *What type of prosthesis should he be fitted for his arm and when?*

Vignette 83: Answer

The gait cycle follows a pattern of phases to provide an energy-efficient means of locomotion. The 2 main phases are stance (62%) and swing (38%). The stance phase of gait is broken down into 3 segments, including initial double-limb support (loading response, hip is flexed 30 degrees and knee is near full extension with slight plantarflexion of ankle), single-limb stance and second double-limb support (preswing), and swing phase (composed of the initial swing [the hip and knee flex and ankle dorsiflexes], midswing, and terminal swing segments).[260] The sequential physical events that make up a stride include foot strike, opposite toe-off, opposite foot strike, toe-off, foot clearance, tibia vertical, and second foot strike. Muscles work in conjunction to make this an effortless process during a normal gait cycle. This involves a delicate balance between eccentric (muscle lengthening while contracting), isocentric (muscle length remains constant), and concentric (muscle shortens) muscle activity.

In the case of our patient, rehabilitation starts with a weight bearing as tolerated protocol but will likely evolve as the patient's pain subsides and strength improves. This will be associated with an element of an antalgic gait. This represents a prolonged stance phase on the uninjured leg in order to protect the painful limb. Conversely, the swing phase of the uninjured extremity is more rapid. A thorough understanding of the basics of the gait cycle make it possible to understand and diagnose more complex abnormalities related to other pathologic conditions (eg, ACL deficiency is associated with a quadriceps avoidance gait—lower quadriceps moment during midstance).

Regarding the upper extremity injury, it is important to understand the function of the shoulder and elbow in regard to choosing an appropriate prosthesis after amputation. A couple things to remember include the fact that recovery from upper extremity amputation is not as good as lower extremity and the remaining segment length is crucial to prosthetic suspension and leverage (optimal length is the junction of the mid to distal third of the forearm). In order to have a higher rate of acceptance and use (approximately 85%), the prosthesis needs to be fitted within the first 30 days compared with when the fitting is delayed (less than 30%). There are 3 basic means to control the upper extremity prosthesis: body power, electric switch control, or myoelectrically.

1. Body-powered device: Garners a terminal device or hook and is best for heavier labor. A harness is worn about the shoulders (harness ring optimally sits at the spinous process of C7); abduction of the scapulae opens the device, and relaxing the shoulders closes the device. Alternatively, elbow flexion and extension are manipulated by shoulder extension and depression.

2. Myoelectric prosthesis: Provides a good cosmetic limb and is best for sedentary individuals. The function of this prosthesis is best with a working elbow and is powered by EMG sensors that are built into the prosthetic socket. It affords the ability to perform overhead activities and can be used in any position.

3. Switch control: The prosthetic contains a length-activated switch within the harness itself. A specific motion is then used to trigger the terminal device, with actions being performed sequentially and not simultaneously.

In our case, the patient is a laborer and is likely to benefit from a body-powered device on recovery. Similarly, during his recovery from the pelvic fracture, he will need a higher/heavier level of function, at least in the first few months of rehabilitation.

Why Might This Be Tested? Gait analysis is often tested in terms of establishing what a pathological condition is, and understanding the basics is important. Similarly, memorizing upper-extremity prostheses and how they function will net you 1 or 2 test questions.

Here's the Point!

Know the gait cycle! An antalgic gait involves a decreased stance phase on the affected limb. Transradial amputations should be fitted for a prosthesis within the first 30 days and will function best with the amputation at the mid to distal third of the forearm.

Vignette 84: Spinal Anatomy Teaser

A 40-year-old female presents with back pain and radiating pain down her right leg. The symptoms began after lifting a heavy box yesterday. She is grossly neurologically intact to motor and sensory function without focal deficit. The only pertinent physical exam finding is reproducible pain when extending the ipsilateral knee 30 degrees. The pain worsens with dorsiflexion of the ipsilateral ankle.

▶ *What is an appropriate initial course of action?*

The patient returns to the clinic 6 weeks later and still has pain, although it is a little better than before. She states that she cannot live with this pain any longer. Her physical examination is still stable and unchanged from before. The patient has been compliant with her therapy regimen, and an MRI is ordered.

▶ *Based on her clinical symptoms, where would her disk pathology be if the herniation resembled that seen in Figure 84-1?*

▶ *Which nerve root level would you anticipate being affected based on the type of herniated disk seen in Figure 84-1?*

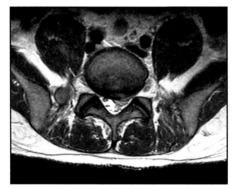

Figure 84-1. Axial MRI of the lumbar spine at the L3-L4 disk space.

▶ *Based on her clinical symptoms, where would her disk pathology be if the herniation resembled that seen in Figure 84-2?*

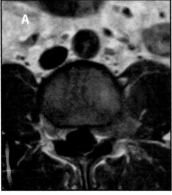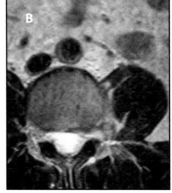

Figure 84-2. (A) Axial T1- and (B) T2-weighted MRIs of the lumbar spine at L5-S1.

► *Three scenarios of motor, sensory, and reflex deficits are listed in Table 84-1. Which nerve root level would you anticipate being affected based on the type of herniated disk seen in Figure 84-2?*

Table 84-1.		
THREE MOTOR, SENSORY, AND REFLEX DEFICIT SCENARIOS		
Motor	*Sensation*	*Reflex*
A	Tibialis anterior	Anteromedial leg	Quadriceps
B	Gastrocnemius	Sole of foot	Achilles
C	Extensor hallucis longus	First web space	

Vignette 84: Answer

The patient has lumbar disk herniation. To treat disk herniation, various studies demonstrate benefits from nonoperative measures acutely. Unless a patient demonstrates cauda equina or profound motor loss, they deserve a trial of nonoperative measures, which includes physical therapy, a brief period of rest, and some formula of pain medication (NSAIDs, muscle relaxants, narcotics). For the most part, x-rays can be obtained after a course of nonoperative management because most will get better with 4 to 6 weeks of management. The most recent large, multicentered study, the Spine Patient Outcomes Research Trial lumbar herniation arm, demonstrated improvement clinically in both nonoperative and operative patient groups. At 4 years, patients who underwent surgery may have a slightly better outcome; however, this result is confounded by many patients who crossed over from the nonoperative group to the operative group in this study.[261]

Once surgery is agreed on as the definitive treatment modality, the results are highly successful. However, patients should be counseled that the reherniation rates average around 10% to 20%.[68,69,262,263] There is little evidence to suggest that a minimally invasive approach for a microdiskectomy fares worse than a traditional open procedure. However, it is widely accepted that a subtotal diskectomy decreases the risk of recurrence but increases back pain compared with a fragmentectomy.[263]

The first step in localizing the pathology is deciding which nerve root is affected. S1 function is assessed by plantarflexion and eversion of the foot. Extensor hallucis longus strength is dictated primarily by L5 function, whereas tibialis anterior strength is associated with L4. Quadriceps strength is indicative of L3 and L4, whereas iliopsoas is dictated by L1 and L2. In terms of sensation, the S1 nerve root innervates the posterior calf, the lateral foot, and the sole. The L5 nerve root involves the lateral calf and the first dorsal webspace. L4 involves the medial ankle and the anterior shin. Lastly, L4 is the predominate root for the knee reflex and S1 for the ankle reflex.

Once the nerve root is identified, one needs to determine the location of compression. At the disk level, 3 regions can be identified, including central, lateral recess, and foraminal. Because the nerve roots in the lumbar spine take off from the spinal cord more cranial than their exiting foramen, at each disk level, there is an exiting nerve root and a traversing nerve root. For example, at the L4-L5 disk space, the L4 nerve root exits the foramen and L5 traverses the disk space in preparation of exiting at the L5-S1 disk space. The most common disk herniation is a posterolateral herniation, which compresses the traversing nerve root; at the L4-L5 disk space, the L5 nerve root is compressed while the L4 nerve root has already exited the foramen. A far lateral disk herniation compresses the exiting nerve root, so at the L4-L5 disk space, it compresses the L4 nerve root while it exits or after it exits the foramen. These types of disk herniation are more common in older patients, typically at the L3-L4 and L4-L5 levels.

Why Might This Be Tested? Lumbar disk herniation is a common problem. Fortunately, many patients can be treated nonoperatively. Two types of disk herniation exist: far lateral herniation and, most commonly, posterolateral disk herniation. Interpreting MRI findings will help decipher which type of herniation the patient is suffering from, and sound knowledge of the spinal anatomy will allow one to answer the question correctly.

Here's the Point!

Determine if the herniation is a posterolateral or far lateral herniation in order to figure out which nerve root is affected. Posterolateral = traversing nerve root. Far lateral = exiting nerve root. Know your anatomy. Enough said!

Vignette 85: Soccer Player Hears a Pop in the Knee!

A 20-year-old female soccer player is running behind a play when the ball is reversed, and as she cuts sharply to follow the play, she immediately feels a pop in her right knee and slides to the ground. The patient experiences an acute onset of pain and swelling with difficulty weight bearing when helped off the field. The team's athletic trainer later notes swelling of the injured knee. The patient presents to the clinic later that week.

▶ *What is the most likely diagnosis?*

▶ *What are the patient's treatment options?*

Vignette 85: Answer

In this patient, the most likely diagnosis is an ACL tear. The hints are young, female athlete, pop, and early knee effusion. In order to further assess this patient, a physical examination would include Lachman's test, which should always be compared with the unaffected knee (translation of >10 mm indicates ACL injury), as well as the pivot shift test. Lachman's is the best test to rule in or rule out ACL injury, whereas the pivot shift test has a high positive predictive value but lower sensitivity.[264] The pivot shift test better assesses the rotational stability of the injured knee.[265] Plain x-rays are typically ordered to rule out any fractures (patella, tibial plateau, or distal femur), whereas MRIs are ordered to assess ligamentous and cartilaginous structures. A good-quality MRI will show ACL tears in more than 95% of cases, although imaging studies are rarely needed because history and clinical exam are often enough to make the diagnosis.

For patients with partial ACL tears with no instability, with complete tears in which the patient has more of a sedentary lifestyle or will decrease athletics activities, and when the epiphyseal plate is still open, nonoperative treatment is usually pursued. Nonoperative treatment involves rehabilitation and physical therapy, especially closed-chain therapy, which strengthens the hamstring and quadriceps to improve knee stability. Some studies have suggested that the incidence of OA is higher in those undergoing nonoperative management of an ACL injury, although others have shown no difference. Patients who choose conservative treatment may eventually have surgery for ACL repair due to continued knee instability.[73]

There are multiple graft options for patients who undergo surgery. The most commonly used grafts are bone–patellar tendon–bone autograft, allograft, and quadrupled semitendinosus/gracilis hamstring autograft. The main advantage of a patellar autograft is the improved incorporation of the graft because of the bone-to-bone healing; disadvantages include anterior knee pain, patellar fracture or tendon rupture, and cosmetic concerns. A quadruple-bundled semitendinosus/gracilis autograft involves quadruple bundling of the semitendinosus with the gracilis. The advantage of this includes less postoperative pain. Disadvantages include slower incorporation of the graft into bone, increased KT-1000 (MedMetric), and decreased knee flexion strength. Allografts have become more popular recently and are indicated in patients older than 40 years, with more sedentary lifestyles, who need an earlier return to activity, have medical comorbidities as the operating time is decreased, or have a poor autologous graft site. Advantages include decreased morbidity due to no harvest site, earlier return of motion, and improved cosmesis; disadvantages include slower graft incorporation and the potential for disease transmission.[266]

For single-bundle ACL reconstruction, the intra-articular landmarks of the tibial ACL footprint include lateral to the slope of the medial eminence, medial to the posterior border of the anterior horn of the lateral meniscus, and 7 mm anterior to the PCL (Figure 85-1). The femoral tunnel footprint has been described at the intersection of the intercondylar ridge and the bifurcate ridge on the medial aspect of the lateral femoral condyle (Figure 85-2). The most common complications with ACL surgery are aberrant tunnel placement (usually too anterior, resident's ridge!) and stiffness after early surgical reconstruction. Anterior tunnel placement limits knee flexion, and arthrofibrosis often plagues early ACL surgeries.

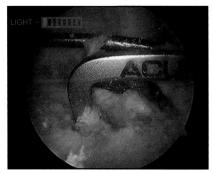

Figure 85-1. Arthroscopic view of the tibial guide for the tibial ACL footprint.

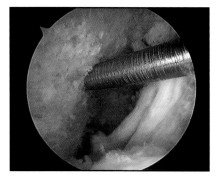

Figure 85-2. Arthroscopic view of a flexible guidewire in the femoral ACL footprint at the intersection of the intercondylar ridge and the bifurcate ridge.

Recently, there has been increased interest in double-bundle ACL reconstruction with the idea of providing translation and rotational stability; however, anatomic single-bundle ACL reconstruction may provide similar stability without the increased technical demands of the double-bundle ACL reconstruction (Figure 85-3).[267]

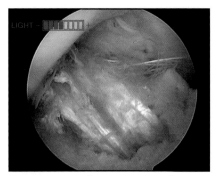

Figure 85-3. Arthroscopic view of an anatomic ACL reconstruction with hamstring autograft.

Why Might This Be Tested? ACL tears are one of the most common sports injuries, and ACL injuries are common on exams. Their presentation and treatment are important concepts, especially in regard to tunnel placement.

Here's the Point!

ACL tears are common sports injuries that should be assessed with Lachman's test and pivot shift test. Surgical management gives good results with all graft options when placed correctly (avoid anterior graft tunnels).

Vignette 86: I Fell From the Roof and Shattered My Ankle

A 43-year-old male presents to the emergency department with right lower extremity pain and deformity after a fall from a roof 16 feet above ground level. He denies any loss of consciousness following the accident, but he is unable to bear weight on his right lower extremity. He is a construction worker and smokes on average 1 to 2 packs of cigarettes per day. On exam of his right lower extremity, there is obvious deformity and shortening of his right lower extremity, most noticeably at the ankle. On palpation of the lower extremity, the lower leg compartments are full but compressible. Sensation is intact distally, and pulses of dorsalis pedis and posterior tibial arteries are palpable. AP and lateral x-rays of the distal tibia and fibula are shown in Figure 86-1.

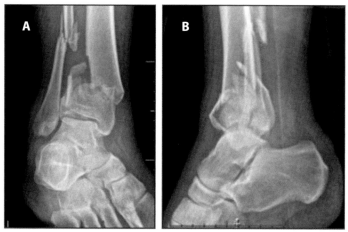

Figure 86-1. (A) AP and (B) lateral x-rays of the right ankle.

▶ *What is the diagnosis?*

▶ *What are other associated injuries?*

▶ *What is the management for this injury?*

Vignette 86: Answer

The patient has a pilon (ie, tibial plafond) fracture. These injuries are the result of a high-energy axial compression mechanism or low-energy rotational injury. The high-energy injuries are associated with increased comminution and significant adjacent soft tissue damage.

Associated injuries include a fracture to the contralateral extremity and/or foot, but a fracture anywhere from the ipsilateral foot to the lumbar spine should be ruled out because the transmitted axial force could result in associated fractures.[268,269] Unlike proximal tibia and diaphyseal tibia fractures, compartment syndrome following a pilon fracture is rare, reported to occur in 0% to 5% of cases. Nonetheless, alert patients should be evaluated routinely for pain (usually out of proportion to examination) with passive stretch to screen for compartment syndrome.

The management of soft tissue and osseous injuries is the primary determinant of fracture healing and functional restoration of the traumatized extremity. As such, the patient's skin is carefully inspected for abrasions, open wounds, and fracture blisters, and a thorough vascular exam of the injured extremity is performed. It is vital to recognize that a variety of underlying comorbidities can affect the ultimate treatment of open fractures as well as the local soft tissues. Thus, obtaining information regarding a patient's medical comorbidities (diabetes mellitus, collagen vascular disease, chronic venous insufficiency, nutritional deficiencies) and use of nicotine (peripheral vascular disease) is of great value. Moreover, knowing the patient's highest level of education, occupation, and workers' compensation status is necessary because these factors, in addition to the aforementioned medical issues, have been shown to affect functional outcome. Previous fractures or surgical incisional scars should be documented. A standard ankle x-ray series and full-length tibia and fibula x-rays are required to fully evaluate the injured extremity and begin surgical planning.

After initial assessment and stabilization, a decision must be made regarding when to obtain a CT scan and whether to perform staged vs definitive surgical fixation. CT scans help define the extent of articular involvement and assist with planning the surgical approach. In patients who are candidates to undergo staged fixation, the CT scan should be obtained after temporizing spanning external fixation to better illustrate fracture fragment orientation and displacement. In patients with relatively simple fracture patterns with mild-to-moderate displacement in the setting of mild soft tissue damage, it is reasonable to obtain a CT scan prior to surgical intervention because these patients will likely be candidates for single-stage definitive fixation.

Nonoperative management should be considered only for nondisplaced fractures or in patients with severe contraindications to surgery because studies elucidate poor outcomes in such a population. The following goals of operative intervention proposed by Ruedi and Allgower in 1969 remain applicable today: (1) reduction and stabilization of associated fibular fracture to restore the length of the lateral column and correct valgus deformity in the distal tibia, (2) anatomic restoration of the tibial articular surface, (3) autologous bone grafting of metaphyseal defects to prevent collapse, and (4) buttress plating of the medial tibia to prevent varus angulation and neutralize rotational forces.

It is well known that complications, such as infection, wound breakdown, malunion, and nonunion, create grave situations that may lead to amputation, particularly in patients treated with early ORIF. Current management and operative techniques, which have evolved over the past 20 years, have led to a specific protocol followed in pilon fracture management. Management consisting of initial external fixation with or without fibular fixation and followed by delayed ORIF is the standard strategy for most pilon fractures.[269] Although a recent study demonstrated that low wound complications rates could be obtained following early definitive operative fixation, the majority of the patients in the study had a soft tissue envelope that was amendable to early surgical intervention.

Plating the fibula at the time of placing an ankle-spanning external fixator remains controversial. Although equally good results have been reported with or without fibular plate fixation at the time of external fixator application, debate remains among surgeons as to when the fibula should be fixed. Some authors argue that addressing the fibula restores length and rotation and assists in the reduction of the tibia. The problem with fixing the fibula initially, however, is related to wound complications and fibula malreduction, which leads others to favor fibula fixation at the time of definitive tibial ORIF.[269] Methodology used for definitive treatment of the tibia is predicated on surgeon experience, the amount of comminution, and the degree of soft tissue damage. As such, pilon fractures can be definitively fixed with Ilizarov or hybrid ring external fixators, minimally invasive plate osteosynthesis, periarticular locked plating, or some combination thereof. Discussing the merits of each method is beyond the scope of this vignette.

Pilon fractures are devastating injuries and can result in diminished patient function and numerous complications. With modern practices, superficial infections have been reported in 5% to 17% of cases, and there is always risk of deep infection, osteomyelitis, and nonunion. Although posttraumatic arthrosis is extremely common after injury, its effect on clinical outcome remains unclear. Most patients who sustain a pilon fracture develop ankle pain and diminished function, as well as an overall negative effect on general health. Contrary to other intra-articular fractures, quality of reduction has not been shown to positively affect patient outcomes. As such, priority must be given to the soft tissue injury to minimize complications. As mentioned previously, medical comorbidities, nicotine use, level of education, occupation, and workers' compensation status have all been shown to effect outcome.

Why Might This Be Tested? Diagnosis and initial workup for pilon fractures is essential for every practicing orthopedic surgeon. Early application of an ankle-spanning external fixator, with or without fibula fixation, is now the standard. The patient should then be followed until resolution of the soft tissue injury or should be referred to a more experienced traumatologist for definitive fixation.

Here's the Point!

Pilon fractures occur as a result of high-energy axial compression or low-energy rotational injuries. Clinical factors that should be taken into account with these injuries include tenseness of the skin, presence and nature of fracture blisters, degree of comminution, and planned stabilization technique and its invasiveness. The standard of care has evolved to a staged treatment with early application of an ankle-spanning external fixator, with or without fibula fixation, followed by definitive fixation of the tibia once soft tissue swelling resolves.

Vignette 87: Doc, I Hurt My Shoulder at Work Lifting This Heavy Box

A 63-year-old male presents with a 3-week history of left shoulder pain. The pain started after lifting a heavy box over his head at work. He localizes his pain to the lateral aspect of his shoulder and has pain at night. The pain is partially relieved with NSAIDs. He had no symptoms prior to 3 weeks ago. Initially, he was started on some rotator cuff–directed physical therapy with reasonable success. However, due to persistent pain and the fact he was not yet at 100%, he returned to the office. Subsequent radiographic evaluation was obtained, including plain x-rays and MRIs of the shoulder (Figures 87-1 and 87-2).

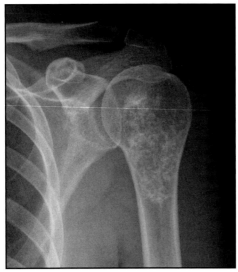

Figure 87-1. AP x-ray of the left shoulder.

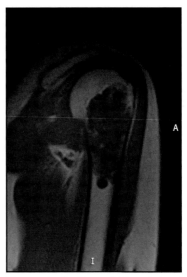

Figure 87-2. Coronal T1-weighted MRI slice of the left shoulder.

▶ *What is the diagnosis?*

▶ *What are the treatment options?*

Vignette 87: Answer

Enchondromas are one of the most common neoplastic entities encountered. The true incidence is unknown because most are asymptomatic and found incidentally (as in our case, the majority of the pain was from rotator cuff tendinitis). Enchondromas are asymptomatic, but patients often present with pain. It is important to confirm an alternate source of pain, commonly OA or meniscal pathology in the knee, greater trochanteric bursitis in the hip, and rotator cuff tendonitis in the shoulder. The features can have significant overlap with CHS, and the presence of unexplained pain is worrisome for a more aggressive process. Approximately 50% of solitary enchondromas are found in the hands. The other common locations include the proximal and distal femur and proximal humerus.

Radiographically, there is an obvious chondroid matrix, usually with intratumoral mineralization and stippled calcifications (remember, popcorn calcifications = cartilage tumor). In the hands, enchondromas may not have any matrix, but rather just appear as lytic lesions. Enchondromas can appear similar radiographically to low-grade CHS. It is important to look for findings that may suggest an aggressive lesion, such as poorly defined borders, cortical breakage, periosteal reaction, a soft tissue extension, or growth over time (in our case, although it is a large lesion, there are no cortical breaks or soft tissue extension). Enchondromas in smaller bones (hand) can appear radiographically aggressive. If there are no worrisome features, advanced imaging studies are unnecessary.

Histologically, enchondromas and low-grade CHSs are indistinguishable. The diagnosis must be made in context of the radiographic studies and clinical presentation. Microscopically, the tumor is simply low-grade cartilage in irregular nests. It is hypercellular compared with normal cartilage, but nuclear atypia is rare. (You have to pay attention to the vignette; enchondromas are typically found incidentally, and CHSs are a cause for the workup.)

The treatment of a radiographically low-grade cartilaginous neoplasm is observation with serial x-rays. Typically, these lesions are monitored for 2 years to document stability. Serial monitoring of benign-appearing lesions that are not symptomatic is the typical recommendation for many tumors and tumor-like conditions (enchondroma, osteochondroma, bone infarcts, nonossifying fibroma, unicameral bone cysts). When surgery is needed, curettage and bone grafting is usually performed. A small number of enchondromas (< 1%) can undergo malignant degeneration, and complaints of new, unexplained pain in the area should be taken seriously and imaged.

Why Might This Be Tested? Enchondromas are a common benign cartilage tumor. They are often histologically similar to CHS, so they are typically on standardized tests to assure you know the difference. The treatment and prognosis are radically different, so know the 2 entities.

Here's the Point!

Enchondromas are benign cartilage tumors that often present as an incidental finding (the history distinguishes them from CHS) during the workup of knee or shoulder pain. These lesions can be watched and monitored without further treatment. On rare occasion, they can undergo malignant transformation, so pay attention to the history of new-onset pain around a known enchondroma.

Vignette 88: Is This Really a Baker's Cyst or Something Else?

A 42-year-old male has moderate activity-related pain and swelling in the posterior aspect of his knee. He states that a doctor told him he had a Baker's cyst 2 years ago. He does not have pain at rest and he does not report any fevers or weight loss. Plain x-rays show no specific findings and are inconclusive. Subsequently, an MRI and biopsy are performed (Figures 88-1 to 88-3).

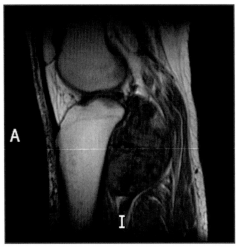

Figure 88-1. Sagittal T1-weighted MRI cut of the knee.

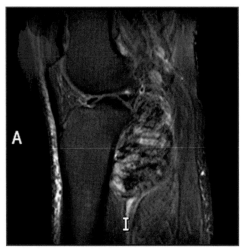

Figure 88-2. Sagittal T2-weighted MRI cut of the knee.

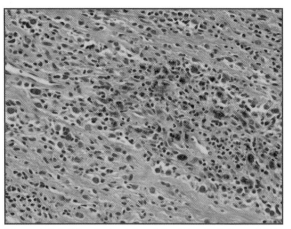

Figure 88-3. Histology slide of the biopsied tissue (400x magnification).

▶ *What is the diagnosis?*

▶ *What are the options for treatment?*

Vignette 88: Answer

Pigmented villonodular synovitis (PVNS) is a primary disease of the synovium. There has been much debate over whether this is a neoplastic or inflammatory condition. Reactions similar to PVNS have been observed after simulation of a hemarthrosis, such as would be seen after trauma or in hemophilia. However, most patients report no history of trauma. PVNS does not behave completely like a neoplastic condition either, but chromosomal abnormalities (5q33 abnormality and increased CSF1 gene expression) have been identified in the tumor mass.

PVNS is typically monoarticular and affects the knee most commonly. Other sites include the hip, ankle, shoulder, and elbow. Most patients are in the third or fourth decade of life at diagnosis. The clinical course can be slow and indolent, mimicking other intra-articular pathology, such as meniscal tears or inflammatory arthritis. Patients are often between 30 and 50 years old, with no sex predilection noted.

The 2 forms of PVNS are focal and diffuse. Focal PVNS is also known as GCT of the tendon sheath and is most commonly seen in the anterior aspect of the knee. These patients often complain of mechanical symptoms. Diffuse PVNS can affect the entire synovial lining. In the knee, this includes the anterior and posterior compartments and the medial and lateral gutters and extends into the surrounding bursal tissue. Bony erosions are common, and degenerative changes may be seen in prolonged disease.

Although plain x-rays may show periarticular erosions and joint space narrowing, MRI is typically more revealing. Due to the large amount of hemosiderin (key word), the signal tends to be dark, but heterogeneous, on T1- and T2-weighted images. MRI should be analyzed carefully to assess the extent of disease for management decisions and preoperative planning. A joint aspiration classically yields brownish-tinged bloody fluid. Histologically, diffuse, expansile sheets of mononuclear cells with areas of hemosiderin-deposition are characteristic of this tumor. The mononuclear component is composed of small histiocyte-like cells and ovoid- to spindle-shaped cells with pale eosinophilic cytoplasm. Hemosiderin-laden macrophages are characteristic.

The treatment of nonrecurrent PVNS is surgical excision. There is some debate about whether arthroscopic or open synovectomy is superior. Regardless of the method, the goal is a complete synovectomy because the recurrence rate is known to be higher after partial synovectomy. In the presence of bony erosion, large amounts of posterior disease, and extension into the surrounding bursal areas, open excision is preferred. The recurrence rates have been reported to range from around 10% to nearly 50%.

Recurrent disease is more challenging. Adjuvant treatment with external beam radiation (3500 to 4000 cGy) and intra-articular injection of radioisotopes may be useful after surgical resection or in isolation. Imatinib, a tyrosine kinase inhibitor, has been shown to be effective in PVNS; however, the optimal indications and duration of treatment remain undefined. TJA should be considered in multiply recurrent painful disease and in the presence of significant joint degeneration.

Why Might This Be Tested? This is a relatively common disorder and can be confused for many other syndromes and injuries. With many giant cells on histological exam, it may be mistaken for other tumors, such as GCT and ABC. Treatment is potentially controversial, so it makes for a good topic for questions.

Here's the Point!

With PVNS, look for hemosiderin on the histology; you will see it inside of multinucleated giant cells. Recurrent hemarthrosis is common, and patients typically have mechanical pain and limited motion. Treatment is a complete synovectomy (open or via scope). Recurrence is common if not complete, and radiation can be used as an adjunct.

Vignette 89: Pigmented Villonodular Synovitis

A 35-year-old obese male with a history of a traumatic fall onto the left hip 3 years ago without fracture or dislocation presents with recurrent diffuse left hip pain. The pain has progressed over the past 3 years and is made worse with physical activity. On physical examination, the patient has severe pain throughout the entire left hip during ROM testing. There is no notable local erythema or effusion noted, but the examination is limited due to his body habitus. The patient is neurovascularly intact with negative anterior and posterior impingement tests. An initial x-ray and histological slides obtained at the time of surgery are shown in Figures 89-1 to 89-3.

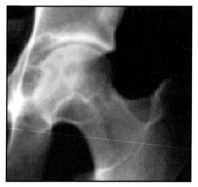

Figure 89-1. Plain x-ray of the hip showing cystic erosions but a preserved joint space.

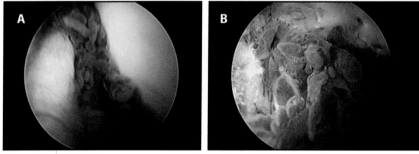

Figure 89-2. (A, B) Macroscopic appearance of the hip joint synovium.

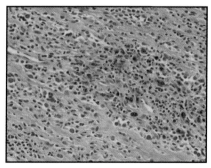

Figure 89-3. Microscopic appearance of the hip joint synovium.

▶ *What is the differential diagnosis?*

▶ *What history and physical exam findings are important to help determine the diagnosis?*

▶ *What other tests should be ordered?*

▶ *What test findings help lead to the final diagnosis?*

▶ *What are the treatment options?*

Vignette 89: Answer

PVNS is a proliferative monoarticular synovial process characterized by recurrent hemorrhage, mononuclear stromal cells, histiocytes, and giant cells. PVNS most commonly occurs in patients aged 30 to 50 years (but can also occur in teenagers) with equal sex distribution. PVNS can occur focally or diffusely and can also be intra- or extra-articular as with a GCT of a tendon sheath. The disease process is thought to be reactive (associated with an earlier traumatic event, like our case) rather than neoplastic.[270-274]

Common clinical findings include pain, swelling, effusion, erythema, and decreased ROM with reported mechanical (locking and/or catching) joint symptoms. PVNS most commonly affects the knee (80% of cases) in addition to the hip, shoulder, and ankle, but the extra-articular form is more commonly found in the hand and wrist. Recurrent atraumatic hemarthrosis is the classic presentation of the disease (rust-color effusions). Differential diagnosis for PVNS includes reactive or inflammatory synovitis, hemophilia, or synovial chondromatosis, but it can also be mistaken for DJD, labral tears, and femoroacetabular impingement if adequate workup is not obtained.

Synovial chondromatosis is a metaplastic proliferation of hyaline cartilage nodules in the synovial membrane and commonly occurs in patients aged 30 to 50 years with a 2:1 male:female ratio. Presenting symptoms are similar to those with PVNS and also commonly occur in the knee, hip, and shoulder. Plain x-rays show variable findings of bony erosions and calcification, whereas CT shows intra-articular loose bodies and MRI can reveal lobular lesions with calcification. Gross pathology shows osteocartilaginous loose bodies, and histology shows hyaline cartilage nodules in various phases of calcification. Advanced imaging and histology can clearly differentiate PVNS from synovial chondromatosis.

Typical findings of PVNS on plain x-rays and CT show cystic erosions on both sides of the joint with advanced disease (see Figure 89-1). T1- and T2-weighted MRI may reveal a focal low-signal nodule within the joint or a diffuse process with low signal intensity. The low signal intensity is caused by hemosiderin (key word with PVNS!) deposition in the joint. MRI may also show a fat signal within the lesion and extra-articular extension of the mass.

Gross pathology from lesions often shows red-brown–stained synovium with numerous papillary projections. A more detailed histologic analysis reveals a mononuclear stromal cell infiltrate in the synovium (see Figure 89-2). Histology may also show hemosiderin-filled macrophages, multinucleated giant cells, mitotic figures, and foam cells, although these findings are not necessary for final diagnosis (see Figure 89-3).

Treatment of PVNS consists of arthroscopic and/or open removal of focal lesion(s), whereas diffuse forms of the disease require aggressive total synovectomy arthroscopically or via an open approach. An anterior arthroscopic synovectomy with an open posterior lesion removal may be used to help remove extra-articular disease. Extra-articular lesions of tendon sheaths are treated with marginal excision. The occurrence of subsequent lesions after surgery indicates incomplete synovectomy, but open and arthroscopic techniques have been shown to have high recurrence rates (up to 30% to 50% local recurrence rate). TJA is indicated in cases of advanced PVNS with concurrent DJD. External beam radiation (3500 to 4000 cGy is recommended) may also be used in select cases of multiple lesion recurrences and can reduce the recurrence rate by 10% to 20%.

Why Might This Be Tested? Hip synovial disease often has a variable presentation and can be easily confused with DJD, labral tears, femoroacetabular impingement, and a number of other conditions. PVNS is a commonly tested subject, and it's important to know the locations of occurrence, radiographic findings, histologic assessment, and treatment.

Here's the Point!

PVNS is a common disorder, and the diagnosis is confirmed with histology findings (hemosiderin-filled macrophages, multinucleated giant cells, mitotic figures, and foam cells). Differentiate from other disorders and look for the hemosiderin!

Vignette 90: Doc, Everything Hurts!

A 52-year-old female presents with bilateral knee pain that continues to worsen. The pain has progressively worsened over the past 8 to 10 months, and she has self-medicated with NSAIDs with limited success in controlling her pain. She has a history of multiple other joint complaints and is significantly disabled by her foot, hand, and wrist involvement dating back approximately 2 to 3 years. The patient complains of generalized malaise, weakness, and stiffness in the morning when she first awakes. She denies any rashes or skin changes other than some nodules that periodically arise on the extensor surfaces of her upper and lower extremities. A 50-pack-per-year history of smoking and no alcohol use is elicited upon questioning her social history. She has not been treated for this condition and is seeking your assistance in establishing a diagnosis. Her bilateral knee x-ray is shown in Figure 90-1.

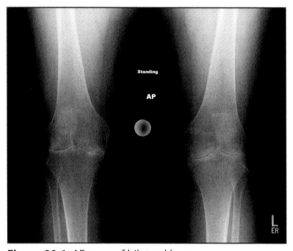

Figure 90-1. AP x-ray of bilateral knees.

▶ *What is her diagnosis?*

▶ *What is the differential diagnosis?*

▶ *What tests should be ordered to establish the diagnosis?*

Now that you have established the diagnosis, the patient wants to know what her options are for treatment.

▶ *What are the patient's initial treatment options?*

▶ *Discuss the risk, benefits, and alternatives of nonoperative management for her condition.*

Three years later, the patient reports back with continued knee pain and states that conservative management is no longer helping her at all and she is seeking surgical treatment options.

▶ *What are her surgical options?*

▶ *What is the best way to handle her perioperative medication regimen?*

Vignette 90: Answer

Part I

The patient's diagnosis is RA. RA is the most common inflammatory arthropathy in the United States, with approximately 25 and 54 cases per 100,000 persons for males and females, respectively.[275] Historically, this disease was devastating, with 20% to 30% of untreated patients becoming permanently disabled within 3 years of diagnosis.[275] The etiology and pathophysiology of RA appear to be related to a combination of environmental and genetic factors, with a 30% concordance rate for monozygotic twins and 80% of White patients with RA expressing the HLA-DR1 or DR4 subtypes. In a nutshell, this is an autoimmune disease in which the patient's own body attacks itself, and joint damage is associated with proliferation of the synovium, synovial macrophages, and fibroblasts. Gradually, there is formation of an invasive, inflamed synovial tissue or pannus that destroys adjacent cartilage and bone as a locally and systemically destructive cocktail of agents are released (cytokines, ILs, proteinases, and growth factors).

To establish the diagnosis, one needs to look at the clues described in the vignette, including female sex, age (onset 30s to 50s), smoking, pain and morning stiffness in multiple joints, weakness, malaise/prodromal symptoms (8% to 15% of cases have symptoms that start within a few days of an infectious illness), hand/wrist involvement, RA nodules (on extensor surfaces), and x-rays that show severe articular destruction with minimal osteophyte formation and diffuse periarticular osteopenia. Other associated risk factors include consumption of more than 3 cups of coffee daily, positive family history, and silicate exposure.[275] However, high vitamin D intake, tea consumption, and oral contraceptive use have been shown to confer a protective effect. The following 7 criteria have been established by the American Rheumatism Association: morning stiffness, arthritis of 3 or more joints, hand involvement, symmetric arthritis, rheumatoid nodules, serum RF positive, and radiographic changes.[275]

The differential diagnosis includes OA, septic arthritis, SLE, gout, scleroderma, fibromyalgia (trigger points commonly found), hemochromatosis (skin changes), polymyalgia rheumatica, sarcoidosis (granulomas), seronegative spondyloarthropathies (psoriasis, Reiter syndrome, inflammatory bowel disease), Still's disease (sore throat, splenomegaly, leukocytosis), thyroid disease, and viral arthritis.[275]

Now that we think we know what we are dealing with, it is important to order the right—or at least best—tests that will confirm the diagnosis. The first tests we start with are the orthopod's go-to tests: ESR and CRP. The ESR is an indirect measure of systemic inflammation and is affected by many factors that artificially increase (inflammatory disease: RA, SLE, infection, increased proteins [myeloma, tissue necrosis], trauma, tumor, heart attack, pregnancy, age, obesity) or decrease (increased plasma viscosity, abnormal red cell shape [sickle cell disease, decreased plasma proteins], hepatic failure/malnutrition, and trichinosis) this value.[276] Elevated levels (typically normal range, 0 to 20 or 30 depending on the laboratory) are common with RA, and results greater than 100 are almost always associated with underlying pathology. The CRP is the second test and is a protein that is produced by the liver under the influence of IL-1 and IL-6. This typically arises early in an acute inflammatory scenario, peaks within 4 to 5 days, and then returns to normal relatively quickly. For some reason, this test has not been standardized for values, so always check the normal ranges for your laboratory.

More specialized tests that we leave for the rheumatologist to order but should know about include the following[276]:

- RF: This is an IgM antibody directed against the Fx portion of the patient's own IgG. IgA RF may predict a more severe disease course but is often not measured. It can be measured with a latex agglutination test (positive is > 1:40 titer), nephelometry (normal, < 20 IU), or enzyme-linked immunosorbent assay (ELISA). RF is not a perfect test, but it follows these guidelines: the higher the level, the worse the prognosis; positive in 70% to 90% of patients with RA and positive in other rheumatologic diseases, aging, idiopathic pulmonary fibrosis, cirrhosis, and sarcoidosis.

- Antinuclear antibodies (ANA): Done in 2 stages. First, the fluorescent antinuclear antibody test is done. If it's positive, a more specific ANA test (ELISA) is done to classify the autoimmune syndrome. A negative test is helpful in ruling out an autoimmune disorder.

- Anticyclic citrullinated peptide (anti-CCP2 is the most common assay): Citrullination of proteins can occur with many processes; however, in RA, there is a somewhat unique ability to form antibodies to these products. It appears to be as sensitive as RF (64% to 89%) but more specific (up to 99%).

- Anticardiolipin antibodies and lupus anticoagulant: Mostly used to evaluate for SLE and a hypercoagulability state.

- HLA B27: When this antigen is present, it indicates a high risk of spondyloarthropathies. Eighty percent of those with Reiter's syndrome carry the antigen, as do approximately 90% of those with ankylosing spondylitis (AS).

- Uric acid: May be used to determine if gout is a possibility.

- Lyme disease: Should be ordered if clinically suspected. This would be a person in the northeast or upper Midwest of the US—just another reason to live in a warmer climate! The initial test is an ELISA and is then confirmed by a Western blot analysis.

For our patient, an ESR, CRP, RF, and ANA would have been appropriate to establish the diagnosis based on the history, clinical exam, and x-rays. A joint aspiration can also be done and typically will show 5000 to 25,000 WBCs, with up to 85% PMNs in the absence of crystals and negative cultures.

Why Might This Be Tested? Making the correct diagnosis is important in these cases, and many vignettes will relate to inflammatory arthropathies. You need to know the correct tests and how to work these patients up so you can interpret vignettes correctly.

Here's the Point!

Know the diagnosis of RA, laboratory tests, 7 criteria of the American Rheumatism Association, and physical exam findings.

Part II

Once the diagnosis of RA is determined, all patients should be referred to a rheumatologist for treatment before considering surgical management. The goal is to initiate DMARDs within 3 months of the diagnosis. Therapeutic goals include preservation of activity, quality of life, and affected joints while controlling systemic complications from these DMARDs. Early initiation of DMARDs is important to prevent joint destruction and modify the course of the disease. Initiation of therapy typically involves the use of an oral NSAID, low-dose oral or intra-articular glucocorticoids, and a DMARD. Typically, the first-line DMARD is methotrexate. Recent trends are toward the use of multiple DMARDS to attempt to induce remission started in conjunction or in a staged manner. Other treatment options when DMARDs are not tolerated or radiographic findings are absent include hydroxychloroquine, penicillamine, sulfasalazine, or minocycline.[275,277] The following describes the available medications to treat RA:

1. NSAIDs: Inhibit cyclooxygenase-1 and -2 and are used to reduce joint pain and swelling in RA. This reaction blocks the transformation of arachidonic acid to prostaglandins, prostacyclin, and thromboxanes.[277] These patients must be observed closely for GI complications because they are almost 2 times more likely to have a serious complication with these medicines that are typically thought to be benign. (For those of you who remember: Alonzo Mourning. Enough said!)
   a. Adverse reactions: GI upset, ulcers, kidney dysfunction, hypertension, perioperative bleeding
   b. Perioperative management: Discontinue 5 half-lives before surgery. Aspirin should be stopped 7 to 10 days prior to surgery.

2. Glucocorticoids: Also serve as an anti-inflammatory agent, and doses of prednisone or an equivalent of 10 mg or less are effective in treating RA and may slow down joint destruction. Side effects at higher doses include osteoporosis, ON, cataracts, and Cushingoid symptoms. Those taking oral steroids should take 1500 mg of calcium and 100 to 800 IU of vitamin D daily. Intra-articular injections can also be helpful to treat symptoms of inflammation locally.
   a. Adverse reactions: GI upset, osteoporosis, ON, cataracts, diabetes mellitus, Cushingoid symptoms, wound-healing complications, infections
   b. Perioperative management: Dose based on surgical stress and perioperative stress dosing. Prevents adrenal insufficiency. Minimally stressful surgeries less than 1 hour and under local

anesthesia do not need treatment; mild procedures (arthroscopy) should get 25 mg of hydrocortisone; moderate procedures (ACL reconstruction) require 50 to 75 mg with a tapering of doses; severe procedures (arthroplasty) require 100 to 150 mg hydrocortisone and a 1- to 2-day taper. For intra-articular injections, suggest waiting 6 to 12 weeks after injection for surgery (particularly arthroplasty procedures).

3. DMARDs: Most common medications include:

   a. Methotrexate: A folate analog that inhibits neovascularization, reduces inflammation, and decreases cytokine production (IL-1, IL-8, and TNF). RA flares can often occur within 4 weeks of discontinuation of the drug therapy.

      i.   Adverse reactions: Nausea, diarrhea, fatigue, mouth ulcers, alopecia, abnormal LFTs, low WBC and platelets, pneumonitis, liver disease, Epstein-Barr virus–related lymphoma

      ii. Perioperative management: Originally reported that medication should be stopped 2 weeks prior to surgery and restarted 2 weeks after surgery. However, a recent study has shown a lower infection rate and absence of RA flares if the medicine is not stopped at all. Those with kidney disease or develop kidney dysfunction should use methotrexate with caution, particularly if associated with a moderate- to intensive-type of procedure.

   b. Hydroxychloroquine (Plaquenil): An antimalarial drug, low potency and toxicity.

      i.   Adverse reactions: Nausea, headaches, abdominal pain, myopathy, retinal toxicity

      ii. Perioperative management: May continue through all procedures.

   c. Sulfasalazine (Azulfidine): Has an unknown mechanism of action in RA

      i.   Adverse reactions: Nausea, diarrhea, headache, mouth ulcers, alopecia, contact lens staining, reversible oligospermia, abnormal LFTs

      ii. Perioperative management: May continue for all procedures; beware, may increase INR in conjunction with warfarin administration.

   d. Intramuscular gold: Mechanism of action as anti-inflammatory is debatable.

      i.   Adverse reactions: Mouth ulcers, rash, leukopenia, thrombocytopenia, proteinuria, colitis

   e. Cyclosporine (Gengraf, Neoral): Immunosuppressant agent that binds to protein cyclophilin of lymphocytes, particularly T-cells

      i.   Adverse reactions: Paresthesias, tremor, gingival hypertrophy, hypertrichosis, hypertension, renal disease, sepsis

   f. Azathioprine (Imuran): A purine analog immunosuppressive drug.

      i.   Adverse reactions: Nausea, leukopenia, sepsis, lymphoma

   g. Infliximab (Remicade): A TNF antagonist; structurally it is a chimeric IgG1 anti-TNF-α antibody.

      i.   Adverse reactions: Infusion reactions, infections, tuberculosis reactivation, demyelinating disorders

      ii. Perioperative management: May continue for minor procedures and hold for moderate to intensive procedures for 1 week and restart 10 to 14 days after surgery.

   h. Adalimumab (Humira): A recombinant human IgG1 antibody that has been shown to have an additive effect when combined with methotrexate treatment.

      i.   Adverse reactions: Infusion reactions, increased infection risk, tuberculosis reactivation, demyelinating disorders

      ii. Perioperative management: May continue for minor procedures and hold for moderate to intensive procedures for 1 week and restart 10 to 14 days after surgery.

   i. Etanercept (Enbrel): A TNF-receptor fusion protein that works quickly with symptoms and often responds within 2 weeks of treatment onset.

      i.   Adverse reactions: Infection, injection site reactions, demyelination

      ii. Perioperative management: May continue for minor procedures and hold for moderate to intensive procedures for 1 week and restart 10 to 14 days after surgery.

   j. Leflunomide (Arava): Competitive inhibitor of intracellular enzyme required for pyrimidine synthesis. Inhibits IL1-A and TNF-α and targets rapidly dividing cells. Slows progression of joint damage radiographically.

      i.   Adverse reactions: Nausea, diarrhea, rash, alopecia, leukopenia, hepatitis, thrombocytopenia, teratogen

ii. Perioperative management: Can continue for minor procedures but would hold for 1 to 2 days preoperatively for moderate and intensive procedures and restart 1 to 2 weeks later. Beware, may elevate levels of warfarin.

k. TNF antagonists: Lower levels of TNF-α, which are elevated in the synovial fluid of RA patients.

l. Anakinra (Kineret): An IL-1 receptor antagonist that has shown some response with or without concomitant methotrexate management

i. Adverse reactions: Infections, decreased neutrophils, headaches, nausea, hypersensitivity

ii. Perioperative management: Continue for minor procedures. Hold 1 to 2 days prior to surgical procedure and restart 10 days after for moderate and intensive procedures.

RA is a lifelong illness, and combination therapy is likely to lead to a 30% to 40% remission rate with extended treatment. ESR, CRP, and radiologic assessment may be used to determine the effectiveness of the treatment. American College of Rheumatology improvement criteria include American College of Rheumatology 20, 50, or 70 based on the percentage improvement in the following: tender and swollen joints, global disease activity, pain levels, disability scores, laboratory test values.[275] Complications of untreated RA include anemia, cancer, cardiac complications (pericarditis), cervical spine disease, eye problems, fistula formation, infections, hand deformities (boutonniere and swan neck), respiratory complications, rheumatoid nodules, and vasculitis.

Why Might This Be Tested? RA is well treated with medications, and more questions are being directed toward medical management, mechanism of action, and side effects of these medications.

Here's the Point!

RA is not treated surgically nearly as much as in the past. Know the DMARDs, what they are, what they do, and what side effects they may cause.

Part III

At this point, her surgical options are as follows: synovectomy ± adjunct treatment (radiation shown to be helpful), TKA, or arthrodesis. For this case, the patient has significant degenerative changes and likely would not be a great candidate for synovectomy. However, a recent meta-analysis found that the degree of degenerative changes did not affect outcomes of synovectomy as much as anticipated.[278] They concluded that advanced radiographic changes are not a contraindication to synovectomy. They also found that synovectomy provides relief for 75.2% of patients at an average of 6-year follow-up, with no significant difference in symptomatic relief with open or arthroscopic debridement. It was noted that arthroscopic synovectomy led to a higher rate of recurrence compared to open procedures. Similarly, in approximately 45% of cases, there was progression of the RA despite the synovectomy; this emphasizes the need for continued medical management in this patient population.[278]

Arthrodesis is essentially contraindicated because the patient typically has multiple adjacent and contralateral joints that are affected by RA. Fusion would be an absolute salvage procedure in this patient. However, if you were to go ahead with arthrodesis, the limb should be positioned as follows: 0 to 7 degrees of valgus and 10 to 15 degrees of flexion. For this case, TKA is the best option with the most sustainable period of pain relief. Patients with RA need to follow the recommendations in Part II of this vignette regarding medication management in the perioperative time frame. Successful outcomes have been reported for patients with RA; however, the overall success in improving health-related quality of life is controversial.

Intraoperatively, poor bone stock and osteoporotic bone is the rule, and surgical planning should take this into consideration regarding implant constraint and augmentation options. Cruciate-retaining or -substituting implants can be used with high levels of clinical success. Skin management during TKA is crucial because the immunosuppressant agents often render the skin friable, and one should not hesitate to immobilize the knee for 1 to 2 weeks before initiating motion if the skin closure is tenuous. Unicompartmental or bicompartmental knee arthroplasties are not an option in the setting of RA.

See Part II for the list of medications and how they should be handled in the perioperative period. Unfortunately, you just need to memorize this management; note that it has changed drastically from the prior urban legends of stopping for 6 weeks around the surgery. You need to know the guidelines for stopping medications, but remember methotrexate, corticosteroids, and NSAIDs (selective agents) are okay to continue up to the day of surgery and start immediately postoperatively but that the other DMARDs should be started or stopped based on their half-lives.

Why Might This Be Tested? RA is typically treated medically, but when surgery is needed, these medications need to be handled appropriately. The question writers seem to like complications, and the DMARDS are ripe for the answering in the perioperative period.

Here's the Point!

All TNF-α antagonists should be stopped prior to surgery. Arthrodesis and so-called partial replacements are not options with RA patients; it is TKA or synovectomy.

Vignette 91: What's Wrong With My Elbow?

A 79-year-old female with multiple medical problems sustains a fall from a standing height onto her dominant left arm and has immediate pain and deformity at the elbow. In the emergency room, she has an obvious deformity, with diffuse swelling and ecchymosis centered at the elbow. Her neurovascular exam is grossly intact but limited by her ability to comply. She lives in an assisted living facility but completes all of her own activities of daily living and light shopping. Her x-rays show a comminuted, low distal humerus fracture with intra-articular extension and displacement.

▶ *What other imaging may be beneficial?*

Additional imaging studies are obtained that show a low transcondylar component with at least 4 fragments of intra-articular comminution.

▶ *What are the primary treatment options for this patient? How would you counsel the patient between these 2 options?*

▶ *If you select to perform ORIF, what approach would you use and what are the surgical principles?*

▶ *How would you rehabilitate it depending on what treatment method is chosen?*

Vignette 91: Answer

Traction x-rays are useful for distal humerus fractures to better demonstrate where the fracture lines and fragments are located. Delineating the number and location of fragments not only helps with fracture classification but with treatment as well. CT is also of great benefit, especially for intra-articular injuries to assist with preoperative planning of surgical approaches and implant needs. In this case, the CT scan revealed a low transcondylar component with at least 4 intra-articular fragments.

Distal humerus fractures are relatively uncommon injuries but are technically demanding to treat surgically (classification systems are listed in Table 91-1). For a comminuted intra-articular fracture such as this, low-demand patients (physiologically older patients, with minimal requirements for lifting or use of assistive devices) used to be treated with "bag of bones" nonoperative treatment, which resulted in some motion, typically through a nonunion site. It was later shown that outcome could be improved by anatomic reduction and stable internal fixation with early ROM, especially in younger patients.[279,280]

For low-demand elderly patients, TEA has become an increasingly popular treatment option.[281,282] This is due to the difficulties encountered with ORIF secondary to osteoporotic bone, metaphyseal comminution, and a poor or compromised soft tissue envelope.[280] In several series reviewing elderly patients, ORIF of comminuted intra-articular injuries has led to between 25% and 45% fair and poor results, with up to 25% requiring conversion to TEA. Improved functional scores and lower reoperation rates have been demonstrated in series of TEA for this type of distal humerus fracture, and in a recent randomized, controlled trial, McKee et al[282] found faster operative times and improved functional scores at all time points up to 2 years in TEA vs ORIF. ROM and complications were not statistically different. However, long-term studies of TEA in this setting are not available, and patients must be willing to comply with the 5- to 10-lb lifetime lifting restrictions that accompany a TEA. Postoperatively, patients are typically splinted in extension for several days and begin early active flexion and gravity-assisted extension with a resting extension splint for between exercises. A more conservative rehabilitation protocol may be considered depending on the quality of the triceps at the time of repair.

If ORIF is chosen for this injury, the most preferred approach for fixation would be an olecranon osteotomy because it gives the best distal exposure for articular reduction. Triceps-splitting and triceps-sparing approaches to the distal humerus are more useful for unicondylar or simple fracture patterns without intra-articular comminution. The surgical principles for ORIF of intra-articular injuries such as this include first performing anatomic reduction and preliminary fixation of the articular segment with a combination of K-wires and screws. Once the articular segment is stable as a single fragment, it is reduced to the shaft fragment, and bicolumnar plating is performed in an attempt to maximize the number of screws and threads that cross the fracture for optimal purchase. Traditionally, this was performed with 90-90 plating, although parallel locked plating of the medial and lateral columns has now been shown to have increased rigidity. Bone grafting is commonly required for metaphyseal defects. The olecranon osteotomy is repaired with a tension band or plate construct. Assuming stable fixation has been achieved, early active and active-assisted ROM within 4 to 7 days of surgery should be started. Passive ROM is typically delayed 4 to 6 weeks.

Why Might This Be Tested? Although uncommon, distal humerus fractures are technically demanding to treat and are frequently encountered by trauma surgeons, upper extremity surgeons, and general orthopedic surgeons. Although good results of ORIF have been shown in the younger population, distal humerus fractures in the expanding elderly population present unique challenges, and treating physicians should be aware of the data regarding ORIF vs TEA.

Here's the Point!

Distal humerus fractures with a simple fracture pattern may be amenable to a triceps-splitting or triceps-sparing approach, whereas more complex intra-articular injuries are best exposed with an olecranon osteotomy. ORIF is typically performed with articular reduction, followed by bicolumnar locked plating and early ROM. TEA as a primary treatment for distal humerus fracture in elderly patients appears to provide improved functional results, although the long-term safety profile is unknown.

Table 91-1.

DISTAL HUMERUS FRACTURE CLASSIFICATION SYSTEMS

Single-Column Fractures	Milch Classification	Treatment
Medial condyle	Type I: medial to the trochlea ridge; Type II: through trochlea ridge	Nondisplaced: immobilize in pronation; displaced: operative fixation
Lateral condyle	Type I: lateral to the trochlea ridge; Type II: through trochlea ridge	Nondisplaced: immobilize in supination; displaced: operative fixation
Bicolumnar Fractures	**Jupiter Classification**	**Treatment**
High T fracture	Transverse fracture at or above the olecranon fossa	ORIF: restore articular surface; elderly/poor bone stock: TEA
Low T fracture	Transverse fracture just above the trochlea	ORIF: restore articular surface; elderly/poor bone stock: TEA
H fracture	Trochlea is a free fragment	ORIF: restore articular surface; elderly/poor bone stock: TEA
Medial lambda	Looks like the Greek symbol with the proximal fracture exiting medially	ORIF: restore articular surface; elderly/poor bone stock: TEA
Lateral lambda	Looks like the Greek symbol with the proximal fracture exiting laterally	ORIF: restore articular surface; elderly/poor bone stock: TEA
Mulitplane	T-type fracture+coronal plane fracture	ORIF: restore articular surface; elderly/poor bone stock: TEA
Capitellum Fractures	**Bryan and Morrey Classification**	**Treatment**
Type I	Hahn-Steinthal: complete fracture of the capitellum	Splint if nondisplaced; ORIF if >2-mm displacement
Type II	Kocher-Lorenz: sleeve fracture from the articular surface	Splint if nondisplaced; ORIF if >2-mm displacement
Type III	Comminuted	Splint if nondisplaced; ORIF if >2-mm displacement
Type IV	McKee's modification: coronal shear fracture (includes capitellum and trochlea)	Splint if nondisplaced; ORIF if >2-mm displacement
ORIF=open reduction and internal fixation; TEA=total elbow arthroplasty.		

Vignette 92: What to Do for My Broken Hip?

A 67-year-old female with a history of Parkinson's disease and osteoporosis presents after a ground-level fall on the day of presentation with immediate groin pain and inability to bear weight on the right lower extremity. Prior to injury, the patient was very active and had just returned from a walking tour of Buenos Aires with no assistive devices or hip pain. On examination, the skin was intact and the patient had a normal neurovascular exam. X-rays of the hip are shown in Figure 92-1.

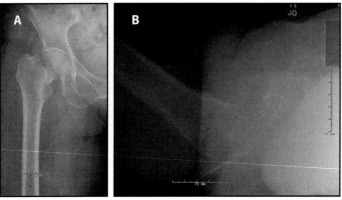

Figure 92-1. (A) AP and (B) lateral x-rays of the right hip.

▶ *What risk factors does this patient have for this injury?*

▶ *What are the treatment options?*

▶ *How does the patient's age and functional status influence treatment?*

▶ *When should surgical treatment be pursued?*

The patient underwent a right THA. The postoperative x-ray is shown in Figure 92-2.

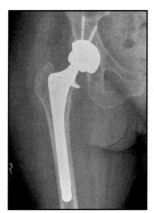

Figure 92-2. Postoperative x-ray showing a right THA.

▶ *What complications is this particular patient at risk for postoperatively?*

Vignette 92: Answer

This patient is at an increased risk for femoral neck fracture due to her age, sex, race, and underlying diagnosis of osteoporosis. These injuries occur in a bimodal distribution, with high-energy mechanisms in younger individuals and low-energy mechanisms (classically a ground-level fall) in elderly individuals. Because the femoral neck is an intra-articular structure, it lacks periosteum and is surrounded with synovial fluid, both of which limit callus formation and healing potential. In addition, the blood supply to the femoral head (know this name: lateral epiphyseal artery from the medial femoral circumflex) travels through the femoral neck and is often disrupted with fracture displacement, placing these patients at risk for avascular necrosis. These fractures are thus classified into the following 2 big categories: displaced or nondisplaced.[283-285]

Treatment options for femoral neck fractures depend on the physiologic age of the patient, ambulatory and functional status, preexisting hip arthritis, and fracture displacement. In young individuals after high-energy trauma, ORIF with 3 cannulated screws in an inverted triangle formation should be performed on an emergent basis for displaced and nondisplaced fractures (beware: in these cases, fracture lines are usually more vertical and difficult to treat). In elderly individuals, ORIF can be considered for nondisplaced or valgus impacted fractures. The addition of a capsulotomy is controversial but thought to help with lowering the incidence of ON related to increased capsular pressures of an associated hematoma. In elderly patients with displaced fractures, treatment is controversial. In low-demand, debilitated, elderly patients with significant medical comorbidities, it is reasonable to consider hemiarthroplasty as an option. In higher-demand, active patients, THA could be considered and is a more cost-effective option. In patients with preexisting hip degeneration, THA should be considered. In elderly patients, operative treatment should be performed as soon as possible to allow early mobilization, which has been associated with a decreased risk of mortality (certainly within 48 hours). In addition, extensive cardiology clearance has been proven to not be cost-effective in managing these patients.

Complications after surgical treatment of a femoral neck fracture vary depending on the treatment selected. ON can occur in patients treated with ORIF, with higher rates in patients with a greater degree of initial displacement or a nonanatomic reduction (use Lowell's lines—s-shaped curve of head and neck transition—for assessment of reduction). Nonunion can also occur after fixation, partially in displaced fractures or those with a varus malreduction. Hemiarthroplasty and THA can suffer those complications typically associated with hip arthroplasty, including periprosthetic sepsis, aseptic loosening, prosthetic wear, and periprosthetic fracture. THA after a femoral neck fracture has a higher rate of instability than arthroplasty performed for OA and a higher rate of instability than hemiarthroplasty performed for femoral neck fracture. This patient is at particular risk for this complication due to the history of Parkinson's disease. The surgeon may wish to avoid the posterior surgical approach, which has also been associated with postoperative instability.

Why Might This Be Tested? Femoral neck fractures are frequently seen and treated by all residents and thus commonly appear on standardized tests. There are multiple potential areas for questioning, including risk factors, treatment options, surgical technique, and complications.

Here's the Point!

Femoral neck fractures occur more commonly in elderly patients, females, and those with osteoporosis. Treatment should occur as quickly as possible to allow early mobilization. Options include ORIF, hemiarthroplasty, and THA, depending on the physiologic age of the patient, the ambulatory and functional status of the patient, preexisting hip arthritis, and fracture displacement.

Vignette 93: Trampoline Accident

A 9-year-old female fell off of a trampoline at home. She landed on her left upper extremity, which is her nondominant arm. After the fall, she had trouble moving her elbow, and a mild deformity was noted by her parents. She presented to the emergency department with elbow pain. An x-ray obtained in the emergency room is shown in Figure 93-1.

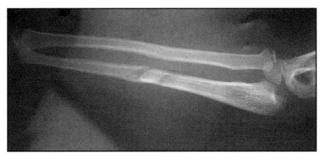

Figure 93-1. X-ray obtained in the emergency room.

▶ *What is the diagnosis?*

▶ *What is the treatment?*

Vignette 93: Answer

The patient has a Monteggia fracture, which is classically defined as a radiohumeroulnar dislocation with a concomitant ulnar fracture.[286] The x-ray shows a fracture of the ulnar shaft and an associated anterior radial head dislocation. This fracture can occur with plastic ("bending fracture") deformation of the ulna or a distinct, complete ulna fracture. The fracture or plastic deformation causes a shortening or relative shortening of the ulna, resulting in radial head dislocation. Radiographically, the radial head should line up with the capitellum on all views. On our x-ray, it is clearly anterior to the capitellum. The most common classification used has been described by Bado[286]:

- Type I: Ulna angulation/fracture and anterior radial head dislocation (apex anterior), more common in children and young adults
- Type II: Ulna angulation/fracture and posterior radial head dislocation (apex posterior), more common in middle-aged and elderly patients (beware radial head fracture)
- Type III: Ulna angulation/fracture and lateral radial head dislocation (varus angulation), more common in children
- Type IV: Ulna and proximal one-third radius fractured

Initial treatment can include closed reduction, casting, and close monitoring. This technique commonly suffices for the cases of ulna plastic deformation. Type I fractures are treated with a long-arm cast in flexion and supination. Type II cases are casted in some extension and Type III are reduced in extension and casted in 90 degrees of flexion/supination. Flexion and supination will enhance the fracture stability by relaxing the biceps and tightening the interosseous membrane. More often in complete fractures, the reduction will not be maintained and, despite an A for effort, will necessitate an ORIF of the ulna. Remember, kids are not small adults; they will tolerate immobilization longer without residual stiffness, so don't be afraid to cast for a longer period of time.

The ulna is the key to this fracture pattern, and length must be restored even in patients with plastic deformation. Once the ulna is out to length, the radial head should reduce spontaneously. If the fracture is transverse or due to plastic deformation, the ulna can be fixed with an IM nail. For fractures associated with a comminuted ulna, oblique, or spiral fracture, fixation with a plate and screws is needed to avoid shortening of the ulna resulting in recurrent dislocation (some advocate removal of plate and screws 6 to 12 months after surgery).[286]

Missed Monteggia fractures may be difficult to diagnose because children will often function well with a dislocated radial head. The problem is that if left dislocated, fibrous tissue will form, and closed reduction becomes almost impossible. In addition, the ulna will start to heal, and length may be difficult to restore. Long-term concerns with chronic dislocation include instability, cubitus valgus, and poor ROM.[286] Ultimately, these chronic fractures should be viewed as an ulnar malunion, and correction requires osteotomy with reconstruction of the annular ligament.[286]

Why Might This Be Tested? Missed Monteggia fractures are a leading cause of elbow fracture–associated litigation. It is imperative to check that the radial head aligns with the capitellum on all views. Always check the joint above and below a radial or ulnar shaft fracture.

Here's the Point!

Monteggia fractures can be easily missed because the elbow in a child may function well despite a radial head dislocation. The ulna length is the key to treating these fractures. Comminution = plating, whereas simpler fracture patterns can be treated with IM fixation.

Vignette 94: Doc, I Am Feeling Clumsy Lately

A 60-year-old female with a history of long-standing RA presents with neck pain and difficulty with fine motor movements. She is able to ambulate but feels a little clumsy lately. She has been on prednisone and several disease-modifying drugs for the past 10 years. Her hands have been severely affected with contractures and ulnar drift of her fingers with little progression over the past 2 years. She has had 2 THAs and is here for cervical spine clearance before undergoing a TKA.

▶ *Her lateral plain x-ray and representative sagittal MRI slice (Figures 94-1 and 94-2) demonstrate what pathology?*

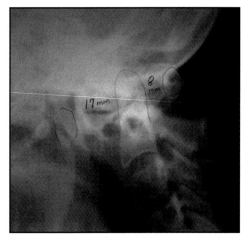

Figure 94-1. Lateral x-ray of the cervical spine.

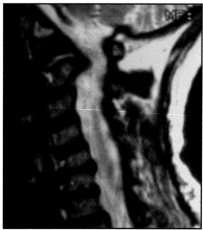

Figure 94-2. Sagittal MRI slice of the cervical spine.

▶ *What structure is not competent?*

▶ *What are predictors of neurological recovery?*

Vignette 94: Answer

RA is a chronic inflammatory disorder that affects the spine in up to 90% of patients. Ligaments and bones are commonly destroyed by the pannus and inflammatory process, leading to pain, subluxation, and neurological damage. Within the cervical spine, the upper cervical spine, occiput to C2, is commonly involved, as these joints are synovial in nature. Three characteristic patterns of instability result: atlantoaxial impaction (ie, basilar invagination or cranial settling found in 40% of cases), atlantoaxial subluxation (AAS) and subaxial subluxation (20% of cases). The most common subluxation is AAS, representing two-thirds of RA-afflicted cervical spines. AAS results from an incompetent transverse ligament or erosion of the dens. AAS can be documented on plain x-rays by measuring the anterior atlantodental interval (AADI). The AADI is the distance from the anterior aspect of the dens to the posterior aspect of the midportion of the anterior ring of C1. The normal value in adults is 3 mm. An AADI greater than 5 mm represents instability. In this patient, the AADI is 17 mm and the posterior atlantodental interval (PADI) is 6 mm.

The AADI, however, is an unreliable predictor of paralysis because of poor correlation between the AADI and cord compression seen on MRI. The PADI has been found to be a better predictor. The PADI better represents the space available for the spinal cord and is the distance between the posterior surface of the dens and the anterior edge of the posterior ring of C1. The critical lower limit is 13 mm, which has a 97% sensitivity to predict paralysis.[287] Surgical indications include neurological deterioration and intractable pain with spinal instability. Other factors include AAS with a posterior AADI interval less than or equal to 14 mm, impaction with odontoid migration greater than 5 mm rostral to McGregor's line, subaxial subluxation with sagittal canal diameter less than or equal to 14 mm, or a cervicomedullary angle less than 135 degrees.[288]

To assess which patients benefited from surgery, Boden et al reported no neurological recovery if a preoperative PADI of 10 mm or less was present, whereas neurological recovery of at least one Ranawat class (Table 94-1) is likely to occur if PADI preoperatively is greater than 10 mm and complete motor function recovery if PADI is greater than 14 mm. If atlantoaxial impaction was present, neurological recovery only occurred if PADI was greater than 13 mm.[287,288] Surgery is generally indicated for an unstable spine (>9- to 10-mm motion on flexion/extension x-rays), myelopathy, and progressive neurologic impairment. Depending on findings, C1-C2 fusion vs occiput-C2 fusion may be indicated.

Table 94-1.	
RANAWAT CLASS	
Grade	*Characteristics*
I	Paresthesias and pain noted on history
II	Weakness noted on subjectively and upper motor neuron findings
III	Documented weakness and upper motor neuron findings A: Ambulatory B: Nonambulatory

Why Might This Be Tested? The natural history of RA is one of significant disease progression, but the presentation of patients with RA with cervical involvement is variable, with only some patients developing neurological compromise. Predictors of neurological recovery dictates when surgery is recommended as a prophylactic manner; these predictors are typically tested.

Here's the Point!

RA commonly affects the cervical spine. Any patient with RA should get preoperative lateral flexion-extension cervical spine x-rays prior to being intubated for general anesthesia. Presentation of RA with cervical involvement is variable; however, 3 characteristic findings can be found, including AAS, cranial settling, and subaxial subluxation. Myelopathy and progressive deficits = surgery/arthrodesis.

Vignette 95: Twisting Knee Dislocation in a Figure Skater

A 19-year-old female with a history of bilateral anterior knee pain was practicing various maneuvers for her upcoming collegiate figure skating competition. She felt like her knee dislocated while performing a spin move. She felt immediate pain with the twisting of the knee, tensed her quadriceps, and felt the knee pop back into place. She developed significant swelling in the knee and was brought in for evaluation due to the fear of this happening during her competition.

▶ *What is the most likely diagnosis?*

▶ *What is the relevant anatomy and subsequent risk factors for this type of injury?*

▶ *What does a typical initial examination reveal?*

▶ *What radiographic studies should be ordered?*

▶ *What are the initial treatment options?*

▶ *What are the chances for recurrent episodes?*

▶ *What is the treatment for recurrent episodes?*

Vignette 95: Answer

Our patient suffered an acute patellar dislocation with spontaneous reduction with quadriceps contraction. First-time lateral patellar dislocations occur equally in men and women at an incidence of 5.8 per 100,000.[289] These patients have a 14% to 44% chance of additional dislocations after nonoperative management. Recurrent instability for these patients increases to 50% after one dislocation. Women are more commonly affected.

Instability of the patellafemoral joint is a multifactorial issue that relies on articular geometry, the vectors of muscles pulling around the knee, and soft tissue stabilizers. Patellofemoral joint structural constraint is rooted in the complex 3D geometry of the trochlear groove. The height and slope offered by the lateral trochlea is the most important osseous constraint offered during knee flexion. Therefore, trochlear dysplasia, or a shallow, flattened groove, is a risk factor for instability.

The Q angle (formed by a line drawn from the anterosuperior iliac crest to the center of the patella and the line from the patellar center to the tibial tubercle) also contributes to patellar stability. On average, males have a smaller Q angle (10 ± 5 degrees) than females (15 ± 5 degrees). During full extension, the tibia externally rotates (thereby increasing the Q angle), the patella disengages from the trochlea, and the posterior forces of the quadriceps and patellar tendon are the weakest. Hence, the mechanism for patellar dislocation is often a noncontact pivoting force with the knee in extension and the lower leg in external rotation (skating twist in our case).

Patients with patella alta have a higher risk for instability because there is a reduced patellar contact area/constraint and the degree of flexion that the patella engages the trochlea is higher (normal 20 degrees).[290] Another contributing factor to instability is a distance over 2.0 cm between the tibial tubercle and trochlear groove.

The medial patellofemoral ligament (MPFL) is the major passive restraint to lateral translation of the patella. Contributing to the soft tissue restraint are the vastus lateralis and medialis obliques (VMO) muscles. An imbalance of strength changes the vector of force across the knee, which may lead to instability (subluxation or frank dislocation). Of note, the VMO is the first muscle to lose strength and the last to strengthen after injury to the extensor mechanism.

A patient with a first-time patellar dislocation will have a tense and painful hemarthrosis. The medial aspect of the patellofemoral joint will be painful due to the torn medial retinacular soft tissues. Because the quadriceps is often inhibited after PF dislocation (due to pain and hemarthrosis), the patient may not be able to perform a straight-leg raise; aspiration and injection of intra-articular local anesthetic may improve the ability to examine the injured knee. The examiner must passively translate the patella medially and laterally. Normal translation should not allow the center of the patella to move to either edge of the trochlear groove. A patient has lateral patella apprehension if he or she has pain or apprehension during this maneuver (pay attention to facial expressions as you examine the knee).

Lateral patellar tilt should also be assessed by trying to laterally tilt the patella to the horizon. This is possible if the lateral retinaculum is tight.

One must obtain PA weight-bearing views of both knees at 45 degrees of flexion along with good lateral and Merchant views. On the lateral x-ray, one must assess trochlear dysplasia and patella alta (Insall-Salvati index: patella tendon length to patella length should be 1 [>1.2 is alta and <0.8 is baja]; Blumensaat's line: with knee flexed 30 degrees, the inferior border of the patella should rest near this line). Trochlear dysplasia is demonstrated by a supratrochlear spur, double contour (hypoplastic medial condyle), and the crossing sign (contour of the trochlea overlaps the anterior cortex). Axial views obtained with a CT scan help with determining version of the limb, patellar tilt (excessive is >20 degrees), as well as distance between the tibial groove and tibial tuberosity.

MRI is often useful for determining the integrity of the medial-sided structures and other osteochondral injuries (Figure 95-1). There may be associated bone bruising of the medial facet of the patella and lateral femoral condyle. There may also be loose bodies in the knee after a significant dislocation event.

Nonoperative treatment is the mainstay for managing first-time dislocations unless there is evidence of loose bodies from osteochondral injury. The goals of treatment include strengthening the VMO, decreasing swelling, and gradually improving knee ROM.[291] This includes patellar bracing and formal physical therapy. If conservative management fails to address patellar instability, surgery is warranted. Recurrent patellar instability is not adequately addressed by lateral release of the retinaculum alone. The MPFL can be

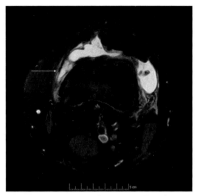

Figure 95-1. Axial T2-weighted MRI of the knee after acute patella dislocation showing injury to the MPFL (arrow), loose bodies from osteochondral injury, and a large effusion.

repaired in most cases or require MPFL reconstruction in chronic instability. If there is an underlying osseous deformity, specific reconstructive procedures may be required to correct specific risk factors: patella alta (distalization of the tuberosity), trochelar dysplasia (trochleaplasty), excessive version (femoral/tibial derotation and osteotomy), and excessive tibial tuberosity lateralization (medial tibial transfer).

Why Might This Be Tested? Anterior knee pain is a common source of office visits for young women. In cases of recurrent patella instability, MPFL reconstruction has been described with good clinical outcomes.

Here's the Point!

First-time dislocations of the patella should be managed with nonsurgical treatment unless there is a loose body in the knee. Successful management of recurrent dislocation hinges on determining and correcting the soft tissue injuries, bony abnormalities, and muscle imbalance.

Vignette 96: Is It Me or Is My Thigh Swollen?

A 15-year-old female has a 3-month history of increasing left thigh pain. The pain is not responsive to rest or medication. On exam, her thighs appear asymmetric and the left side has a firm, fixed mass on palpation. A plain x-ray is shown in Figure 96-1. An MRI and biopsy specimen of the lesion are shown in Figures 96-2 and 96-3.

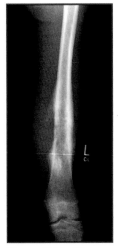

Figure 96-1. AP x-ray of the left distal femur.

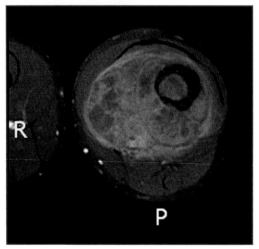

Figure 96-2. Axial T1-weighted fat-suppression MRI section of the left thigh through the mass.

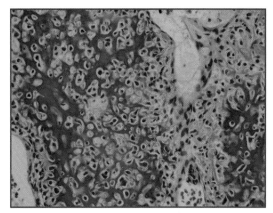

Figure 96-3. Histology section of the lesion (400× magnification).

▶ *What is the diagnosis?*

▶ *What are the appropriate imaging studies to order next?*

Vignette 96: Answer

Osteosarcoma is the most common primary sarcoma of bone, with roughly 1500 new cases in the United States each year. Its distribution is bimodal, with the first peak in adolescents and young adults and the second in older individuals. The second peak represents secondary osteosarcomas, arising in previously irradiated tissue and Paget's disease. Patients with hereditary retinoblastoma are susceptible to developing osteosarcoma due to alterations of the RB1 tumor suppressor gene. Li-Fraumeni syndrome, a p53 deficiency, is associated with a number of malignancies, including osteosarcoma.

The most common sites of osteosarcoma are the metaphyses of the distal femur, proximal tibia, and proximal humerus; less commonly, it will present in the diaphysis of long bones or the axial skeleton. The presentation is typically increasing pain, not related to activity, and occurring at rest and at night (if you see night pain in the thigh in an adolescent, think osteosarcoma). A deep, firm, fixed mass will typically be present. Ten percent may present with a pathologic fracture.

The radiographic appearance is a destructive bone lesion with poorly defined borders and areas of bone formation, lysis, periosteal reaction (classically a Codman triangle), and a soft tissue mass. All tumors must be imaged with MRI of the entire affected bone because a skip metastasis—a discontinuous site of disease in the same bone—may be present. MRI is also useful to assess the soft tissue component, determine its location to neurovascular structures, and plan the surgery and reconstruction if limb salvage is possible. Patients are staged with a chest CT to look for pulmonary metastases and a bone scan to look for other sites of osseous disease. Twenty percent of patients present with metastatic disease.

There are several subtypes of osteosarcoma (Table 96-1), categorized as IM or surface-based lesions. Eighty percent are conventional osteosarcoma, a high-grade IM lesion, and often present as a stage IIB lesion (Table 96-2). The cells can be primarily osteoblastic, chondroblastic, or fibroblastic. Telangiectatic osteosarcoma can have a radiographic appearance indistinguishable from a stage III ABC. Histologically, telangiectatic osteosarcoma will have malignant cells in the septa between cysts, which will not be seen in ABC. Small cell osteosarcoma histologically appears to have areas of classic osteosarcoma, and other areas that appear similar to Ewing's sarcoma. The final subtype of IM osteosarcoma is low-grade IM, which may initially appear similar to fibrous dysplasia but with cortical destruction.

Parosteal osteosarcoma, a surface lesion, is a low-grade lesion classically seen as a radiodense tumor arising from the posterior cortex of the distal femur (proximal tibia and humerus, too). Histologically, there is a bland-appearing "school of fish" fibrous stroma around neoplastic osteoid. Its treatment is surgical alone, and there is no role for chemotherapy in an isolated lesion. Periosteal osteosarcoma is also surface based and typically chondroblastic, and radiographically it can have a sunburst pattern. The last subtype is high-grade surface osteosarcoma, which is histologically identical to conventional osteosarcoma.

Immunohistochemical staining is not as useful in osteosarcoma as it is in other entities, and there is no characteristic translocation or staining pattern. However, 70% of osteosarcomas have some chromosomal abnormality. The diagnosis depends on the identification of osteoid—a dense pink, amorphous, intercellular material. At low power, the pattern of growth can be described as a "basket-weave" or "lacy" osteoid. At higher power, significant nuclear atypia and pleomorphism are apparent.

Conventional osteosarcoma is treated with neoadjuvant chemotherapy, surgical resection and reconstruction, and adjuvant chemotherapy. The tumor is fairly radioresistant, and radiation is reserved for palliation and unresectable lesions. The most accurate prognostic factor is the response to therapy, as demonstrated by the histological findings of the resected specimen. A good response is more than 90% of tumor necrosis. Five-year survival is 60% to 78% for patients without evidence of metastasis at the time of resection.

Limb salvage is possible in about 90% of cases. In tumors distal to the knee, a below-knee amputation will often be a better option than an attempt at limb salvage. After resection of the tumor, the osseous deficiency can be reconstructed in many ways depending on the site and extent of the resection. For intercalary tumors not requiring joint resection, an allograft or prosthesis may be placed to span the defect. When a joint is sacrificed, which is the most common scenario, an osteoarticular allograft, allograft-prosthetic composite, arthrodesis, or oncology endoprosthesis may be considered. A challenging reconstructive scenario is a femoral or proximal tibial lesion in a young patient (younger than 12 years). Often, resection of the sarcoma requires removal of an adjacent growth plate, and a standard reconstruction would result in a significant limb-length inequality at skeletal maturity. Here, amputation, rotationplasty, and growing prostheses are the reconstructive options.

Table 96-1.

KEY WORDS, CHARACTERISTICS, AND FINDINGS OF COMMON OSTEOSARCOMAS

Osteosarcoma Type	Key Words	Location/ Demographics	Radiology/Labs
Intramedullary "classic"	Most common; most often diagnosed as stage IIB; 10% to 20% with mets, most often to the lungs; retinoblastoma tumor suppressor gene predisposes to osteosarcoma; Rx: typically chemotherapy and limb salvage resection	Second decade of life (children and young adults); typically around the knee, proximal humerus, or pelvis	Blastic and destructive lesion; Codman's triangle; sunburst pattern; MRI to assess for skip mets; alkaline phosphatase may be 2 to 3 times higher than normal
Parosteal	Low-grade tumor; often a painless mass; Rx: wide local resection; often chemo not needed; 95% long-term survival with local control	Found on the surface of long bones in the metaphyseal region; histology can be confused with fibrous dysplasia	Mass seems stuck to the cortex and is heavily ossified; typically pictured posteriorly on distal femur
Periosteal	Rare, surface form of osteosarcoma; 20% to 35% risk of pulmonary mets; intermediate prognosis for survival; Rx: chemo and limb salvage resection	Patient 15 to 25 years old; found in diaphysis of long bones (tibia and femur); histology is predominately chondroblastic	Sunburst or hair on end lesions noted; no involvement of the IM canal
Telangiectatic	Looks a lot like an ABC; genetics: associated with tumor suppressor genes (RB-1 and p53) and oncogenes (HER2/neu, c-myc, c-fos); Rx: chemo and limb salvage resection	Males > females; proximal humerus, proximal femur, distal femur, proximal tibia are common locations; histology: lakes of blood, malignant cells, some but not a lot of osteoid	X-rays show lytic, expansile lesion; MRI shows fluid levels; labs: increased LDH and alkaline phosphatase

ABC = aneurysmal bone cyst; IM = intramedullary; LDH = lactate dehydrogenase; MRI = magnetic resonance imaging.

Table 96-2.

ENNEKING (MSTS) STAGING FOR MALIGNANT BONE TUMORS

Stage	Grade	Tumor
IA	Low	Intracompartmental
IB	Low	Extracompartmental
IIA	High	Intracompartmental
IIB	High	Extracompartmental
III	Any	Metastasis

Why Might This Be Tested? There are many types of osteosarcomas, and each one has particular characteristics that are often tested. It is also the most common primary bone tumor and is associated with disease conditions, such as Paget's disease and postirradiation tumors. So much to test on this topic! Definitely review Table 96-1.

Here's the Point!

Osteosarcomas are spindle cell neoplasms that produce bone (osteoid). Know the pertinent facts from Table 96-1. If you see young patients with unexplained thigh pain, start thinking osteosarcoma.

Vignette 97: Winter Ice Claims Another Ankle!

A 42-year-old male sustained a slip and fall in his icy driveway this morning. Upon presentation to the emergency department, he was found to have a gross deformity of the right ankle. Pulses were palpable and symmetric. Radiographic evaluation revealed a displaced, trimalleolar ankle fracture with complete disruption of the ankle mortise.

▶ *What factors determine the stability of an ankle fracture?*

▶ *What fracture patterns are most likely to require surgical intervention?*

A closed reduction was performed under local anesthesia, and a plaster splint was applied for immobilization.

▶ *What is the appropriate time frame for surgical stabilization?*

▶ *What factors are most critical in determining surgical outcome?*

Vignette 97: Answer

Ankle fractures are the most common intra-articular fractures of any weight-bearing joint. Much of the recent attention devoted to ankle fractures in the literature can be attributed to the landmark 1976 article by Ramsey and Hamilton, which showed that malreduction of an ankle fracture leads to abnormal tibiotalar contact stresses and invariably to posttraumatic arthritis. Therefore, the goals of treatment are to anatomically reduce the joint surfaces, restore congruency to the ankle mortise, and prevent arthritis.

The scope of this vignette is not broad enough to attempt to review the entire focus of ankle anatomy, ankle fracture classification, and operative techniques. Rather, we will strive to nail down some of the high-yield points in ankle fracture evaluation and management.

An ankle injury is considered unstable when the normal constraints to ankle motion are disrupted, permitting non-physiologic movement of the talus. In the setting of such instability, ORIF has been shown to confer better outcomes in all fracture patterns when compared with closed treatment. (All patients do better with hardware!) It is critical to remember that the primary stabilizer of the ankle under physiologic loading is the deltoid ligament. In the absence of a medial injury, the talus is stable; in other words, if the talus is subluxed, the medial structures are, by definition, violated.

In the setting of an unstable fracture in which there is a medial injury, the talus is typically displaced laterally. This is usually manifested by an increase in the medial clear space as seen on the AP x-ray. The presence of medial clear space widening, rather than fracture displacement, has been shown to be the most critical criteria for deciding on surgery vs nonoperative management for isolated lateral malleolus fractures. With a distal fibular fracture, in the presence of medial swelling, ecchymosis, and/or tenderness to palpation, a stress x-ray (gravity stress test, external rotation stress, or valgus stress view) is recommended to evaluate the integrity of the deltoid ligament.

The timing of surgery, as is the case with the surgical management of any acute fracture, is determined by the status of the soft tissue envelope. The tissues about the ankle are notoriously unforgiving, and delaying surgery for several days or the application of a spanning ankle external fixator are often wise options in the setting of profound swelling. Fracture blisters are often present within 24 to 48 hours and have been shown to be problematic in the setting of wound healing when noted to be blood filled (as opposed to serous filled).

Stable, isolated lateral malleolar fractures have been shown conclusively to do well with nonsurgical management. In bimalleolar-equivalent fracture patterns, better outcomes have not been demonstrated in the setting of deltoid ligament repair; therefore, ORIF of the lateral malleolus is adequate as the sole fixation. Medial exploration and repair is reserved for circumstances when the mortise does not reduce (incarcerated deltoid ligament) with fixation of the distal fibula alone. Isolated medial malleolus fractures and bimalleolar fractures are practically always treated surgically. In the case of trimalleolar injuries, the posterior malleolus, an avulsed fragment with ligamentous attachment to the posterior-inferior tibiofibular ligament, must be assessed intraoperatively. Although this will often reduce anatomically with fixation of the distal fibula fracture, the fragment traditionally requires fixation when noted to comprise 25% to 30% of the articular surface of the tibial plafond (or displaced > 2 mm). Much has been made in the recent ankle literature in implicating malreduction of the posterior plafond fragment in the setting of trimalleolar ankle fractures as a player in the etiology of future ankle arthritis.

Syndesmotic injuries can be subtle and difficult to interpret radiographically. Although it is universally agreed upon that suprasyndesmotic (Weber C) injuries with an obvious tibia-fibula diastasis require fixation, little else is clear in the literature surrounding syndesmosis injuries. Boden postulated the syndesmosis is stable in (most) cases in which the fibula fractures occurs within 3.5 to 4.5 cm of the ankle joint. A better technique is to assess the integrity of the syndesmosis intraoperatively, via the Cotton test, by directly visualizing the movement of the fibula after fracture fixation has been performed. However, the literature does not provide clarity under the heading of surgical technique: 3 vs 4 cortices, 3.5- vs 4.5-mm screws, metal vs biological screws vs suture button repair, activity status after surgery, and with screw removal vs screw retention. For this reason, these concepts are less likely to be tested on the exam. Lack of recognition of syndesmotic injuries at the time of surgery has also been attributed to early-onset ankle arthritis in the recent ankle literature. Ankle fusion and ankle replacement are considered as salvage procedures for posttraumatic ankle arthritis.

Rates of osteochondral injuries in operatively treated ankle fractures have been reported in the literature to be seen in as many as 75% of cases. Many new studies advocate the use of arthroscopy in the surgical treatment of unstable ankle fractures (arthroscopic reduction and internal fixation), yet routine arthroscopy of ankle fractures does not appear to confer better outcome at this time.

With respect to postoperative management, although there are theoretical advantages to early weight bearing after ORIF, most studies have shown minimal to no benefit to starting immediate weight bearing or ROM exercises. A favorite ankle fracture question centers around the fact that it takes 9 weeks for patients to have a return to baseline in total braking time when driving.[14]

Why Might This Be Tested? Ankle fractures are common and often underappreciated with regard to their complexity. A high index of suspicion must be maintained in order to accurately diagnose subtle cases of ankle (and syndesmotic) instability.

Here's the Point!

To prevent early-onset posttraumatic ankle arthritis, the articular surface and ankle mortise (particularly the posterior malleolus and syndesmosis!) must be anatomically reduced.

Vignette 98: Looks Like a Truck Ran Over My Foot

A 66-year-old insulin-dependent diabetic female presents to the emergency department with profound swelling of the foot. She does not recall any specific traumatic episode over the past several days. Her physical examination is significant for midfoot swelling, erythema, rigid pes planus, and abduction of the forefoot. Pulses are palpable. Her foot is insensate. X-rays reveal complete dislocation of TMT joints 1 through 5.

▶ *What is most likely the etiology of this condition?*

▶ *What are the most common clinical presentations seen with this condition?*

▶ *How is this condition staged?*

▶ *In what circumstances is surgical intervention recommended?*

Vignette 98: Answer

Charcot neuroarthropathy is a condition commonly seen in patients suffering from diabetes mellitus or other causes of peripheral neuropathy. It is a progressive, destructive, noninfectious process often affecting the weight-bearing joints (foot/ankle) in patients with sensory neuropathy. Although diabetes mellitus (as in our patient) is by far the most common underlying etiology (up to 70% of patients with diabetes mellitus have sensory neuropathy) seen in patients with Charcot joints, other potential causes include alcoholism, myelomeningocele, leprosy, renal dialysis, and congenital insensitivity to pain. Patients with type 1 diabetes mellitus and Charcot disease typically present at a much younger age than those with the type 2 condition. Charcot arthropathy can be bilateral in about 10% to 35% of patients.

The pathogenesis of a neuropathic joint is believed to be from a single traumatic episode or repetitive microtrauma in an ambulatory patient who suffers limited sensation. Normal protective mechanisms, such as activity restrictions and immobilization, are absent in such patients. Failure to seek medical attention is commonplace. Autonomic dysfunction may contribute to bony destruction as enhanced blood flow results in bone resorption and loss of bony architecture. Furthermore, the release of inflammatory cytokines (TNF-α, IL-1) has recently been implicated in the disease process for Charcot.

The clinical features of Charcot neuroarthropathy varies with the time of presentation. In acute cases, the foot is red, hot, and swollen, and it is difficult to differentiate between Charcot and infection. Distal pulses are typically bounding, and most patients will experience no, or little, pain. The clinical and radiographic findings are much worse than the patient describes (foot looks like it was run over by a truck in the absence of trauma). In subacute or chronic cases, markedly less swelling is seen. Ankle and foot deformity is common as the midfoot bony architecture is lost; the longitudinal arch collapses, the foot widens, and the classic rocker-bottom deformity results. The dynamic effect of the tendo-Achilles complex is lost, and an equinus contracture occurs. With chronic deformity, ulceration of the skin occurs, rendering the patient susceptible to developing deep infection. The overall goal of treatment is to obtain a stable, plantigrade foot without ulceration so patients can resume their ambulatory status without pain or loss of function.

Stage 0 disease (not originally described in the Eichenholtz classification) refers to the typical exam findings seen in the acute presentation of Charcot in the absence of any findings on plain x-rays (a simple way to differentiate between Charcot and cellulitis is to elevate the leg and observe whether the dependent erythema seen in Charcot disease resolves). Treatment in this early phase consists of protected weight bearing, patient education, and emphasis on meticulous foot care (often a daunting task).

In stage 1, the fragmentation phase, osteopenia, fracture, subluxation, or fulminant dislocation is seen. Surgery is not recommended for stage 1 disease; rather, strict immobilization in a total contact cast is used. The total contact cast is meant to provide an even distribution of pressure across the plantar foot. Frequent follow-up is needed for serial x-rays and cast changes. Total contact casting involves cast changes every 2 to 3 weeks for a total of 4 to 6 months and has been shown to have a 75% success rate when used along with protected weight bearing. At the end of treatment, the cast can be changed to an orthotic walker or custom shoe orthosis as tolerated.

In stage 2, the coalescence stage, healing is evident clinically and radiographically as swelling dissipates and x-rays show union of fracture fragments. During this phase, patients are transitioned from a total contact cast to a removable bivalve AFO (BAFO).

Stage 3, the reconstruction phase, is characterized by complete bony healing. Here, fixed deformity of the foot and ankle is often recognized due midfoot, hindfoot, or ankle instability. In the absence of significant deformity, ulceration, or equinus, the patient is fitted with custom inlay shoes.

As complications in the closed management of patients with Charcot neuroarthropathy develop, one must entertain surgical intervention. In advanced cases, soft tissue breakdown occurs, leading to ulcerations, deep infection (osteomyelitis), and severe, uncontrolled deformity. Osteomyelitis is a common occurrence with longstanding ulcer formation and is often difficult to distinguish from longstanding Charcot disease. MRI is not specific for one condition vs the other, and a WBC-labeled scan is often useful in making such a determination. With recurrent forefoot ulcer formation, an isolated Achilles tendon lengthening has been shown to achieve excellent clinical results. In recurrent ulcer formation in the hindfoot or midfoot secondary to bony prominences and minor deformity, exostectomy can be effective. In a non-plantigrade rocker bottom-type deformity of the foot, arthrodesis is recommended to salvage the viability of the limb. With bone infection, aggressive debridement of the infection must be undertaken. In the absence of restoring the mechanical axis to its native state, amputation is a considerable risk.

It is also important to anticipate the possibility of complications related to the development of Charcot in diabetic patients with ankle fractures. An added measure of caution must be applied to the rigidity of fixation (syndesmotic fixation, locked plating constructs, etc) and the duration of immobilization. In neuropathic patients, unstable fractures should still be treated with ORIF provided there is sufficient vascularity (cast treatment is likely to lead to varus angulation, skin compromise, etc).

Why Might This Be Tested? Charcot neuroarthropathy is a common consequence of missed injury or microtrauma in patients with diabetes mellitus or forms of neuropathy. It must be differentiated from infection, which is often difficult to do.

Here's the Point!

Failure to arrive at an early diagnosis, immobilize the patient, and correct the deformity may lead to recurrent ulcer formation, osteomyelitis, and ultimately, loss of limb. WBC-labeled scanning is recommended because physical exam, plain x-rays, and MRI are often insufficient to make the proper distinction.

Vignette 99: Hey, Watch Me Pop My Elbow Out!

A 16-year-old female gymnast sustained a simple elbow dislocation after a fall from the uneven bars 4 years ago. She has had 3 subsequent dislocations, with the first 2 being traumatic but the most recent occurring while pushing up from a seated position. A closed reduction was achieved each time with sedation in the emergency department. She denies any pain in the elbow between dislocation episodes but feels like there are some movements that make her feel like her elbow is going to "give out."

▶ *What are the important parts of the physical examination on this patient?*

The physical exam reveals full symmetric painless elbow ROM from 10 degrees of hyperextension to 150 degrees of flexion. There is no tenderness or swelling about the elbow, and her active elbow flexion and extension are 5/5. She has a positive posterolateral drawer test for pain and apprehension but not for frank subluxation. Stress fluoroscopy in varus demonstrates asymmetric increased gapping at the radiocapitellar joint on the AP view, as well as gapping of the ulnohumeral joint on the lateral projection (Figure 99-1).

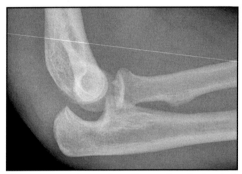

Figure 99-1. Lateral radiograph of the left elbow.

▶ *What structures are likely deficient and causing instability in this case?*

▶ *Is advanced imaging required?*

▶ *What are the principal treatment options?*

Vignette 99: Answer

This patient has posterolateral rotatory instability (PLRI) secondary to multiple elbow dislocations. Unlike MCL insufficiency, which typically presents with medial elbow pain in the throwing athlete and laxity on valgus stress but not true elbow dislocation or subluxation, PLRI represents insufficiency of the LCL complex, the primary stabilizer to varus stress.[292] It is insufficiency of the posterior lateral ulnar collateral ligament (LUCL) fibers of the LCL complex that truly contribute to this instability rather than the anterior fibers that blend into the annular ligament, and it is the LUCL that gets reconstructed surgically in cases of chronic instability. PLRI is more of a problem with routine activities of daily living than MCL insufficiency because varus loads to the elbow are common with any shoulder abduction. Although PLRI is often seen after elbow dislocation or fracture/dislocation, it is also reported secondary to cubitus varus deformity and lateral epicondylitis after multiple steroid injections or vigorous surgical debridement.[293]

Physical examination in the setting of chronic PLRI is often benign. ROM is typically full or shows slight loss of extension. The patient may be minimally tender over the LUCL. Although frank instability is difficult to detect in the awake patient, especially if the patient is muscular, provocative stress testing of the LUCL will typically at least elicit apprehension compared with other diagnostic stress testing.[292,293] The posterolateral drawer test is best performed with the patient supine, the arm adducted, and the shoulder forward flexed 90 degrees. The examiner places one hand at the lateral elbow and provides medially directed pressure while the other arm takes the elbow through a flexion/extension arc while supinating the forearm with axial load and valgus stress. This tends to produce pain or actual subluxation in supination and extension. If the elbow subluxates, the examiner may feel it clunk into a reduced position with pronation and flexion.[292,293] True subluxation is much easier to reproduce in the anesthetized patient and should always be checked for in the operating room prior to surgery for lateral instability.

Plain and stress x-rays with a good clinical history and physical exam is typically all that is required in most cases. MRI can be helpful in ruling out other soft tissue pathology and will typically show attenuation of the ligament and fluid signal between the ligament and the common extensor origin. CT plays a role in cases of fracture malunion or significant posttraumatic HO.

Although subtle instability or gapping in the acute setting of a simple elbow dislocation can resolve with activation of the anterior musculature, chronic instability, such as in this case, is principally treated surgically. Typically, the lateral ligament complex is attenuated and of too poor quality to repair primarily to the epicondyle as one can often do in the acute setting. The treatment is thus secondary reconstruction, most commonly with palmaris longus autograft or hamstring autograft or allograft. Although a detailed description of the surgical technique is out of the scope of this vignette, the procedure is done through a lateral approach with drill holes through the humerus near the isometric point and through the ulna along the supinator crest to try to best recreate the anatomic origin and insertion of the LUCL. There are multiple acceptable fixation options.[293]

Postoperatively, the elbow is protected in an orthoplast splint or hinged elbow brace for 6 weeks, but early ROM with the arm adducted to prevent varus stress under the supervision of a therapist is started to prevent stiffness. With proper surgical technique and graft placement, recurrence rates are very low and patients typically regain nearly full elbow and forearm ROM, occasionally with small flexion contractures.

Why Might This Be Tested? PLRI is a classic presentation with popularized physical exam techniques that reproduce LCL insufficiency. (Subtle instability can be difficult to differentiate from lateral epicondylitis and radial tunnel syndrome; it may not present with classic findings.) When the diagnosis is correct, LUCL reconstruction yields excellent clinical results, typically in a young, active patient population.

Here's the Point!

Unlike MCL insufficiency, LCL insufficiency presents as more of a problem with routine activities. Have a high index of suspicion for this condition in patients with instability episodes, mechanical symptoms, or previous treatment for lateral epicondylitis. Be aware of how to perform provocative testing for PLRI. LUCL reconstruction with tendon graft is the treatment of choice and has excellent results.

Vignette 100: I Can't Walk Very Far Anymore. Is This Just Old Age?

A 67-year-old female patient community ambulatory with a cane presents with a long-standing history of right knee pain that has worsened over the past 6 months. Pain is worse in the morning and is exacerbated by walking more than 2 blocks, and there is associated swelling. She has no significant past medical or family history. Lateral, AP, and Rosenberg x-rays are obtained (Figure 100-1).

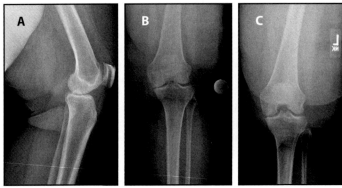

Figure 100-1. (A) Lateral x-ray of the left knee showing superior and inferior patellar facet osteophytes. (B) AP x-ray of the left knee showing medial joint space narrowing, subchondral sclerosis, and cysts. (C) Rosenberg x-ray of the left knee showing medial joint space narrowing, subchondral sclerosis, and notch osteophytes.

▶ *What is the patient's underlying diagnosis?*

▶ *What is the etiology of OA?*

▶ *What is the pathophysiology of this disease process?*

▶ *What are the treatment options?*

Vignette 100: Answer

The patient's underlying diagnosis is OA, a noninflammatory disease process and the most common type of arthritis. It is the most common cause of disability allowance and the second most common cause of disability after ischemic heart disease.[294] It is a disease process resulting from a complex interaction between genetic and environmental factors. With an increasingly large aging population coupled with a difficult obesity epidemic, the effect of OA continues to rise.

Primary causes of OA refer to an intrinsic defect, such as mutations in genes resulting in skeletal malformation syndromes or in genetic polymorphisms of genes leading to increased susceptibility to developing OA. Secondary causes refer to environmental factors that lead to early cartilage degeneration and/or progressive deterioration, such as trauma or infection. However, there must be a complex interplay of primary and secondary factors given that not all patients with a chondral insult will go on to develop OA; they are able to maintain a bone and cartilage homeostasis. Aging, weight, sex, and biomechanical instability are known risk factors for disease progression.[294]

Progressive deterioration and loss of the articular cartilage results in formation of periarticular osteophytes that are engineered by the body to deal with the added load and strain.[295] The osteochondral interface continues to degrade, leading to further cartilage loss and eventual subchondral microfracture and, finally, subchondral cyst formation. Furthermore, the subchondral layer becomes progressively sclerotic as it attempts to compensate for the cartilage loss. This bone, although thicker, appears to be more compliant than the subchondral bone of a normal joint, which challenges prior dogma that this sclerosis leads to a stiffer joint.[296] Sclerostin, an inhibitor of the Wnt pathway of bone formation, is decreased in areas of bony sclerosis, allowing for continued increased localized bone formation in response to the greater mechanical loading from loss of the normal joint structure. In contrast to the subchondral cortical bone, the subchondral trabecular bone demonstrates osteoporotic changes, possibly as a result of stress-shielding from the thickened cortical plate.

Microscopically, histology will show the loss of superficial chondrocytes, evidence of replication, and degradation of the tidemark (the demarcation line between calcified and articular cartilage). The calcified cartilage is penetrated by vascular elements and mediated by VEGF, resulting in progressive migration of the calcified cartilage deeper into the articular cartilage zones. These new vascular elements have also been found to express nerve growth factor, potentially contributing to symptomatic OA pain. The end result is thinning of the subchondral cartilage, which alters joint biomechanical forces.[297] In addition, VEGF shows increased expression in the synovium, especially in patients with RA, allowing for a more exuberant synovial contribution to the overall inflammatory response. However, unlike RA, the synovium is a minor player in the cascade of joint degradation, with the articular surface being the primary driver of cartilage degradation and resultant OA (Figure 100-2).[298] Furthermore, more than one chondrocyte may be found in each lacuna (chondrocyte cloning), and these chondrocytes are hypertrophic in appearance. Fissuring can also be seen with a pagetoid appearance of the subchondral bone.

The biology will show the cartilage to have increased water content, decreased PG content with molecules that have shorter chains, and an increased chondroitin:keratan sulfate ratio, leading to overall collagen abnormalities that are further enhanced by MMPs.

The molecular biology pathways involve a cascade of cytokines and degradative enzymes. Chondrocyte insult triggers the release of IL-1, which is also released by synoviocytes, neutrophils, and other inflammatory cells that may be influenced by the mechanism of injury. IL-1 will increase the production, activation, and/or release of degradative enzymes, such as cathepsin B and D, MMPs (collagenase, gelatinase, stromelysin, plasmin), and ADAMTS (a disintegrin, and metalloproteinase with thrombospondin motifs). Tissue inhibitor of metalloproteinases inhibit the action of these metalloproteinases.[298] Symptomatic pain appears to also be mediated by chemokines released by the synovium, specifically CCL19, as well as nerve growth factor from the neovascular channels formed in the subchondral bone promoted by VEGF and other joint chemokines monocyte chemotactic protein and monocyte inflammatory protein (Figure 100-3).[299]

Physical exam findings include an enlarged joint, crepitus, and decreased ROM. X-rays may show the 4 cardinal signs of OA: joint space narrowing, osteophyte formation, subchondral cysts, and sclerosis. Subchondral cysts form as microfractures in the subchondral surface and allow an influx of synovial fluid that has no channel for egress. Advanced imaging will show an eburnated surface.

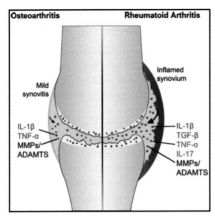

Figure 100-2. Diagram comparing the cytokines involved in OA vs RA. Synovial inflammation is the primary driver of joint degradation in RA, whereas the subchondral surface initiates the cascade of articular cartilage loss in OA. (Adapted from Sun HB. Mechanical loading, cartilage degradation, and arthritis. *Ann N Y Acad Sci.* 2010;1211:37-50.)

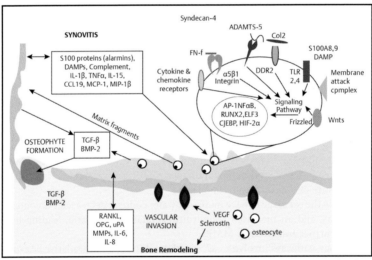

Figure 100-3. Diagram of the complex molecular interactions involved in cartilage degradation and OA pathogenesis. (Adapted from Loeser RF, Olex AL, McNulty MA, et al. Microarray analysis reveals age-related differences in gene expression during the development of osteoarthritis in mice. *Arthritis Rheum.* 2012;64[3]:705-717.)

Conservative treatment options include activity modification, the use of an assist device, weight loss, and quadriceps strengthening (particularly for knee OA), NSAIDs, acetaminophen, and judicious use of corticosteroid injections. The evidence supporting viscosupplementation injections is poor, with recent AAOS evidence-based clinical practice guidelines reflecting this.[300] Surgical options include joint arthroplasty, resection arthroplasty, or arthrodesis, depending on the joint involved. In the knee, for single-compartment OA in a relatively young patient, unicompartmental arthroplasty or HTO is also an option.

Why Might This Be Tested? OA is a noninflammatory arthritis influenced by genetics and environmental factors that leads to significant pain and loss of mobility. Predictable changes in cartilage are often the target of questions and need to be memorized.

Here's the Point!

Several degradative enzymes mediate the progressive loss of cartilage. The effects of aging and OA on cartilage are generally opposite except for PG content, which decreases in both conditions. In OA, the water content is increased, PG content is decreased, keratin sulfate concentration is decreased, and PG degradation is significantly increased.

Vignette 101: Inflammatory Arthropathies

A 35-year-old male presents with an insidious onset of low back pain and stiffness that is worse in the mornings. There is pain that radiates down from his lower back through the buttocks and into the upper thighs bilaterally with the absence of bowel or bladder dysfunction. The pain is persistent, not relieved with positional changes, and associated with some chest pain with deep inspiration. He has no significant past medical history and does not drink alcohol or use tobacco products. He reports that his father and brother suffer from a similar type of lower back pain. On physical examination, the patient has pain with taking a deep breath and a mild kyphotic deformity noted grossly. The patient has a slight heart murmur and pain with flexion, abduction, and external rotation testing. There is a loss of the normal lumbar lordosis, ROM of the spine appears diffusely limited, and there is pain on palpation of the lower back and into the sacrum. Neurologic examination is normal with preservation of deep tendon reflexes symmetrically.

▶ *What is the diagnosis?*

▶ *What is the appropriate management of this disorder?*

▶ *What other consequences might be seen in the future?*

▶ *If the patient complained of urinary difficulties and conjunctivitis, what would the diagnosis be?*

Vignette 101: Answer

Okay, this is an easy one—the diagnosis is AS. AS is a seronegative inflammatory disease that typically affects the axial skeleton, particularly the sacroiliac joints. Typically, autofusion of spinal segments lead to a fixed hyperkyphotic posture and subsequent hip and knee contractures. In this vignette, there were few distractors and several phrases that were clubbing you over the head with the AS diagnosis. AS has a predilection for the male sex (M:F = 3:1) in the second through fourth decades of life. In North America, there are typically 1 to 2 cases per 1000 people, and 15% to 20% have a positive family history of the disease.[301] Eighty percent to 95% of patients are HLA-B27 positive, and carriers of the gene have a 16% to 50% increased chance of developing AS. One theory is that AS is an autoimmune disorder that occurs after an infection with *Klebsiella pneumoniae* in individuals who are HLA-B27 positive.[301] The pathophysiology of AS includes inflammation and bony destruction at the site of tendon insertions (enthesopathy). The inflammation leads to ankylosis and loss of motion, particularly in the spine, leading to syndesmophyte formation and the classic presentation of a "bamboo spine." Systemic inflammation associated with AS can lead to inflammatory bowel disease, psoriasis, uveitis/iritis, pulmonary fibrosis, aortitis, and genitourinary problems.[301]

The history described in the vignette is characteristic for AS, with back pain and stiffness that typically occurs in the morning or with extended periods of sitting, recumbency, and/or standing. When the costovertebral joints are impacted, breathing may become painful and further compromised as a greater spinal kyphosis develops. Buttock and SI joint involvement (positive flexion, abduction, and external rotation test) are hallmarks, and neurologic examination is typically normal at the initial presentation. Things to assess clinically include the occiput-to-wall distance, gaze angle, and chin-brow angle. ESR, CRP, and RF are routinely tested to make the diagnosis, and HLA-B27 testing can be used as well. Typically, the ESR and CRP are mildly elevated, RF is negative, and HLA-B27 is positive. X-rays often show signs of sacroiliitis that include progressive sclerosis, joint space widening, and eventual fusion of the joints. Typically, a Ferguson view is needed to better visualize the SI joints (AP pelvis with tube directed 30 degrees cephalad).[301] Ossification about tendinous insertions is often seen diffusely as well. Fusion of the spine (bamboo spine) with syndesmophytes that are bilateral and have insertions at the upper and lower margins of the adjacent vertebrae (compared with diffuse idiopathic skeletal hyperostosis, which has larger, asymmetric, and nonmarginal insertions of the syndesmophytes).[301] Protrusio acetabula may occur, and similar radiographic findings may occur in other spondyloarthropathies, such as psoriatic arthritis, reactive arthritis, arthritis associated with inflammatory bowel disease, and undifferentiated spondyloarthropathy.[301]

Initial management for these patients includes the standard NSAIDs, rest, ice, and stretching. However, once the back pain/SI pain is diagnosed as AS, then RA-type medications can be used to manage the pain found with this inflammatory arthropathy. Similar to RA, early initiation of DMARDs (sulfasalazine, methotrexate, and TNF-antagonists) may delay disease progression and lessen the pain. Hip disorders occur in 30% to 50% of patients and are often (90%) bilateral in nature. Standard THA can be used to treat AS involvement of the hips with consideration for pre- or postoperative HO prophylaxis. Corrective spinal osteotomies may be required to improve sagittal plane balance and correct chin-to-chest deformities and varying levels of kyphotic deformities. Beware—fiber optic intubation is recommended for these patients (yes, that means add another 30 minutes to your anesthesia time). For AS patients with increasing back pain, it is important to suspect a fracture, even in the setting of minimal trauma and normal-appearing x-rays. Missed fractures typically present as a rapidly progressive kyphosis, and AS patients have a high rate of neurologic injuries with fractures.[301]

In the case of urinary symptoms and conjunctivitis, the diagnosis is Reiter syndrome. This classic triad of urethritis, arthritis, and conjunctivitis was described in 1916 and still shows up on tests today! This syndrome is associated with HLA-B27 and a preceding infectious process, such as nongonococcal venereal disease or infectious diarrhea. The patient population is similar to AS, with a predilection for males between the ages of 15 and 35 years. Often, Reiter syndrome is a clinical diagnosis and is managed conservatively at initial presentation. Infections should be managed appropriately, and NSAIDs should be used to treat pain and inflammation. If symptoms are refractory and a definitive diagnosis has been established, then DMARDs can be used. Follow-up is suggested because up to 25% can develop into a chronic disabling illness.[302]

Why Might This Be Tested? Question writers love the triads, genetic factors, and radiographic descriptions. AS and Reiter syndrome frequently make an appearance on these tests as an answer or a distractor.

Here's the Point!

AS is associated with HLA-B27 and is treated like RA in refractory cases. Treat back pain seriously in these patients so as not to miss a fracture. Reiter syndrome = urethritis, conjunctivitis, and arthritis.

Vignette 102: My Pinkie Finger Is Not Working!

A 58-year-old female with a longstanding history of RA affecting the hand and wrist noticed a sudden inability to actively extend the small finger 5 weeks ago. Last week, she noticed an inability to extend the ring finger as well. There was no history of trauma. Her antirheumatic medications are currently optimized. She has noticed limited wrist and forearm ROM over the years and pain with forearm rotation. Physical exam reveals complete lack of active MCP extension in the ring and small fingers. The long and index fingers extend normally. There is prominence of the distal ulnar dorsally and limited wrist and forearm motion with pain on the latter. The ring and small fingers can be passively extended fully, but after doing so, the patient cannot hold them actively in an extended position. Observation of tenodesis in passive wrist flexion reveals no increased extension of the ring and small finger. X-rays show diffuse degenerative disease of the radiocarpal and intercarpal articulations as well as the DRUJ with dorsal migration/prominence of the ulna (Figure 102-1).

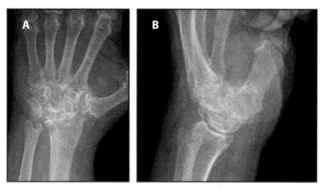

Figure 102-1. (A) AP and (B) lateral x-rays of the affected wrist.

▶ *What is the patient's underlying diagnosis, and how does it typically progress?*

▶ *What other diagnoses are in the differential?*

▶ *What is the treatment and how does it differ depending on progression?*

Vignette 102: Answer

The underlying diagnosis in this rheumatoid patient is attritional rupture of the common extensor tendons, or Vaughan-Jackson syndrome.[303] The classic pathology is inflammatory synovitis of the DRUJ. The resultant dorsal migration of the distal ulna and pannus formation at the DRUJ causes attritional rupture that typically first affects the small finger extensors, extensor digiti minimi, and extensor digitorum communis (EDC) at the level of the wrist, followed by gradual progression in a radial direction, as in this case. PIP and DIP extension will often still be present to some degree from the intrinsics. Tendon ruptures in general in the rheumatoid patient occur where a tendon passes close to a bony prominence, such as the distal ulna in this case, Lister's tubercle for the extensor pollicis longus, or the scaphoid volarly for flexor tendon ruptures.[304] Invasive tenosynovitis alone can cause rupture of the extensor tendons under the extensor retinaculum or the flexor tendons in the carpal tunnel in some cases.[304] Attritional rupture of the flexor pollicis longus, Mannerfelt-Norman syndrome, is the most common flexor tendon rupture in RA.

The differential diagnosis is critical in this case and primarily includes 3 other conditions in patients with RA. The first is a lack of MCP extension (EDC function) secondary to ulnar subluxation of the EDC into the valley between the digit's metacarpal head and its ulnar neighbor, caused by incompetence of the radial sagittal band. In this case, upon passively extending the digit fully, the EDC will usually be recentered over the MCP joint, and the patient will often be able to hold it in that position actively, ruling out tendon rupture. The second condition is dislocation of the MCP joint, typically of the proximal phalanx volarly. This results in an obvious deformity at the MCP, inability to passively extend the MCP joint (unique compared with the other 3 conditions), and an evident dislocation on a lateral x-ray. The third condition is posterior interosseous nerve compression in the proximal forearm secondary to elbow synovitis. These patients classically have greater loss of active long and ring finger extension compared with the small and index fingers and should have normal passive digital extension with tenodesis in wrist flexion; both findings differ from a case of attritional rupture.

Treatment of Vaughan-Jackson syndrome is surgical and should be undertaken quickly so that further rupture does not occur as the destructive pannus creeps radially. Regardless of how many tendons are affected, treatment classically consists of distal ulna resection and DRUJ synovectomy to eliminate the core problem,[305] followed by any of several tendon transfers depending on how many tendons are ruptured.[303,304,306] Although there is no universal agreement on which transfers should be used, the most simple would be side-to-side transfer of a ruptured small finger common extensor to an intact ring finger extensor, with the addition of extensor indicis proprius transfer and flexor tendon sublimis transfer as 2, 3, and 4 tendons are ruptured.[306]

Our patient could classically be treated with distal ulna resection, DRUJ synovectomy, side-to-side transfer of the ring finger extensor to the intact long finger extensor, and extensor indicis proprius transfer to the small finger EDC. Patients need to be aware of the extensive rehabilitation required, including likely 6 weeks of a combination of a static resting splint and dynamic splinting with extension outriggers.

Why Might This Be Tested? It is a condition with a well-defined anatomic basis and several differential diagnoses that also have sound anatomic basis. The treatment is relatively well defined by principle, although the finer points of which transfer to perform are a bit variable.

Here's the Point!

Lack of finger extension in a rheumatoid patient can arise due to several different pathologic processes, which should be differentiated based on careful history taking, physical examination, and x-ray review. If the diagnosis of attritional rupture is made, the treatment is surgical (typically, distal ulna resection and tendon transfer) and should be embarked upon quickly to avoid further ruptures.

Vignette 103: Protect Those Hands!

A 28-year-old laborer was using a grinder when he sustained a degloving injury to the volar aspect of his dominant right long finger between the PIP and DIP joints. His physical exam reveals no significant contamination, brisk capillary refill, and intact 2-point sensation distal to the zone of injury. His wound measures 1.5 cm long by 1 cm wide, and there is exposed flexor tendon, but he demonstrates good function of the profundus and sublimis tendons.

▶ *What regional or advancement flap option is most indicated for this injury?*

▶ *How would this recommendation change if it were the fingertip or the dorsal aspect of the digit?*

▶ *What else can be considered for volar injuries to the thumb tip?*

Vignette 103: Answer

This patient has a clean degloving injury of the volar aspect of a digit (non-thumb). If this was simply partial thickness with no exposed tendon, neurovascular bundle, etc, the treatment of choice would likely be healing by secondary intention with regular dressing changes if healing can be achieved within 2 to 3 weeks. If the wound takes longer than that to heal, the risk of digit contracture and infection increases. Full-thickness skin grafting (good cosmetic result and do not contract like split-thickness grafts) is an option, but the morbidity of graft harvest and increased risk of infection and graft fissuring make secondary healing superior within the aforementioned time restraints.

In a case such as this with exposed tendon, neither secondary healing nor skin grafting is an ideal option because the tendon requires vascularized adipose tissue and skin to maintain gliding and optimize healing. Small- to medium-sized defects volarly on the digit at this level are most commonly treated with a cross-finger flap from an adjacent digit and skin grafting of the donor site. The flap is divided 2 to 3 weeks later once it incorporates at the recipient site. Volar defects at the tip of the digit also commonly have the option of a thenar flap. This is primarily used for the index and long finger because it is difficult for the ring and small fingers to reach the thenar eminence appropriately. The thenar flap is especially useful in young females who may be displeased with the donor site from a cross-finger flap.

Transverse amputations or those with dorsal greater than volar tissue loss are amenable to a V-Y flap, although the same principle applies to secondary healing being most effective with no exposed bone. Dorsal full-thickness defects of the digits, when small, can be treated with a reverse cross-finger flap, although kite flaps based on the dorsal metacarpal artery system (DMCA) are popular and in this setting are more versatile than the reverse cross-finger flap. The most common is a flap derived from the first DMCA vessel between the thumb and index rays for coverage of the thumb or dorsal index finger. The vessels become smaller and less consistent as one progresses ulnarly within the DMCA system.[307] Digital artery island flaps based on a single digital artery are versatile, can be made almost the entire length of the digit, and can be distally based for fingertip coverage or proximally based to cover long defects of an adjacent digit volarly or dorsally.

The thumb also has the unique advantage of having the Moberg flap as an option for thumb tip defects given its volar and dorsal perfusion and better tolerance of flexion contractures than the other digits. The first DMCA flap and groin flap for larger defects are the other workhorse flaps for the thumb. More proximally based regional flaps include the radial forearm flap for the dorsal hand and lateral arm flap for versatile free flap hand coverage.[308]

Flaps can be classified based on blood supply to include axial pattern (a single arteriovenous [AV] pedicle), random pattern (no single AV system), and venous flaps (vein-to-artery anastomosis). Flaps can also be classified according to tissue types: cutaneous (skin and subcutaneous tissue), fascia/fasciocutaneous (flaps with fascia), muscle/musculocutaneous (involve perforators and may involve overlying skin), and bone/osteocutaneous (free fibula). All free flaps are axial pattern flaps and should have the anastomoses attached outside of the zone of injury.

Although countless flaps have been described for the hand, both regional and distant, the former represent the most common and likely to be tested. Also be aware that dermal regeneration matrix products are become increasingly popular as substitutes for flaps, although their indications are still being defined and they are unlikely to be tested at this time.

Why Might This Be Tested? Many of the flaps discussed here are well described for tissue loss in specific areas (volar vs dorsal, fingertip vs more proximal, thumb vs non-thumb) and thus are commonly tested.

Here's the Point!

Err toward healing by secondary intention for defects, especially smaller ones, without exposed bone, tendon, joint, etc. Skin grafting is another option for larger defects. Defects with exposed deep structures classically require rapid coverage with vascularized tissue, usually in the form of a flap. Know the common ones and what type of defect they are usually used for.

Vignette 104: That Darn Throw Rug!

A 62-year-old male with a medical history of diabetes mellitus and bilateral THAs presents to the emergency room after sustaining a ground-level fall while tripping on a rug at home. The patient's index THA was performed for primary OA. The patient had recently undergone a left revision THA for aseptic loosening 6 weeks prior to presentation. His postoperative course was uncomplicated, and the revision THA proceeded without complication. A posterior approach and a long, fully coated femoral component were used for the revision. The postoperative x-rays demonstrated no evidence of intraoperative fracture and good component alignment (Figure 104-1). The patient progressed to ambulate with a walker without pain.

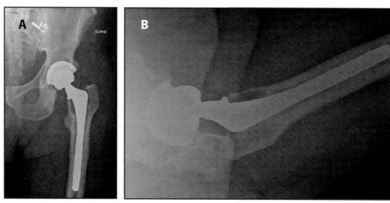

Figure 104-1. Postoperative (A) AP and (B) shoot-through lateral x-rays after the index revision procedure.

Upon presentation to the emergency room, the patient reported significant proximal anterior thigh pain. His neurovascular exam was within normal limits, but he had significant pain with left hip ROM. X-rays show a Vancouver B2 periprosthetic femoral fracture (Figure 104-2).

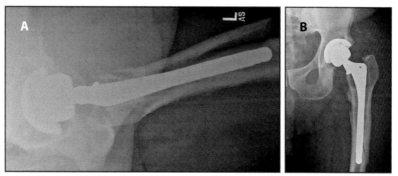

Figure 104-2. (A) Shoot-through lateral and (B) AP left hip x-rays after a ground-level fall onto the hip.

▶ *What is the incidence of periprosthetic fracture following THA?*

▶ *What are the risk factors for periprosthetic fracture following THA?*

▶ *What are the treatment options for a periprosthetic hip fracture?*

▶ *What complications are most common postoperatively?*

Vignette 104: Answer

Despite an appropriate indication for revision (aseptic loosening), acceptable femoral and acetabular component positioning, and appropriate postoperative rehabilitation, this patient sustained a Vancouver B2 periprosthetic fracture (Table 104-1 [must memorize this classification because it drives your treatment]). The incidence of postoperative periprosthetic fracture has been estimated to range between 1.5% and 4%.[309,310] A number of risk factors have been implicated in the etiology of periprosthetic fractures, including osteoporosis, component malpositioning, revision surgery, bony remodeling following prior THA, and unrecognized intraoperative fracture.

Table 104-1.		
VANCOUVER CLASSIFICATION		
Type	*Fracture Location*	*Subtype*
A	Trochanteric region	• Ag: Greater trochanter • Al: Lesser trochanter
B	Around or just distal to stem	• B1: Stable prosthesis • B2: Unstable prosthesis with adequate bone stock • B3: Unstable prosthesis with inadequate bone stock
C	Well distal to stem	

It is important to keep the fundamental goals of treatment in mind when addressing these potentially difficult patients, including fracture fixation, hip stability, early return to function, protection of the abductors, and restoration of limb lengths. In order to accomplish these goals, an appropriate algorithm should be followed, which is where the Vancouver classification comes into play. Its relatively straightforward categories have proven to be helpful in selecting a treatment strategy for patients with periprosthetic fracture. The most difficult aspect of the classification can be in determining implant stability because prior x-rays are not available for comparison. High rates of failure have been implicated when inappropriately deeming an unstable implant as stable (for testing purposes, lean toward a loose implant, especially if the femur was cemented in place or is a proximal fit stem).[311]

Workup includes orthogonal x-rays at the time of evaluation, as well as both the original operative note and any previous x-rays of the prosthesis whenever possible, to evaluate for evidence of loosening. ESR and CRP are routinely obtained to screen for a concomitant infectious process, and, intraoperatively, a cell count and frozen section are obtained to confirm the absence of an infection (this can drastically alter treatment options). Skeletal traction, ideally a tibial traction pin, should be considered in unstable fracture patterns and when surgery may be delayed for greater than 24 to 48 hours.

According to a recent AAOS Instructional Course Lecture, Vancouver A fractures are typically associated with osteolysis-related avulsion fractures.[312] In the setting of a stable implant, they are ideally treated with polyethylene liner exchange, ORIF (using cables and/or suture fixation in a tension band construct), and possible bone grafting. Postoperatively, the patients will require protected weight bearing and restricted abduction; if repair is unsuccessful, a constrained liner may be required to maintain hip stability. Be careful with testing because every now and then the acetabular component will also be grossly loose on the x-ray and may need revision (pay attention and don't be distracted by the femur fracture). Vancouver type C fractures represent fractures distal to the implant and are treated with ORIF.

Vancouver type B fractures, however, represent a range of stable and unstable components with variable bone stock. The treatment of B1 fractures is generally thought to include ORIF with plate fixation and possible allograft strut augmentation (remember to check implant stability; if unstable, a fracture will not heal, and the fixation will fatigue and ultimately break).

Vancouver B2 and B3 fractures are a challenging problem because they represent loose implants with variable amounts of bone loss. These fractures are largely treated with revision THA, although allograft-prosthetic composite and megaprosthesis are options with severe bone loss, particularly in low-demand patients. The technique and fixation used depends on the fracture pattern, surgeon preference, and patient factors. Cemented, cementless, and impaction grafting techniques have been described, but cemented implants have demonstrated high rates of nonunion (cement interferes with fracture healing) and refracture postoperatively. In the majority of cases, cementless fixation with a long-stemmed, fully coated (Wagner- or cylindrical-style) or a modular arthroplasty system will provide an adequate solution for such periprosthetic fracture surgeries. Adequate fixation requires distal fixation 2 cortical diameters past the tip of fracture. Monoblock and modular femoral components (Figure 104-3) have shown good outcomes with regard to fracture union and patient outcomes.[309,313]

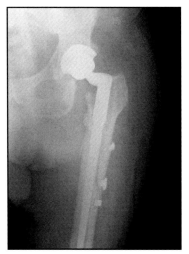

Figure 104-3. Postoperative x-ray with a modular, tapered stem and cable fixation of the fracture. The stem is used as an endoskeleton to reduce femur fragments to it.

The primary disadvantage of monoblock stems is their lack of modularity, which may predispose to postoperative instability (perhaps the most common major complication following revision for fracture) and component subsidence. Modular systems allow the surgeon to acquire distal axial and torsional stability independent of proximal component positioning, which may aid with postoperative instability. Additional fixation may be provided with cerclage cables or possibly with allograft struts. Modular stems are not recommended for use when there is limited or no proximal support because taper fracture and corrosion can occur. In such cases, a megaprosthesis or allograft prosthetic composite should be used with preservation of proximal bone if possible to aid with abductor and hip flexor function.

Postoperative complications include instability, infection, limb-length discrepancy, abductor muscle deficiency, limp, refracture, and nonunion. Notably, modular systems are thought to help minimize the risk of instability and limb-length discrepancy, although not distinctly proven. Despite one's best efforts, dislocation remains a concern, and the use of postoperative bracing has not been reported to lower these risks.

Why Might This Be Tested? Periprosthetic fractures are a common problem faced by orthopedic surgeons. There are multiple potential areas for test questions, including classification, treatment options, surgical techniques, and complications.

Here's the Point!

Periprosthetic fractures are classified using the Vancouver Classification system, which is descriptive and useful in determining treatment. The choice of treatment in type A, B1, and C fractures is typically straightforward, with ORIF as the workhorse technique. Vancouver B2 and B3 fractures are more difficult to treat and allow for several different treatment strategies.

Vignette 105: Why Does My THA Hurt After a Cardiac Cath?

A 65-year-old man presents with a medical history of diabetes mellitus, hypertension, coronary artery disease, and bilateral hip OA. The patient had undergone bilateral THAs in 1997 (left hip) and 1999 (right hip). The right hip required the use of a constrained liner secondary to abductor muscle deficiency. Both hips had performed well, and he had not experienced any complications until 2 weeks following a recent cardiac catheterization (Figure 105-1). He presented to the emergency room 24 hours later with complaints of malaise, right hip pain, subjective fevers, and swelling. Upon evaluation, the patient's examination showed minimal swelling about the anterolateral aspect of the hip, painless ROM, no erythema, and a well-healed surgical incision. Preliminary laboratory analysis demonstrated a serum WBC of $12.77 \times 10^3/\mu L$ (normal range, 4.0 to 10.0 cells/μL), ESR of 86 mm/hr (normal range, 0 to 17 mm/hr), and CRP of 217.5 mg/L (normal range, 0 to 8.0 mg/L).

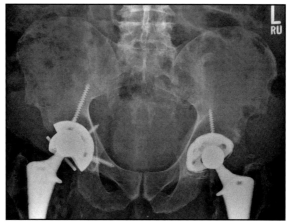

Figure 105-1. AP pelvis x-ray prior surgical revision for infected THA.

▶ *How are periprosthetic joint infections categorized?*

▶ *What are the diagnostic tools used to detect a periprosthetic joint infection?*

That evening, a fluoroscopically guided hip aspiration was performed, which returned purulent fluid. The synovial fluid analysis demonstrated 122,400 WBC/mm^3 with 98% neutrophils.

▶ *What are the treatment strategies for an acutely infected total joint?*

After much discussion, it was determined that this was an acute hematogenous infection, and the patient underwent irrigation and debridement with head and liner change. Intraoperative cultures grew *S epidermidis*. On postoperative day 10, the patient's hip incision had increasing drainage and erythema. The wound continued to drain, with increasing erythema and discomfort for the patient over the next 10 days despite IV antibiotics.

▶ *What are the treatment strategies for PJI now?*

Vignette 105: Answer

PJI is unfortunately one of the most common complications following joint replacement and is estimated to occur in about 1% to 2% of cases.[283] Risk factors for PJI include depression, alcohol abuse, urinary tract infections, rheumatologic diseases, cardiopulmonary disease, and peripheral vascular disease.[314] A number of efforts have been undertaken to minimize the risk of periprosthetic infections, including the routine use of preprocedure antibiotic prophylaxis when undergoing GI, genitourinary, dental, and cardiac procedures. Preoperative preparation has become increasingly important, with protocols involving MRSA screening (nasal ointment management, home chlorhexidene showers, and the addition of vancomycin at the time of surgery) and further evidence to prove the efficacy of preoperative skin preparation (chlorhexidene wipes).

PJIs are typically categorized by the timing and the mechanism of infection (acute postoperative, acute delayed [hematogenous], or chronic).[315] Clinical findings, such as pain, limited ROM, and wound drainage/erythema, suggest infection. Screening laboratory tests include ESR and CRP, which may then suggest synovial fluid aspiration (send for cell count with differential and cultures) if elevated. Current evidence suggests that a WBC count greater than 1700 cells/μL (range, 1100 to 3000 cells/μL) or a neutrophil percentage greater than 65% (range, 64% to 80%) is highly suggestive of a chronic infection.[316] In the acute setting (within 4 to 6 weeks after surgery), the current literature suggests higher synovial WBC counts may be necessary to diagnose PJI (27,800 cells/μL following TKA and 12,800 cells/μL following THA).[317,318]

At present, there is no consensus diagnostic criterion for the diagnosis of PJI, but the Musculoskeletal Infection Society has presented a comprehensive definition that incorporates the many diagnostic metrics currently available (Table 105-1).[319] Other potential for novel diagnostic markers include IL-6, IL-8, α2 macroglubulin, and VEGF, but they are currently cost-prohibitive and restricted to certain specialized centers.[315] Leukocyte esterase test strips, commonly used for urinalysis, have also proven to be highly predictive of PJI (80% to 93% sensitive and 88% to 100% specificity).[319]

Table 105-1.

CRITERIA FOR A PERIPROSTHETIC JOINT INFECTION

- There is a sinus tract present with direct communication to the prosthesis

- A pathogen is successfully cultured from at least two separate tissue or fluid samples obtained from the affected prosthetic joint; or

- At least four of the following six criteria exist*:
  o Elevated serum erythrocyte sedimentation rate (ESR) and serum C-reactive protein (CRP) concentration
  o Elevated synovial white blood count
  o Elevated synovial neutrophil percentage (PMN%)
  o Presence of purulence in the affected joint
  o Isolation of a microorganism in one culture from the affected joint/synovial fluid
  o Histologic analysis yielding greater than five neutrophils per high-power field in five high-power fields observed at 9400 magnification

*Despite excellent accuracy, there may be cases in which PJI exists with fewer than four of the above criteria.

Adapted from Parvizi J, Zmistowski B, Berbari EF, et al. New definition for periprosthetic joint infection: from the Workgroup of the Musculoskeletal Infection Society. *Clin Orthop Relat Res.* 2011;469(11):2992-2994.

Once the diagnosis of PJI has been elucidated, the characteristics of the infection and the patient's health must be determined. These include the duration of symptoms and the patient's immune status, overall health, and history of prior joint infections. Patients unfit for surgery may be considered candidates for long-term antibiotic suppression, but this remains a controversial approach to PJI. Patients with acute onset of symptoms (< 2 weeks) may be considered candidates for a one-stage procedure (ie, irrigation and debridement with head and liner exchange), but reinfection rates are high. Some have advocated a full one-stage procedure in which all components are removed and then new implants placed at the same setting (several variations on this theme now exist, such as interval wound vac and local antibiotic infusion with reimplantation after an abbreviated course of antibiotics). Two-stage exchange is characterized by the explantation of infected components, interval placement of an antibiotic spacer, and a subsequent revision arthroplasty following a 6-week course of parenteral antibiotic therapy. This remains the gold standard for PJI in North America, particularly for chronic infections. It should be noted that a high rate of failure has been documented in the setting of a failed irrigation and debridement and subsequent 2-stage exchange arthroplasty.[320] In this case, an attempt at treating this infection with a washout was made; the relatively early failure likely indicates this was a chronic smoldering infection. Two-stage exchange is indicated if chronic suppression cannot be achieved.

Why Might This Be Tested? PJI is a common complication following primary and revision arthroplasty. A number of high-quality studies have clarified the diagnostic criterion for PJI and helped clarify the optimal treatment. These studies, as well as AAOS practice guidelines, make this topic easily testable.

Here's the Point!

When approaching a patient with a presumed diagnosis of a PJI, there are a number of tools at your disposal (eg, serum inflammatory markers, synovial fluid analysis, and microbiological studies). Well-established guidelines exist to help in the diagnosis and treatment. Acute infections may warrant a trial irrigation and debridement, whereas chronic or recurrent infections may require a 2-stage procedure.

Vignette 106: Doc, Why Am I So Knock-Kneed?

A 55-year-old woman with RA presents with a several-year history of worsening knee pain and deformity. The pain is diffuse, nearly constant, and exacerbated by any activity. Nonoperative treatments, including DMARDs, NSAIDs, corticosteroid/viscosupplementation injections, and physical therapy, have failed to provide any significant relief. Recent x-rays are shown in Figure 106-1.

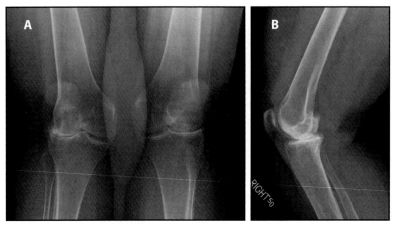

Figure 106-1. (A) AP and (B) lateral x-rays of valgus arthritis with involvement of other compartments.

▶ *What is the diagnosis?*

▶ *What nonoperative treatments are available?*

▶ *List the potential surgical options for this patient.*

After all forms of nonoperative management have been exhausted, TKA is settled on as the treatment of choice for our patient.

▶ *What sequence of steps should be performed to create coronal balance of the valgus knee?*

▶ *What must be considered when setting femoral component rotation in a valgus knee?*

▶ *In managing the bony defect laterally, what solutions can be used to create a stable platform for the tibial component?*

Vignette 106: Answer

This patient has tricompartmental DJD (secondary to RA) of the knee, most severely on the lateral side, with a valgus deformity. Valgus deformities are more common in patients with inflammatory arthritis such as RA (although varus malalignment is still more common overall) but can also be present in patients with OA. The valgus deformity is also more commonly found in females.[23] Other situations that can lead to a valgus deformity include posttraumatic conditions (lateral tibial plateau fracture) and metabolic bone disease and after a prior lateral meniscectomy. Such deformities typically involve an element of lateral bone deficiency and tight lateral structures of the knee.

Given the severe involvement of all compartments of the knee, TKA is the only surgical intervention warranted (UKA and osteotomy are contraindicated with inflammatory arthritis). The nonoperative treatments that may provide temporary relief are essentially the same as those for the varus knee. Patients who present with valgus DJD of the knee should be queried about a history of inflammatory arthritis. If they do not carry a formal diagnosis of inflammatory arthritis but have signs such as polyarticular involvement, multiple swollen warm joints, and/or systemic symptoms, further workup is indicated. In cases of RA, arthroscopic synovectomy may be effective for short-term management, and DMARDS can slow or even prevent progression of this destructive process. In addition, patients with inflammatory arthritis have unique anesthetic risks, such as cervical spine instability, that should be identified and evaluated prior to surgery.[321]

When performing TKA in a knee with a valgus deformity, the ultimate goals of surgery remain the same as that in a varus knee: create balanced flexion and extension spaces, a neutral mechanical alignment, and central patellar tracking.[23] To achieve these results, a series of releases of the contracted lateral structures is performed until the soft tissue tension of the lateral knee matches that of the medial side. Authors have differed on the exact sequence and specific technique of the lateral release. In general, the posterolateral capsule is released first, followed by a "pie crusting" release of the iliotibial band (this is especially true if the lateral joint is tighter in flexion than extension), releasing the LCL off its femoral insertion, and lastly the popliteus tendon.[24,322] In rare cases of a severe valgus deformity, one may find extensive attenuation of the medial ligamentous structures. In this situation, an extensive lateral release will balance the medial and lateral compartments but will also create a flexion/extension mismatch that will require use of a semiconstrained or constrained implant.[323] Valgus malalignment is often accompanied by wear and/or hypoplasia of the lateral femoral condyle. It is important to remember that in posterior referencing systems, femoral rotation may be compromised by a hypoplastic or worn lateral femoral condyle, which will abnormally internally rotate the femoral component. Do not place the femur with an internal rotation orientation! Make sure you use Whiteside's line, the transepicondylar axis, and/or the grand piano sign to guide appropriate alignment and resection.[25,26,324]

Osseous defects can be managed based on the size and containment of the area. Small defects (3 to 5 mm) can be managed by filling them with cement or bone graft (autologous at the time of primary TKA). Medium (5 to 10 mm) and large (> 1 cm) defects can be treated with cement reinforced with screw(s) technique ("rebarb"), autologous bone graft, modular wedge augmentation, structural allograft, or metaphyseal sleeve augmentation depending on size and location.

Why Might This Be Tested? Valgus knees are a common subject in test questions because they are rarer than the varus counterpart. The specific order of ligamentous release is controversial, but rotational alignment is crucial in these cases.

Here's the Point!

Valgus knees can lead to internal rotation of the femoral component if appropriate landmarks are not respected. Modern management of ligamentous release involves pie crusting the tight lateral structures. Remember, if peroneal nerve palsy is found postoperatively, flex the knee and loosen the bandage.

Vignette 107: Pesky Snowboarders!

A 9.5-year-old boy fell while snowboarding. The child had immediate pain and deformity to his left thigh and was unable to bear weight on the lower extremity after the fall. He was brought down from the ski slope and taken directly to the emergency room. X-rays obtained at that time showed the midshaft femur fracture (Figure 107-1).

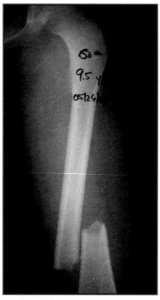

Figure 107-1. X-ray showing a midshaft femur fracture.

▶ *What are the treatment options for a 9.5-year-old child?*

▶ *What would be the recommended treatment if the child were 11 years old?*

▶ *Describe the contraindications to flexible nailing a femur fracture.*

Vignette 107: Answer

The child has a displaced midshaft femur fracture, which is a relatively common injury (incidence is 19.5/100,000 children).[97] Management of these fractures depends on age, patient size, fracture location, and other injuries. Treatment may include spica casting, Pavlik harness, traction, external fixation, ORIF, and IM nailing. In this age range, it is extremely uncommon for the fracture to be nondisplaced. The treatment would be operative intervention. This could include an external fixator and ORIF with a plate or flexible nails. In 2009, the AAOS developed a practice guideline for treating pediatric femoral shaft fractures (14 recommendations made).[98]

Midshaft transverse femur fractures in patients younger than 10 years (typical range is 5 to 11 years old) and less than 100 lb are usually treated with closed reduction and flexible titanium or steel nails. Typically, 2 nails are used that measure about 80% of the femoral canal at its narrowest diameter. Contraindications to flexible nails are patients older than 10 years of age and more than 100 lb, long spiral/oblique fractures, fractures with comminution, or fractures that are too far distal or proximal. The nails are usually inserted in a retrograde fashion with a soft "C" shape molded into the flexible nails. If, however, the fracture is more proximal, one flexible nail may be inserted in a retrograde fashion in a "C" shape and the second can be inserted from distal to the greater trochanter and shaped in an "S" shape.

Retrograde nailing is easier and gives better torsional stability, whereas anterograde insertion is better at resisting shortening. The starting point for the nails should be about 2.5 cm proximal to the distal femoral physis. Timing of the surgery should be expeditious but when the child is stable. Early surgical management is advocated for high-energy trauma, associated head injury, floating knee, and concomitant vascular injury.[99] Occasionally, temporary fixation with an external fixator is required initially with subsequent conversion to an IM nail within 2 weeks to avoid complications (treatment to union with an external fixator is associated with delayed union and refracture).[99] Postoperative care may include casting or placement of a knee immobilizer to add in comfort and support for the fracture. Weight bearing is usually limited for 4 to 6 weeks pending radiographic evidence of healing.

Percutaneous plate fixation is becoming popular. It can be considered in any patient who requires operative fixation. It is considered an "internal external fixation" and therefore bridges the fracture site. It is particularly useful in fractures through bone cysts and with unstable fracture patterns or fractures that are very proximal or distal. Placing the plate percutaneously in a retrograde or antegrade fashion avoids the extensive dissection required for ORIF.

Patients older than 10 years can be treated with a rigid nail; however, the starting point has to be at the greater trochanter rather than a piriformis starting point because of the risk of avascular necrosis with a piriformis starting point in a patient with open growth plates. Insertion of a nail through the greater trochanter is not without risk and may lead to a proximal femoral valgus deformity, femoral neck narrowing, and greater trochanter physeal arrest.[97]

In infants younger than 6 months, a Pavlik harness or spica cast can be used to treat a displaced femoral shaft fracture.[98] In infants younger than 36 months, child abuse needs to be ruled out. Patients younger than 6 years (6 months to 5 years) are typically treated with a spica cast for a period of 6 weeks if less than 2 cm of shortening has occurred. Fractures that are shortened more than 2 cm are typically treated with 2 weeks of traction with serial x-rays to assure acceptable position of the fracture, followed by a spica cast. Waterproof cast padding under a spica cast is acceptable in treating femoral shaft fractures with a lower rate of skin irritation.[98]

Other key points include the following: angular deformity is better tolerated closer to the hip than the knee; remodeling potential is greatest in those younger than 10 years; acceptable alignment in 2- to 10-year-old patients at time of healing is less than 15 degrees of varus/valgus, less than 20 degrees of anterior/posterior angulation, and less than 30 degrees of malrotation; average overgrowth in 2- to 10-year old patients is 0.9 cm; and spica casting can be very difficult for patients and family to care for.[99] The complication of refracture may occur with the use of an external fixator for treatment or after hardware removal.

Why Might This Be Tested? It is important to be aware of the different treatment options in each age group (0 to 6 years, 6 to 10 years, and older than 10 years) as well as the indications and contraindications to each type of treatment.

Here's the Point!

Know the treatment indications: infants/toddlers (0 to 6 years)=spica casting or Pavlik harness; young children (6 to 10 years)=flexible nails; adolescents (older than 10 years)=femoral nail with trochanteric start point. External fixation is a temporary solution, with extended use being associated with delayed union and refracture.

Vignette 108: Look Out for That Ice!

A 67-year-old male with a history of a right TKA approximately 1 year ago was doing well until he slipped on ice, fell on his anterior knee, and suffered a transverse patella fracture. ORIF of the patella fracture was attempted twice with persistent nonunion and hardware failure. Overall, he managed well until the past 2 to 3 weeks, during which he developed increasing complaints of pain and inability to actively extend his knee. X-rays of the patient's injured knee are shown in Figure 108-1.

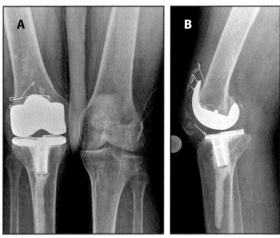

Figure 108-1. (A) AP and (B) lateral x-rays of the right knee.

▶ *Describe the classification for periprosthetic patella fractures.*

▶ *What are the indications for patellar fractures after TKA to be managed nonoperatively?*

▶ *When ORIF results in nonunion, what are the next options?*

▶ *When is revision of the femoral and tibial components warranted?*

Vignette 108: Answer

Ortiguera and Berry described a classification system for periprosthetic patellar fractures, as follows:

I.   Stable implant, intact extensor mechanism (nonoperative treatment has good success if the patella is not dislocated, implant is stable, and extensor mechanism is intact)

II. Disrupted extensor mechanism (repair of the extensor mechanism with partial patellectomy, ORIF, or extensor mechanism allograft)

III. Loose patellar component and

   a.   Reasonable bone stock (component revision or resection)

   b.   Poor bone stock (implant removal and patelloplasty, patellectomy, or extensor mechanism allograft)

   Periprosthetic patella fractures are not uncommon, with prevalence rates ranging from 0.11% to 21.4%. Such fractures are more common after revision surgery and less likely to occur intraoperatively. Risk factors include aggressive clamping during resurfacing, over-resection/reaming (leaving less than 10 to 15 mm of bone), and thermal injury from cement or saw. Patella fracture after TKA can be managed nonoperatively if the component is stable and the extensor mechanism is intact. Given this patient's inability to actively extend the knee, surgical intervention would be warranted in the form of ORIF had there not been 2 prior attempts at repair.[325] Unfortunately, in this situation, previous surgery leading to diminished blood supply and decreased bone stock place the patella at risk for persistent nonunion. In cases with patellar ON (related to fat pad removal and sacrifice of the lateral geniculate artery with a lateral release), less than 10 mm of bone remaining, significant osteolysis, and malposition of the components, ORIF may be at greater risk to fail.

   For those with patellar maltracking, anterior compartment stuffing (under-resection of the patella and anterior placement of the femoral component), or femoral/tibial malrotation/alignment, greater loads are transferred to the patellofemoral joint, predisposing the patient to patella fracture and/or dislocation. Furthermore, components with a central peg have a greater risk of fracture, as do males, metal-backed and cementless components, and patients with osteoporosis and excessive ROM. Of note, ORIF is subject to higher failure rates and postoperative complications, so prevention is a key for periprosthetic patella fractures.

   In our case, an extensor mechanism allograft reconstruction (with an Achilles tendon and calcaneus bone block or with an entire quadriceps/patella/patellar tendon allograft) is indicated.[326] For cases with allograft reconstruction or ORIF, the reconstructions must be protected with absolute knee stability and minimization of anterior knee forces. If components are malrotated or there is a history of patellar maltracking, revision is indicated to a more constrained component. A hinged prosthesis best protects the anterior knee and should be considered. Postoperatively, the knee is held in extension in a cast for 6 to 8 weeks with gradual mobilization over the next 6 to 8 weeks. If tensioning in full extension and postoperative restrictions are respected, results are promising, with an average postoperative extensor lag of less than 5 degrees.

   Why Might This Be Tested? Patella fractures are not uncommon after TKA. The classification system guides management, and these procedures are rife with complications as well as testable material!

Here's the Point!

If the extensor mechanism is disrupted or the component is loose, surgery is warranted. When possible, conservative management is a great option because surgical management, including ORIF of the patella, soft tissue repair, and extensor mechanism allograft, have significant complication rates.

Vignette 109: Upper Extremity Biceps Tendon Injuries

A 55-year-old male who has worked at a furniture warehouse for the past 15 years presents to the clinic with pain in his anterior shoulder that tends to radiate down his arm after a long day of work. The patient reports that he has had the anterior superior shoulder pain for the past 5 years but has recently noticed the radiation of the pain down his arm. The pain previously would remit with ibuprofen and occasional ice, but that does not seem to be working now. The patient also notes that he had similar symptoms when he pitched in high school.

▶ *What is the most likely diagnosis?*

▶ *What is the differential diagnosis in a patient with anterior shoulder pain?*

▶ *What treatment options are available to patients?*

Vignette 109: Answer

The most likely diagnosis in this patient is biceps tendinopathy. The differential diagnosis in a patient with anterior shoulder pain includes impingement syndrome, rotator cuff tears, tendinitis, bursitis, SLAP tears, AC joint injury, arthritis, and adhesive capsulitis.

Biceps tendinopathy is a range of disease, spanning from tendinitis to synovitis of the tendon sheath to degenerative tendinosis with subsequent tendon rupture, and it can occur in a diverse population, affecting both young and old patients. Although the distal and proximal biceps tendons can be affected, the proximal biceps, specifically the long head of the biceps, is usually affected as a part of other shoulder pathology, such as impingement, rotator cuff disease, and SLAP tears, in which inflammation from adjacent structures can then cause associated inflammation in the long head of the biceps. The long head of the biceps originates at the superior edge of the labrum and supraglenoid tubercle, the short head originates at the coracoids process, and the distal tendon inserts at the radial tuberosity. The long head is intra-articular but extrasynovial, and as it courses distally, it sits in the intertubercular groove of the humerus, forming the bulk of the muscle with the short head. The long head of the biceps can be affected as associated inflammation while intra-articular from concurrent shoulder pathology, or it can be isolated tendinitis caused by direct injury to the tendon along its course.[327] Subluxation of the tendon from the intertubercular groove can also cause pain in patients and is usually associated with subscapularis tendon tears.

The patient in the vignette presents as typical biceps tendinopathy, with anterior shoulder pain, which may be along the intertubercular groove that radiates down to the elbow. Patients with biceps tendinopathy typically report a history of repetitive overhead activities, such as laborers, and patients with isolated tendinitis are typically young athletes who play sports with repetitive overhead motions, such as baseball and volleyball. In order to further assess the injury, Yergason's test and Speed's test can be performed, but these do not have high specificity and sensitivity.[328] Yergason's test involves putting the patient in 90 degrees of arm flexion with pronation, and pain is elicited along the intertubercular groove with resisted supination. Speed's test involves putting the patient's elbow extended with the forearm supinated, and resisted arm flexion elicits pain. In patients in whom subluxation of the tendon is a concern, the tendon may be able to be grasped when in subluxation. Because of the association with other shoulder pathology, there may be concurrent findings during the exam that may elicit shoulder pain. In patients with severe disease that results in tendon rupture, a Popeye deformity may be present. Patients who tend to have distal biceps tendon pathology are usually middle-aged and exhibit symptoms more acutely with flexion of the elbow against an increased force. They usually report markedly decreased flexion and supination strength than those with long head rupture.

Plain x-rays should be obtained to rule out other gross deformities in patients. MRI can identify shoulder pathology in addition to pathology in the biceps tendon, but its sensitivity and specificity may be low. Ultrasound is a useful imaging modality in imaging patients, but it shows high user dependence.[328]

For nonsurgical treatment in these patients, the first step is activity reduction, NSAIDs, and ice. If the symptoms persist, corticosteroid injections can be made in the glenohumeral joint first, with later injection into the tendon sheath in the intertubercular groove if symptoms continue. Physical therapy may also play a role in addressing concomitant shoulder pathology and modalities directed at the long head of the biceps.

In patients for whom conservative treatment fails, surgical intervention is the next step. Indications for surgery for the long head of the biceps include partial-thickness tear of 25% to 50%, subluxation of the tendon, and subluxation with a subscapularis tear. In addition, relative indications include type IV SLAP tear, symptomatic type II SLAP tear in a patient older than 50 years, and chronic pain not manageable with nonoperative treatment. The 2 most common procedures are tenotomy and tenodesis. Tenotomy is usually indicated in patients who are older with lower demand or who would not be unhappy with a cosmetic appearance such as the Popeye deformity. Tenodesis is indicated in a younger population, laborers, and patients who require a more active lifestyle. The clinical outcomes have been similar with tenotomy or tenodesis; however, patients who undergo tenotomy have more cosmetic issues and fatigue after repeated flexion and supination. Tenotomy can be performed arthroscopically, with debridement of the tendon. It is important to explore the tendon in the joint and assess for instability. Tenotomy can be performed by incising the tendon at the labrum, with subsequent release of the tendon into the intertubercular groove. Tenodesis can be performed arthroscopically and open. The tendon can be fixed with interference screws distally in the intertubercular groove or proximally in the glenohumeral joint. In an open procedure, the tendon is fixed to the proximal humerus with interference screws.[327,328]

Complications of tenotomy include the previously mentioned Popeye deformity and fatigue with increased use of the muscle, as well as the potential for minor deficits in elbow flexion and supination strength. Complications of tenodesis include continued pain, musculocutaneous nerve palsy, humerus fracture, and possible rupture after tenodesis.

Why Might This Be Tested? Biceps tendinopathy is a common problem in young athletes, laborers, and the older population. It is a part of the differential diagnosis in a patient who presents with anterior shoulder pain, and physicians must also be wary of its concurrence with other shoulder pathology.

Here's the Point!

Biceps tendinopathy is on the differential for anterior shoulder pain, and although most patients are managed with nonsurgical treatment, those for whom surgery is indicated may have different preferences for postsurgical outcomes. Tenotomy and tenodesis are indicated in different patient populations.

Vignette 110: Innocent Bystander Shot in the Belly

An 18-year-old male is shot in the belly during a bank robbery. He is emergently taken to the emergency room, and a diagnostic workup is initiated. It is found that the bullet penetrated the abdomen and is lodged in the L2 vertebral body. His lactic acid level is greater than 3 mmol/L and he has a perforated colon. On thorough physical exam, he has no focal neurological deficits. CT of the L2 vertebral body demonstrates that the spine is mechanically stable. Flexion and extension films demonstrate a stable spine as well.

► *Besides having general surgery manage his colon perforation, what other medical management is necessary for this patient?*

► *What, if any, role does spinal surgery play in this case?*

► *What is the role of antibiotics?*

Vignette 110: Answer

Stabilize the patient medically (fluid resuscitate and make sure well oxygenated), but the bullet can stay if the spine is structurally sound and there is no evidence of progressive neurological deficits. Antibiotic use is controversial but appropriate with organ perforation.

Civilian gunshots and military gunshots are 2 different types of injuries. In civilian injuries, the gunshot wound is low velocity. Nevertheless, the body may be injured from the direct path of the bullet or the concussive effects of the bullet. Frequency of injuries demonstrates 20% of injuries to occur in the cervical region, 50% in the thoracic region, and 30% in the lumbar region.[329] If neurological injury occurs, the neurological injury is at least one level higher than the vertebrae level in 70% of cases. In 20%, the deficit levels are the same, and in 10%, the vertebrae level is 2 levels lower.[330]

The role of bullet removal is controversial, but it is a commonly accepted procedure performed nevertheless. There is no role for laminectomy and bullet removal at the cord injury level but is potentially worthwhile at the level of the conus and caudad to the conus.[331] A possible benefit to decompression at the conus and cauda level may be due to the fact that more nerve roots can be compressed by a bullet, and there is higher potential for axons to regenerate at this level than in the spinal cord. In incomplete spinal cord injury patients, many authors have advocated removal of the bullet; however, the National Institute of Disability and Rehabilitation Research indicates that there is no benefit. If patients experience neurological deterioration, prompt decompression is indicated. Lastly, although rare in low-velocity injuries, if the spine is unstable, surgery via fusion is indicated.

For antibiotics, previous studies advocated aggressive debridement and bullet removal if abdominal viscera had been damaged; however, recent studies demonstrate a course of 1 to 2 weeks of IV antibiotics without debridement was sufficient to prevent late infection or osteomyelitis if GI organs were affected.[332,333] All abdominal injuries are not the same. Similarly, all GI injuries are not equal. Colon injuries have a higher rate of infection than stomach, small intestine, and solid abdominal organ injuries. A recent retrospective review demonstrated that even with at least 5 days of IV antibiotics, there was a significantly higher incidence of spinal and wound infections in patients who sustained a GI injury compared with patients with gunshot wounds to the spine without a concomitant GI injury.[333] Furthermore, operative intervention in the setting of GI injury increases the risk for development of postoperative infections. In summary, most physicians still recommend a course of at least 5 days of IV antibiotics to cover gram-positive, gram-negative, and anaerobic bacterial flora if a patient has a gunshot to the spine and GI injury. In the absence of hollow viscous perforation, antibiotic prophylaxis is not necessary.[334] Lastly, steroids are not indicated in gunshot injuries to the spine.

Lactic acid has been tested recently in regard to guiding fluid resuscitation. In normal patients, lactate is less than 2 mmol/L. Lactate is produced during anaerobic metabolism, and accumulation may be a sign of hypovolemia. Decreased circulation results in decreased oxygenation to tissues, resulting in anaerobic metabolism and lactic acid formation. However, other causes can include necrosis, neoplasia, and liver failure. Lactate has been tested as a sign of under-resuscitation due to the fact that lactate can be elevated before clinical changes are evident on physical exam.

Why Might This Be Tested? With an increased emphasis on spinal trauma, questions related to gunshots to the spine are fair game on standardized tests. Debridement and antibiotic use has changed with emerging data, and the latest recommendations are now being tested.

Here's the Point!

In cases with bullet wounds to the spine, debridement is not necessary unless it is a high-energy injury. Typically, antibiotic treatment alone is sufficient. Progressive neurological deficits, particularly at the conus level and lower, may benefit from decompression surgery, and stabilization is a case-by-case scenario based on spinal column stability.

Vignette 111: Atraumatic Knee Pain in a Soccer Player

A 27-year-old male soccer player presents to the office with a 5-month history of right anteromedial knee pain with activity. For the past several months, symptoms have not improved with conservative measures, such as activity modification and NSAIDs. He denies any known history of trauma and is unable to recall any specific event or activity leading to his current symptoms. On physical examination, he has a small palpable effusion. No significant ligamentous laxity is observed on provocative testing maneuvers. X-rays are obtained of the right knee and subtly suggest a chondral defect on the medial femoral condyle; there is no limb malalignment noted on the mechanical axis views. MRI demonstrates no meniscal pathology but shows a 1×1-cm chondral defect on the medial femoral condyle (Figure 111-1).

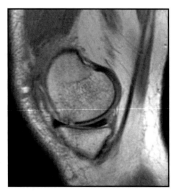

Figure 111-1. Sagittal MRI of the right knee.

▶ *What is the pathoanatomy behind this condition?*

▶ *What history and physical exam findings are important in evaluation?*

▶ *How is this condition classified?*

▶ *What are the treatment options?*

Our patient does very well with his surgery and refers his teammate, who reports similar symptoms. Prior microfracture surgery 18 months ago was unsuccessful for him. An arthroscopic picture of his lesion is shown (Figure 111-2).

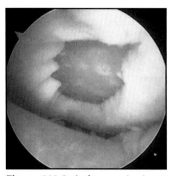

Figure 111-2. Arthroscopic view.

▶ *What are the options for this lesion (measured as 6 cm² intraoperatively)?*

Vignette 111: Answer

The patient has a focal chondral defect of the femoral condyle. Full-thickness chondral defects of the knee are often quite challenging because articular cartilage has a limited capacity for healing/regeneration. Frequently associated with other intra-articular injuries, such as meniscal tears, ACL tears, and patellar dislocations, articular cartilage lesions are routinely encountered during diagnostic arthroscopy. Such chondral defects are theorized to develop from blunt trauma or shear stress that stems from acute injury or repetitive overload.[335-338]

The initial event that leads to chondral injury is an abnormal loading of articular cartilage, typically a contact stress greater than 24 MPa. When this load occurs too rapidly, the chondral matrix is unable to adapt quickly enough. The high focal area of stress results in chondrocyte death and articular cartilage fissuring. Repetitive trauma to the joint helps propagate further injury.

In the office, it is important to ask patients with suspected chondral damage about any prior knee trauma or surgery. Physical exam is useful for detecting ligamentous laxity or posterolateral corner insufficiency, as well as any motion defects or limb malalignment. Weight-bearing AP, lateral, and mechanical axis x-rays should be obtained and evaluated for significant arthritic changes and malalignment (associated limb malalignment is a contraindication for all surgical treatments of chondral injuries unless it is concomitantly addressed). MRI should also be reviewed thoroughly, and the location, size, and associated pathology of all cartilage lesions should be noted. Chondral injury is often best visible on fat-suppressed and specialized fast-spin echo images.

The gold standard diagnostic tool for detecting and evaluating chondral lesions is arthroscopy. Although more than 50 arthroscopic grading scales are in existence, the Modified Outerbridge classification[336] remains the most widely utilized (Table 111-1). Lesions are classified according to depth, but size and location are equally important factors when determining treatment options.

Table 111-1.	
MODIFIED OUTERBRIDGE GRADING SYSTEM FOR FULL-THICKNESS ARTICULAR CARTILAGE DEFECTS	
Grade	*Characteristics*
I	Softening
II	Fibrillation and superficial fissures
III	Deep fissures, no exposed subchondral bone
IV	Exposed subchondral bone
Adapted from Curl WW, Krome J, Gordon ES, Rushing J, Smith BP, Poehling GG. Cartilage injuries: a review of 31,516 knee arthroscopies. *Arthroscopy.* 1997;13(4):456-460.	

Conservative management of chondral lesions is a first-line treatment that should be completely exhausted prior to considering more aggressive options. Nonsurgical treatment includes activity modification, ice, compression, and various pharmacologic measures (NSAIDs and acetaminophen). Other interventions that may be effective include weight loss, corticosteroid injections, viscosupplementation, unloader braces, and physical therapy focusing on quadriceps strengthening.

Surgical treatment of chondral lesions is warranted when conservative management fails to provide adequate relief. Surgical options consist of 2 large categories, including either cartilage reparative procedures (microfracture, chondroplasty/debridement) or cartilage restorative techniques (ACI, osteochondral autograft, and osteochondral allograft).

Given the small size of this patient's lesion (1×1 cm), a cartilage reparative procedure may be sufficient to alleviate symptoms. Cartilage reparative procedures aim to stimulate the underlying marrow to initiate hematoma formation, stem cell migration, and eventual vascular ingrowth. Unlike native hyaline cartilage consisting of type II collagen, these techniques elicit the growth of fibrocartilage made up of type I collagen. Arthroscopic debridement, or chondroplasty, has been shown to temporarily improve symptoms by removing loose flaps or edges of cartilage that mechanically impinge on joint surfaces. As noted by Levy, patients frequently do quite well after this simple intervention, and repeat biopsy specimens suggest that fibrocartilage may regrow in some debrided lesions.[337] Microfracture is a technique that involves the use of surgical awls or small drills to create defects in the sclerotic subchondral exposed bone, thereby promoting the formation of a smooth fibrocartilaginous surface. Important technical adjuncts when performing microfracture include carefully debriding calcified cartilage prior to creating holes and using continuous passive motion with protected weight bearing postoperatively.

The patient's teammate has a larger lesion, and cartilage reparative procedures are generally not helpful. In large chondral lesions, cartilage reparative procedures are generally not helpful. In these instances, an ACI, osteochondral autograft, or osteochondral allograft procedure may be recommended instead of microfracture or debridement. An algorithm for approaching chondral lesions of a given size is shown in Figure 111-3.

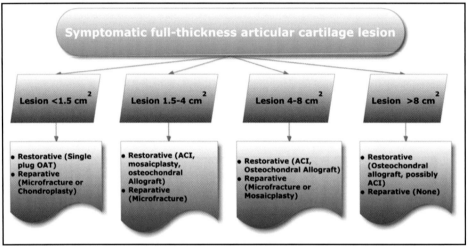

Figure 111-3. Algorithm for treatment of symptomatic articular cartilage lesions indicated for surgical management. (Adapted from Browne JE, Branch TP. Surgical alternatives for treatment of articular cartilage lesions. *J Am Acad Orthop Surg.* 2000;8[3]:180-189.)

Given the large size of this patient's lesion (6 cm^2) and history of failed microfracture, a cartilage restorative procedure is most warranted. Cartilage restorative procedures seek to alleviate the symptoms by reconstructing the microarchitecture of articular cartilage; the end goal is restoration of all biomechanical and physiologic properties of the cartilaginous surface. The primary restorative procedures to consider include ACI, osteochondral autografting, and osteochondral allografting. ACI is generally indicated for younger (aged 20 to 50 years), active patients with an isolated traumatic femoral chondral defect greater than 2 to 4 cm^2. Concomitant ligamentous and meniscal pathology, joint malalignment, and patellofemoral instability should be corrected at the time of surgery. Osteochondral autografting is an appealing option for large lesions but is limited by the donor's finite amount of healthy cartilage available for grafting, as well as morbidity. Osteochondral allografting is an effective alternative to autografting in larger full-thickness chondral lesions (> 10 cm^2), particularly in instances in which the patient has failed a prior cartilage procedure.

Why Might This Be Tested? Chondral lesions of the knee are extremely common and routinely encountered during arthroscopy, and management includes the option of reparative vs restorative techniques.

Here's the Point!

Chondral lesions are best classified according to size, location, and thickness. Full-thickness articular cartilage injuries in young patients with stable knees and normal alignment may benefit from a cartilage reparative or restorative procedure if nonoperative management fails. Smaller lesions (< 1.5 cm^2) are more likely to benefit from cartilage reparative procedures, whereas larger lesions (> 4 cm^2) are more likely to require a cartilage restorative procedure.

Vignette 112: Neck Pain After a 3-Story Fall

A 45-year-old male fell from 3 stories and sustained a presumed injury to his neck; however, the patient is obtunded and does not respond well to physical examination. He has some ecchymosis and tenderness to his upper neck. Palpation of the rest of the spine reveals no stepoffs or point tenderness. AP pelvis, AP chest, and lumbar spine films are adequate and within normal limits.

▶ *What imaging study is required for the cervical spine?*

Plain x-rays are shown in Figure 112-1. In order to better visualize the fracture, a CT scan is obtained (Figure 112-2). The remainder of his spine has been cleared clinically and radiographically for evidence of fracture.

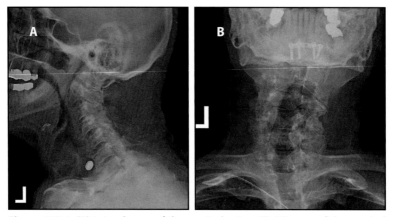

Figure 112-1. (A) Lateral x-ray of the cervical spine. (B) AP x-ray of the cervical spine.

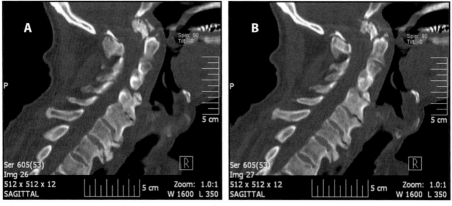

Figure 112-2. (A) Sagittal CT scan section of the cervical spine. (B) Additional sagittal section of the cervical spine.

▶ *What type of spinal fracture is this?*

▶ *What are the treatments for this injury?*

▶ *What are the risk factors for nonunion?*

Vignette 112: Answer

Cervical spine clearance in the trauma setting is a highly published topic in the literature. In the past, cervical x-rays were considered the gold standard, but they have since been supplanted by CT scans as the minimum radiographic study. Growing evidence exists that if patients are at high risk for cervical spine trauma, x-rays are no longer required, and CT scans are the first-line screening modality.[339-343] To simplify matters, patients can be subcategorized into 4 groups. Asymptomatic patients can be cleared clinically without x-rays. An obtunded patient should obtain at least a multidetector CT scan. Controversy arises as to whether this scan suffices, when the CT scan is normal, or whether an MRI is warranted regardless of the CT scan in those cases where a reasonable physical exam is unobtainable. Symptomatic patients require advanced imaging as appropriate (CT and/or MRI). Other patients, including those who are intoxicated or have distracting injuries, can be cleared clinically if the temporary distracting situation will clear up soon or by using the same protocol as obtunded patients.

Our patient sustained a dens/odontoid fracture (C2). The mechanism of this injury is hyperflexion or hyperextension. The most common classification separates these fractures into 3 groups. Type I is an avulsion fracture, type II is a fracture at the base, and type III is within the body. Type II can be further divided to include IIa minimally displaced, IIb posteroinferior to anterior superior, and IIc posterosuperior to anteroinferior. In general, type I fractures are treated with a hard cervical collar. Type III is treated in a cervical orthosis or halo if it is nondisplaced and in a halo if it is displaced. Type II is generally treated operatively because it has a higher risk of nonunion (20% to 80%).

Halo traction is used for reduction and, if acceptable, the patient is treated in a halo for 12 weeks followed by placement in a cervical orthosis. If there is displacement in a halo, delayed union or nonunion, or multiple risk factors for nonunion exist, a C1-C2 fusion vs an anterior odontoid screw is the recommended treatment. Anterior screw fixation is best suited for horizontal or oblique and posterior fractures and is contraindicated in oblique and anterior fractures. Other contraindications include concomitant transverse ligament disruption, atlantoaxial joint injuries, kyphosis, obesity, barrel chest, and osteoporosis.[344]

Risk factors for nonunion include age older than 50 years, displacement greater than 4 mm, and posterior angulation (6 to 7 mm).[344,345]

Why Might This Be Tested? In the adult population, odontoid fractures account for 9% to 15% of cervical spine fractures. Odontoid fractures are the most common individual cervical spine fractures for persons older than 70 years. Therefore, identification, classification, and treatment of these fractures is critical.

Here's the Point!

Many odontoid fractures can be treated nonoperatively. Displaced type II fractures with posterior angulation in elderly patients who smoke are at highest risk for nonunion. Anterior screw fixation is best suited for horizontal or oblique and posterior fractures but is contraindicated in oblique and anterior fractures.

Vignette 113: My Crooked Knee Keeps Me From My Construction Job

A 37-year-old construction worker presents with a history of about 2 years of isolated pain over the medial aspect of the knee. He underwent an arthroscopic medial meniscectomy about 10 years ago after a soccer injury. He states that construction is all he knows, and he is adamant about returning to work without restrictions. On physical examination, the patient has a mild varus deformity (which is correctable on stress testing) of the lower extremity with a ROM of 3 to 120 degrees. With further testing, his ligamentous exam is stable, and he has isolated medial joint line tenderness. An x-ray is shown in Figure 113-1.

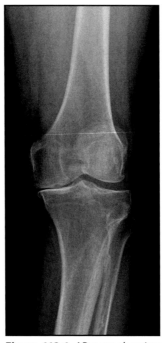

Figure 113-1. AP x-ray showing isolated medial compartment DJD.

▶ *What relative contraindications would prevent this patient from undergoing an arthroplasty procedure?*

▶ *What are his treatment options if not arthroplasty?*

After a long discussion, the patient elects to undergo HTO to correct the deformity of his leg and treat the isolated medial compartment DJD.

▶ *Describe the techniques for HTO and the pros and cons of each approach.*

▶ *In counseling the patient, what can his anticipated outcome include?*

▶ *How does a prior HTO affect a future TKA?*

Vignette 113: Answer

Medial compartment disease in a young laborer = HTO. The patient's age and activity level (they are hitting you over the head with the young laborer in this question) are relative contraindications to arthroplasty, UKA, and TKA. A trial of treatment with a medial unloader brace that shifts weight off the affected compartment (if deformity is correctable, as in this case) may help the patient's symptoms and provide him with expectations of relief from a valgus-producing osteotomy. Knee arthrodesis is a little excessive because he has unicompartmental disease, but it is historically an option in a young, high-demand patient with tricompartmental knee damage (know the correct position of arthrodesis even though it is not commonly performed: 5 to 8 degrees of valgus, 0 to 10 degrees of external rotation, and 0 to 15 degrees of flexion). The other option is an HTO; contraindications include greater than 15 degrees of flexion contracture, more than 2 to 3 mm of medial bone loss, lateral subluxation of more than 1 cm, less than 90 degrees of flexion, ligamentous instability (varus thrust when walking), and inflammatory arthritis (we are safe in our case).

The most commonly used HTO techniques are the lateral closing-wedge and medial opening-wedge procedures. Each of these techniques has unique advantages and disadvantages.[346] The opening-wedge technique is generally felt to be technically easier, given the ability to "dial in" the degree of correction. The opening-wedge HTO appears to affect the joint line less and is easier to convert to a TKA than a closing wedge HTO. The closing-wedge provides a more stable initial construct that allows for immediate weight bearing. It also provides for more bony contact across the osteotomy with a lower rate of nonunion or delayed union.[347] It is important to avoid overcorrection and subsequent patella baja that may limit knee ROM and make exposure for TKA more difficult.

The published results of HTO vary. Clinical success and survivorship improve with careful surgical indications and avoiding under- and overcorrection. The reported survivorship at 10-year follow-up ranges from 50% to 85%.[348-350] Even in some of the best performing series, a failure rate of 32% at 15 years has been reported.[349] Given the large decline with time after an HTO, this surgical procedure is best indicated as a bridge to TKA for younger, more active patients.

Although somewhat controversial, many authors believe that conversion of a failed HTO to a TKA is more difficult than a primary procedure.[351,352] To restore a neutral mechanical axis, augments, stemmed components, and components with increased varus-valgus constraint may be required. The history of prior surgery, as well as increased dissection and operative time, place these cases at increased risk for infection and perioperative complications. Retained hardware can be addressed with a high-speed metal-cutting burr to remove what is in the way. Care must be taken to debride metal shards because they can act as third-body wear in the future; also make sure retained hardware does not alter the alignment of the construct. Lastly, alteration of the joint line and scarring/contraction of the patellar tendon can result in a patella baja that will make exposure and balancing the flexion/extension gaps more challenging.

Why Might This Be Tested? Although not as frequently performed as TJA, osteotomy surgeries are often a source of questions. Relatively clear-cut indications and contraindications exist, making this subject easy to question.

Here's the Point!

Single compartment disease in a young and active patient = HTO. For a varus deformity, it is a proximal tibial osteotomy, and for a valgus deformity, it is a distal femoral osteotomy. It is important to avoid over- or undercorrection because they can lead to early failure. Remember that obesity is a relative contraindication to HTO. TKA after HTO always has a harder exposure and may require extensile techniques.

Vignette 114: Since I Was Shot in the Elbow, I Can't Move My Wrist!

A 33-year-old male sustained a gunshot wound at the level of the elbow joint with a low-velocity missile 10 months ago. No fracture was seen, and he has had no surgery. His wounds have healed well, but he complains of the inability to fully extend the wrist and all digits, including the thumb. He has not undergone therapy or splinting. Physical exam reveals an intact soft tissue envelope and 5/5 elbow flexion and extension but no appreciable function of the wrist extensors, EDC, or extensor pollicis longus. He has diminished sensation on the dorsal aspect of the radial hand and thumb. He has full passive ROM of the digits and wrist flexion and lacks only 10 degrees of passive wrist extension.

▶ *What is the patient's underlying diagnosis?*

▶ *What are the patient's principal surgical options?*

▶ *What are some basic concepts of tendon transfers?*

▶ *What active functions are essential to restore, and what are the commonly used transfers to achieve this?*

▶ *What are the concepts of treatment of radial nerve palsy with humerus fractures?*

Vignette 114: Answer

This patient has evidence of complete radial nerve palsy. Be aware that this is not simply a posterior interosseous nerve (PIN) palsy because such an injury would have intact function of the brachioradialis and ECRL, which are innervated by the radial nerve proper. This would present with weakness and radial deviation upon wrist extension. Although most cases of nerve injury from gunshot wounds are neuropraxias, this patient has shown no recovery of radial nerve function. EMG would be able to confirm the absence of recovery. Typically, an EMG is performed approximately 2 weeks after the injury to allow signs of complete denervation to be detectable and is repeated at 8 to 12 weeks if no clinical recovery is noted. The radial nerve can be very slow to recover, often taking 4 to 5 months or more to start showing signs of recovery.[353]

The patient's primary surgical options at this point are nerve repair vs tendon transfer. Although late nerve repair (>6 months) has a poor prognosis with other peripheral nerve injuries, such as the peroneal nerve, radial nerve repair or grafting can typically be successful even 12 months or more postinjury. Given the slow recovery of the radial nerve and the good outcomes in a delayed setting, one should consider waiting until at least 6 months after injury to explore. The decision between exploration and grafting vs tendon transfer is a difficult one. Nerve repair in this chronic setting would almost assuredly require nerve grafting (usually with sural autograft) and then a waiting period of at least 4 to 6 months for recovery. If it were to fail, the patient would be treated with tendon transfers. Since it is human nature to want instant gratification, the patient must understand this potential time lapse.[354]

Proceeding directly to tendon transfers would provide a faster return to function. There are several important principles of tendon transfers:

- Supple ROM must be maintained during any waiting period, and contracture is much easier to prevent than correct. This would include wrist and finger extension and thumb abduction/retroposition for the radial nerve.

- The donor muscle must be expendable, meaning that there must be another functional muscle performing its same function.

- Muscle strength and excursion have been well studied in the upper extremity and should be matched as well as possible between donor and recipient, realizing that muscles will usually lose one grade of strength after transfer.

- "One tendon–one function" describes how a single tendon should not be transferred to 2 tendons performing different actions or with large differences in excursion because doing so will greatly dissipate the force to both.

- Synergism involves using donors and recipients that are typically paired up functionally in simultaneous action (ie, wrist flexors with finger extensors).

- Appropriate tissue equilibrium describes waiting for swelling to go down and ROM to be supple before proceeding with transfers and also assuring that all transfers are performed in a healthy bed of tissue free of significant scar tissue or poorly vascularized tissue (exposed bone, hardware).[355]

The functions that need to be restored in this setting are wrist extension, digital extension, and thumb extension and abduction. Although numerous transfers have been described, the most common transfers are the pronator teres to extensor carpi radialis brevis, palmaris longus or FDS to extensor pollicis longus, and a wrist flexor (flexor carpi radialis or ulnaris) to the EDC.[354]

Although the topic of radial nerve palsy with humerus fracture is somewhat controversial, most authors agree that for closed fractures with primary (at the time of injury) or secondary (after reduction attempt) radial nerve palsy, early exploration is not recommended because approximately 90% will typically recover. This spares most patients from unnecessary surgery, and the infrequent patient without nerve recovery will usually do well with nerve grafting or tendon transfer. Early exploration should be considered in cases of open fracture, vascular injury requiring repair, or unstable fractures requiring surgical fixation.[353]

Why Might This Be Tested? Radial nerve palsy is common posttraumatically, and the successful classic tendon transfers are commonly tested, as are the principles of tendon transfers. The actual timing of grafting vs tendon transfer is more controversial and less likely to be tested.

Here's the Point!

Traumatic radial nerve palsy with the exception of a sharp (knife) penetrating wound is likely to recover spontaneously, albeit slowly, and is usually treated with observation and then with nerve grafting or classically described tendon transfers if the nerve does not recover. Know the principles of tendon transfers because they are well accepted and apply no matter where transfers are being considered.

Vignette 115: My Hip Fracture—Stable or Unstable?

A 92-year-old male with a medical history of diabetes mellitus and hypertension sustained a ground-level fall on the day of admission with immediate pain in the left hip and inability to bear weight. On examination, the skin was intact and the patient was intact to neurovascular examination. X-rays are shown in Figure 115-1.

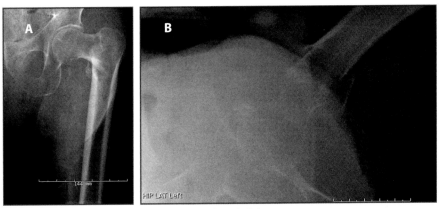

Figure 115-1. (A) AP and (B) lateral x-rays of the left hip.

▶ *How is this fracture classified, and how does this influence treatment?*

▶ *What are the treatment options?*

▶ *What aspects of surgical technique most strongly predict success or failure?*

▶ *Could THA be considered?*

▶ *What factors might complicate THA as a treatment for this condition?*

Vignette 115: Answer

Intertrochanteric fractures most frequently occur in older osteoporotic individuals after low-energy mechanisms. Generally, these fractures are classified as stable (ie, able to resist varus and proximal medial to distal lateral loading after fixation) and unstable (ie, transtrochanteric fractures, fractures with subtrochanteric extension, fractures with comminution of the posteromedial cortex with involvement of the lesser trochanter implying loss of the calcar buttress, or fractures that extend into the lateral femoral cortex, which are reverse obliquity or transtrochanteric fractures by definition). Treatment options include placement of a sliding hip screw, an implant designed to slide so as to compress the fracture site, or placement of a cephalomedullary fixation nail, which is appropriate for stable and unstable fracture patterns because of its shorter moment arm, decreased tensile strength, and filling of the intertrochanteric region. In select unstable fractures, due to comminution of the lateral wall, a sliding hip screw supplemented with a trochanteric stabilization plate or a proximal femoral locking plate may be appropriate.[356-358]

Classically, the iliopsoas and adductors pull the distal fragment into adduction and flexion, resulting in a varus extension deformity. The specifics of the fracture line can cause other deformities; for instance, in a transtrochanteric fracture with medial comminution, the abductors may pull the proximal fragment into varus while the iliopsoas may pull the lesser trochanter proximal and medial.

In cases in which the vascularity of the femoral head is in question, cases with significant preexisting OA, or cases with fracture extension into the neck or the head, a THA can be considered. This procedure can be technically complex because loss of proximal femoral landmarks can introduce difficulties with recreating anatomic limb length and offset. Revision components and distal-fixation stems should be available. In addition, if the fracture line separates the abductors from the shaft, a trochanteric claw plate may be necessary as a supplement to THA to prevent dysfunction, limping, and instability.

Several aspects of surgical fixation have been linked with failure or success. A lower distance between the tip of the implant and the apex of the femoral head (the tip-apex distance), as measured on lateral and the AP x-rays, has been directly correlated with success. In the Baumgaertner et al series, a tip-apex distance of less than 25 mm was associated with a 0% cutout rate, a distance of 25 to 29 mm was associated with a 6% cutout rate, a distance of 30 to 34 mm was associated with a 17% cutout rate, a distance of 35 to 44 mm was associated with a 24% cutout rate, and a distance of more than 44 mm was associated with a 60% cutout rate.[356] Malreduction in distraction and/or varus has also been linked to failure. During placement of a sliding hip screw, left-sided fractures can be malreduced into extension due to the torque of the screw insertion on the proximal fragment (may need a derotational screw or wire). One additional source of trouble when a long nail is used remains the mismatch between the smaller radius curvature of the femur in the sagittal plane and the larger radius of curvature of the implant causing anterior cortical perforation of the implant at the femoral bow. When using a nail, a medial start point reduces the likelihood of a varus malreduction.

Why Might This Be Tested? Intertrochanteric fractures are common, and several biomechanical principles can be tested using the intertrochanteric fracture as an example; thus, this topic is frequently tested.

Here's the Point!

Intertrochanteric fractures occur most frequently in elderly osteoporotic patients after low-energy trauma. These fractures are classified into stable and unstable variants. Stable variants can be treated with a sliding hip screw or a cephalomedullary implant, but unstable variants are often better suited with a cephalomedullary implant.

Vignette 116: This Knee Pain Is Keeping Me From Playing Intramural Soccer

A 20-year-old male presents with a 2-month history of increasing knee pain. He does not recall a traumatic event, although he is a recreational athlete. Neither rest nor NSAIDs relieve the pain as they have in the past for prior knee injuries. A plain x-ray, MRI, and histology from the affected knee are shown (Figures 116-1 to 116-4).

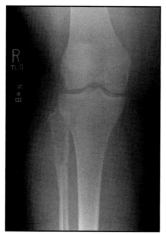

Figure 116-1. AP x-ray of the right knee.

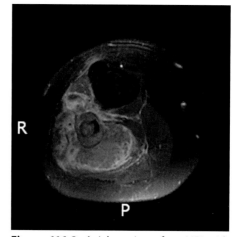

Figure 116-2. Axial section of an MRI with gadolinium.

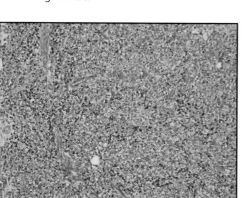

Figure 116-3. Histologic section of the tumor (200× magnification).

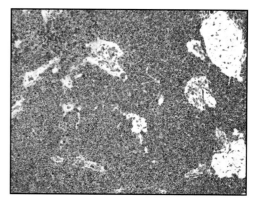

Figure 116-4. Histologic section stained specifically for CD99 (100× magnification).

▶ *What is the diagnosis?*

▶ *What are the treatment options?*

▶ *What are potential treatment-related complications in long-term survivors?*

Vignette 116: Answer

Ewing's sarcoma and the family of primitive neuroectodermal tumors are small-round-blue-cell tumors that have some element of neuroectodermal differentiation. It is the fourth most common (second most common in children) primary malignancy of bone after myeloma, osteosarcoma, and CHS. Eighty to ninety percent of cases occur in patients younger than 20 years (beware: in vignettes, patients will typically fall between 5 and 30 years old), with the peak in early adolescence. Ewing's sarcoma commonly occurs in the metaphyseal-diaphyseal area of long bones (namely the distal femur, proximal tibia, femoral diaphysis, and proximal humerus), as well as the pelvis and ribs. Around one-quarter of cases present with metastatic disease. It often presents like an infection, with pain, fever, and elevated ESR and WBC count.

Radiographically, these present as destructive bone lesions with cortical disruption and abundant periostitis. It is high on the differential in an aggressive, diaphyseal lesion in a skeletally immature patient. The margins are often permeative or moth eaten, and the periosteal reaction to the tumor has a classic onion-skin appearance. The other possible entities given the plain radiographic appearance are osteosarcoma, osteomyelitis, and eosinophilic granuloma. In younger patients, lymphoma, leukemia, rhabdomyosarcoma, and neuroblastoma should be considered. Axial MRI or CT scans commonly show a large enhancing soft tissue mass, often larger than the x-ray would suggest. The staging workup consists of a chest CT, bone scan, and bone marrow biopsy. A positron emission tomography CT scan with F-18 fluorodeoxyglucose may also be useful in identifying other sites of disease, quantifying the tumor activity, and monitoring the response to treatment.

Histologically, the tumor has a characteristic appearance as a sheet of small, round blue cells with little intervening stroma. The cells show scant clear cytoplasm and indistinct cell membranes with round nuclei, fine chromatin, and minimal clear/eosinophilic cytoplasm. Immunohistochemical staining for CD99 is strongly expressed in nearly all cases but is not specific for Ewing's sarcoma. Other immunohistochemical stains that may be positive are S-100, vimentin, and periodic acid-Schiff. The classic genetic abnormality is a t(11:22) translocation, present in 85% of cases, forming a fusion between the EWS and FLI1 genes; know this translocation because it is a favorite of question writers.

In accessible lesions or expendable bones, Ewing's sarcoma is treated with neoadjuvant chemotherapy, surgical resection, and postoperative chemotherapy. Ewing's sarcoma is radiosensitive and may be used for positive margins after surgical resection, although re-resection to obtain negative margins is associated with better outcomes. Most data indicate that surgery is superior to radiation for local control when wide margins can be obtained. These studies have a selection bias toward surgery in more easily resectable and smaller lesions. Bones such as the fibula and clavicle are considered expendable and are nearly universally excised.

Locations such as the spine, pelvis, and entire femur require an extensive surgical resection with significant functional morbidity afterward. In these scenarios, radiation may be used, along with chemotherapy, as the definitive treatment. Bones that are irradiated often require surgical stabilization after radiation therapy because they are susceptible to fracture. Other complications of radiation include joint stiffness, limb-length inequality, and muscle atrophy.

The 5-year survival for localized disease is 65% to 82% and for metastatic disease is 25% to 39%. Long-term survivors of Ewing's sarcoma who have received radiation are particularly susceptible to developing a secondary malignancy in the radiation field. The lag time is typically around 10 years, but it can happen at any time. Development of a second malignancy is related to the size of the radiation dose. Children are more sensitive to the adverse effects of radiation than adults.

Why Might This Be Tested? Pediatric tumors are commonly tested, particularly with the associated genetic translocation (can't say it enough—t[11:22]). There are several small-round-blue-cell tumors that can be confusing and occur in relatively specific age ranges; you just have to know them (Table 116-1).

Table 116-1.
DIFFERENTIAL DIAGNOSIS FOR SMALL-ROUND-BLUE-CELL TUMORS

Tumor	Age Range
Metastatic neuroblastoma and leukemia	Younger than 5 years
Eosinophilic granuloma	5 to 10 years
Ewing's sarcoma	5 to 29 years
Lymphoma	Older than 30 years
Myeloma and metastatic carcinoma	Older than 50 years

Here's the Point!

If you see a small-round-blue-cell tumor in a person aged 5 to 30 years with an associated fever and elevated WBC count and ESR, think Ewing's sarcoma. If the lesion is destructive with an onion-skin pattern in the metaphyseal or diaphyseal region of long bones, then really think Ewing's sarcoma. Treatment is chemotherapy→surgery→chemotherapy (with radiation for nonresectable tumors and those with metastases). Metastatic involvement, spine and pelvic tumors, large tumors, those that do not respond to chemotherapy, and high lactate dehydrogenase levels often portray a poor prognosis.

Vignette 117: Motor Vehicle Accident and Lower Extremity Numbness

A 25-year-old male is a restrained driver involved in a motor vehicle accident. Upon extraction from his vehicle, it is noted that his blood alcohol level is normal and he is fully cooperative. On exam, the patient is assessed as having an incomplete neurologic injury. He has decreased motor strength in the lower extremities with intact rectal tone and sensation. He states over the next few hours that he is having increasing numbness in the ipsilateral leg. He has no other medical problems and is otherwise healthy. He has no other injuries, and his lactic acid level is normal. X-rays, CT scans (Figures 117-1 and 117-2), and MRIs (Figures 117-3) are obtained.

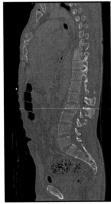

Figure 117-1. Sagittal CT section of the lumbar spine.

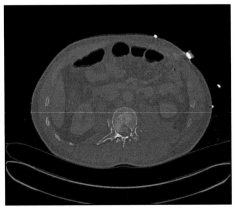

Figure 117-2. Axial CT slice through the zone of injury.

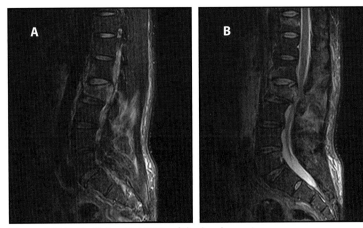

Figure 117-3. (A, B) Sagittal MRIs of the lumbar spine.

▶ *What type of injury is this fracture?*

▶ *What are indications for surgery?*

▶ *How should this patient be managed?*

Vignette 117: Answer

The patient sustained a burst fracture involving the lumbar spine. The L2 vertebral body is affected, and compromise of the spinal canal can be seen on the imaging studies. The L2 and L3 spinous processes also have fractures. The MRI demonstrates disruption of the ligamentum flavum, a key component of the posteroligamentous complex. Thoracolumbar burst fractures are a common cause of spinal injury as the transitional region of kyphosis to lordosis is susceptible to axial loading injuries. The defining features of the burst fracture are compressive failure of the anterior and middle spinal columns. Due to this high level of trauma, it is important with a burst fracture to make sure the remainder of the trauma exam is within normal limits.

In the past, an emphasis was placed on the 3-column concept described by Denis. The anterior column was the anterior longitudinal ligament to the mid-vertebral body, the middle column was from the mid-vertebral body to the posterior longitudinal ligament, and the posterior column was the posterior elements. Two of the 3 columns were considered unstable. By definition, a burst fracture was considered unstable. Recently, emphasis has focused more on the posterior ligamentous complex as a determining factor of whether a burst fracture is stable, while also factoring in neurological status and the mechanism of injury.

Various classifications have been devised to help guide treatment of burst fractures. Most burst fractures are considered to be stable patterns. From the viewpoint of biomechanics, an unstable burst occurs if there is greater than 25 degrees of kyphosis, greater than 50% vertebral body height loss, or greater than 40% canal compromise. These patients should be treated operatively because they are indirect markers that the posterior tension band is disrupted. Recently, the Thoracolumbar Injury Classification and Severity Score system was created to guide management of such injuries. This system combines many of the previous concepts into an algorithm that bases treatment on morphology of the injury, integrity of the posterior ligamentous complex, and neurological status of the patient.[359] Based on the number of points, surgery is advised. The exact scoring system does not need to be memorized, but general concepts are as follows. Incomplete neurologic injury is generally accepted as an indication for surgical decompression. An anterior approach is indicated if neural compression anteriorly results in an incomplete neurologic injury following attempts at postural or open reduction. The posterior ligament complex disruption generally requires a posterior procedure, and an incomplete neurologic injury with posterior disruption generally requires a combined AP approach. Laminectomy alone has not been effective for restoration of neurological function but has been shown to lead to further progression of the deformity and neurologic injury. Furthermore, if the anterior and middle columns demonstrate comminution, kyphosis, and lack of apposition, a short posterior fixation is likely to fail, and anterior strut support or a longer posterior instrumentation should be considered.[360]

Why Might This Be Tested? Most thoracolumbar burst fractures are stable injuries that can be treated nonoperatively.[361] The onus for an orthopedic surgeon is to identify those that are unstable and require stabilization. Know when to operate and when to brace.

Here's the Point!

Patients who have neurological deficit or a mechanically unstable spine require surgical stabilization with or without decompression. An unstable burst occurs if there is greater than 25 degrees of kyphosis, greater than 50% vertebral body height loss, or greater than 40% canal compromise; these patients should be treated operatively because they are indirect markers that the posterior tension band is disrupted.

Vignette 118: Persistent Back Pain After a Fall

A 59-year-old female presents to the office 6 months after a fall down the stairs of her apartment that caused a lumbar compression fracture. She was initially treated with narcotic pain medications, a back brace, and activity restriction but now reports ongoing pain and functional limitations despite being told that her fracture had healed. She has a history of mild intermittent low back pain but has had no previous workup. She is postmenopausal, and a DEXA scan 2 years ago was within normal limits. Her current pain is exacerbated by movement and prolonged sitting and is only minimally relieved with lying down. She would like to get back to walking and playing with her 2 young grandchildren but is becoming increasingly frustrated by her pain.

▶ *What type of spinal orthosis might this patient have been prescribed?*

▶ *Is a brace still appropriate at this time?*

▶ *What are other possible consequences of lumbar braces to consider?*

Vignette 118: Answer

For acute spinal compression fractures, flexion control orthoses can be used to permit upright positioning yet limit forward flexion. Jewett and cruciform anterior spinal hyperextension braces are commonly described rigid flexion-control options for acute compression fractures,[362] whereas lumbar and lumbosacral corsets are commonly prescribed for low back pain and muscle strains. Although corsets may provide a kinesthetic reminder, support the abdominals, reduce excessive lumbar lordosis, and decrease lateral bending, their overall efficacy remains controversial. More restrictive thoracolumbosacral orthosis (TLSO) braces, such as a Taylor brace or Knight-Taylor brace, provide flexion and extension control through additional paraspinal bars, axillary straps, and an interscapular band but are often reserved for postsurgical or nonsurgical management of other stable spine fractures.[363]

In this case, given radiographic confirmation of fracture healing, the clinical situation, and the other physical implications of spinal bracing, orthosis use is not recommended. In general, limiting axial rotation of the spine with bracing may lead to increased motion at the unrestrained cephalad and caudad segments to the orthosis, which can exacerbate an arthritic condition or biomechanical abnormality. TLSOs may further impede gait by shortening stride length, slowing cadence depending on fit, and impairing balance. Although this patient has no known history of a spinal condition, she may have increased fatigue and demand on supporting structures and muscles due to the increased energy consumption associated with bracing. Trunk muscles can also be weakened by atrophy or strained from prolonged use, leading to additional musculoskeletal complications and chronic pain issues. Of note, TLS flexion-control orthoses are the only TLSOs that do not increase intra-abdominal pressure that could further exacerbate lung or pelvic floor conditions. Also, the suprapubic bands used in the Jewett brace can be adjusted and substituted with boomerang bands in women to avoid direct pressure on the bladder. Finally, caution with these braces should be considered in osteoporotic, elderly patients due to the increased hyperextension forces that can be placed on lumbar posterior elements, risking additional fragility fractures.[363]

Why Might This Be Tested? Spinal orthoses are widely available over the counter and are commonly prescribed by various practitioners. General familiarity with the different options and indications can help optimize treatment outcomes and understand other associated complications.

Here's the Point!

Spine bracing can be used to support and stabilize the trunk to allow for fracture healing. Although a variety of options are available, other biomechanical and functional implications of this type of bracing should also be considered.

Vignette 119: Complications in THA

A 65-year-old female presents with endstage OA of the right hip. She has been told that she needs a THA and is interested in moving forward. However, she is concerned with complications that some of her friends have had after surgery. She presents with her husband and daughter for a detailed discussion on THA. The 3 biggest concerns she reports are the need for a blood transfusion, that her legs will not be equal lengths after surgery, and nerve damage.

▶ *Describe how often these potential complications can occur.*

▶ *What protocols can be implemented to prevent such complications?*

Vignette 119: Answer

Blood transfusions after THA can be quite common, with studies regularly reporting about 15% to 25% (and sometimes higher) rates of allogenic transfusions. Allogenic transfusions have the possibility of causing transmission of blood-borne viruses, longer hospital stays, immune-mediated reactions, infection, and higher costs. Common rates of viral transmission are as follows: HIV (1:225,000), HBV (1:200,000), HCV (1:30,000 to 150,000), hemolytic reaction (1:100,000), and fevers in 1% to 3% of transfusions. There are many techniques that can be used to limit the rate of blood transfusions (Table 119-1).

Table 119-1.

STRATEGIES IN BLOOD MANAGEMENT WITH THA

	Preoperative Strategies	Intraoperative Strategies	Postoperative Strategies
Successful	• EPO • Autologous blood donation (in anemic patients)	• Antifibrinolytics (tranexamic acid—topical or IV) • Blood salvage system (best with long surgeries)	• Strict transfusion protocols
Unsuccessful	• Iron supplementation	• Cautery agents (bipolar sealant)	• Reinfusion drains
Undetermined	• Hemodilution	• Topical hemostatic agents	

EPO = erythropoietin; IV = intravenous.

Modalities that can help lower transfusion rates include erythropoietin, which is a natural glycoprotein that kickstarts the human body to generate red blood cells. It is normally produced by the kidneys and is highly effective in reducing blood transfusions in patients with preoperative anemia. Preoperative autologous blood donation is self-explanatory and can be helpful in anemic patients as well. Cell salvage systems can help if there is a large anticipated blood loss from the surgery (> 1000 mL). Tranexamic acid is a synthetic product that competitively blocks the lysine binding sites of plasminogen and inhibits them from attaching to fibrin molecules. This blocks dissolution of clots and reduces the amount of surgical bleeding and transfusion rates into the single digits for primary THA.[364] The dosing of tranexamic acid can change, so I'm not sure if you have to worry about questions on it, but it is typically given as follows: (1) a single or repeated dose of 1 g IV; (2) 20 mg/kg as a single or divided dose IV; or (3) topically with 1 to 3 g mixed into 100 mL and applied to the surface of the hip tissues. Concerns with increased venous thromboembolism (VTE) in the setting of tranexamic acid have been allayed, with several studies showing no greater risk as well as excellent compatibility with all DVT prophylaxis regimens. Strict transfusion protocols can lower transfusion rates by lowering the threshold for transfusion (that means raising the restrictions and only transfusing for a hemoglobin of less than 8.0 g/dL). Maximizing the modalities that work and minimizing those that do not is the topic of discussion with the patient on trying to be as cost-effective in blood management as possible.

In discussing limb-length discrepancy with patients, it is important to review the rate of dislocation (often reported between 1% and 7%), which is often inversely related to limb lengthening (occurs in 10% to 30%).[365] Keeping the leg short may compromise hip stability; conversely, making the leg long helps reduce the risk of dislocation at the expense of a high rate of litigation. Although the overall goal is restoration of exactly equal leg lengths, this can be difficult to achieve intraoperatively. Some consequences of an acquired limb-length discrepancy include compromised hip biomechanics, sciatica, low back pain, dislocation, limp, and need for a shoe lift/special shoe. Limb lengths can be measured from the ASIS to the medial malleolus (true limb-length discrepancy) or from the umbilicus to the medical malleolus (apparent limb-length discrepancy). This can also be measured on plain x-rays (Figure 119-1) and can be predicted on preoperative templating films. For templates, the acetabulum template sets the COR, while the femoral stem is then placed and should line up with this point on the acetabulum (if they do not match up, then the femur is proximal to the COR, and the template will be lengthening the leg; if it is lateral to the COR, it is reducing offset and vice versa). In a recent study, 8.9% of cases had some element of shortening, 0.5% with no limb-length discrepancy and 90.6% with lengthening. Seventy-eight percent of the limb-length discrepancies were less than 1 cm in magnitude.[366] Overall, they found no decrease in functional or clinical outcomes with the limb-length discrepancies. However, it is important to maximize stability and minimize limb-length discrepancy or you will have some unhappy patients. You explain to the patient you will use templating to estimate sizes and target minimal lengthening of the limb while restoring the COR with the chosen implants. Other reports have found that patients can perceive a limb-length discrepancy greater than 6 mm and that such lengthening led to worse hip scores (it is also important to understand that the shorter the patient, the less he or she will tolerate any limb-length discrepancy).

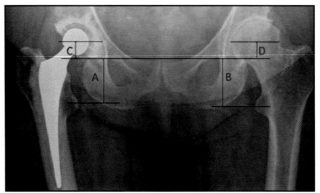

Figure 119-1. Limb-length discrepancy is defined by $(C + A) - (D + B)$.

In discussing nerve injury with patients, it is important to remember the structures that are at risk with the various approaches to THA (anterior = femoral nerve; direct lateral = superior gluteal; posterior = sciatic nerve). Overall, there is a 1% to 2% risk of nerve injury after THA, with higher numbers associated with hip dysplasia and revision surgery.[367] Overall, the most common nerve injured is the sciatic; 3 major types of damage patterns are described in Table 119-2.

Nerve injuries are often related to the surgical approach, with injury to the superior gluteal neurovascular structures when using a transtrochanteric or direct lateral approach (particularly if the dissection extends beyond the 3- to 5-cm safe zone proximal to the greater trochanter). The obturator nerve can be injured when there is penetration of the anterior quadrants of the acetabulum (ie, screws, reamers, cement). The femoral nerve is rarely injured with THA (0.04% to 0.4%) and typically occurs with anterior placement of retractors. Sciatic nerve injury (0.6% to 3.7%, typically cited as 1.5%) comes from retraction, stretch, or direct compression of the nerve, typically affecting the common peroneal and not the tibial branch of the nerve. Typically, those who are going to regain function will do so by 7 months after the injury.[367] Generally, the healthier and younger a patient is, the better the prognosis for nerve function recovery. If a nerve injury occurs, the best way to treat it is to brace to prevent contractures, therapy to keep the affected joints stretched out, and electrical stimulation to keep the muscles functioning. If no recovery at all is noted by 6 to 12 weeks, electrodiagnostic studies can be obtained to determine the extent of the injury.

Why Might This Be Tested? Injuries and complications are ripe for questioning, particularly around an elective surgery. You must know the surgical exposures and anatomy at risk with each approach to the hip. In addition, limb-length discrepancy and preventing one are often tested (most recently in the setting of digital templating), as are blood conservation techniques because there are several that definitely work and several that do not work.

Table 119-2.

SEDDON CLASSIFICATION OF NERVE INJURIES

Neuropraxia	Axonotmesis	Neurotmesis
Often a minor injury: • Conduction block • Anatomically intact nerve • Typically a period of sensation loss	A more severe injury: • Axons are disrupted • Surrounding connective tissues are intact • Wallerian degeneration occurs distal to the site of injury • If the endoneurial structures are intact, regeneration occurs 1 mm/day.	The most severe injury: • Complete disruption of the nerves • Can result in painful neuromas
Recovery: • Likely to have complete recovery	Recovery: • Variable based upon the length of neural regeneration required, host health, and muscle integrity	Recovery: • Worst prognosis for recovery

Adapted from DeHart MM, Riley LH Jr. Nerve injuries in total hip arthroplasty. *J Am Acad Orthop Surg.* 1999;7(2):101-111.

Here's the Point!

Tranexamic acid, erythropoietin, autologous blood donation, and strict transfusion protocols can be used to reduce the rate of allogenic transfusions in THA. Limb-length discrepancies are best prevented with detailed planning, but when one occurs, it is associated with a high rate of litigation. Nerve injuries are rare with primary THA; remember, the common peroneal nerve branch is the one most commonly injured.

Vignette 120: Crick in the Back!

A mother brought in her 4-year-old son because she noticed him leaning to one side while at the beach over the summer. The mother states that he has been extremely active and not complaining of any back pain. He has met all milestones up to this point without noticeable problems. Clinically, the patient shows asymmetry of his shoulders, a curvature of his spine, and asymmetric clonus. There are no focal motor or sensory deficits noted on examination. Examination of the back reveals curvature of the spine and the absence of skin lesions, spots, or abnormalities. There is a family history of "back problems," but they are not sure exactly what the condition is.

▶ *What is the initial study you would order?*

▶ *Why is Figure 120-1 concerning?*

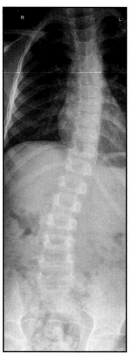

Figure 120-1. AP x-ray of the spine.

▶ *What study should you order next?*

Vignette 120: Answer

The first step in answering the question is making the diagnosis, which is scoliosis in this case. Scoliosis has been divided into 3 categories: infantile (younger than 3 years), juvenile (4 to 9 years), and adolescent (10 years to maturity). In more general terms, early-onset scoliosis occurs in patients younger than 5 years. In addition, scoliosis can be broken down into categories based on etiology (congenital, neuromuscular, or idiopathic).[100] The initial workup should include a thorough physical exam to rule out café-au-lait spots and axillary freckling (found with neurofibromatosis), assess shoulder height differences, complete a thorough neurovascular exam, and check for pelvic obliquity and rigidity (or lack of flexibility) of the curve. Once a diagnosis of scoliosis is suspected, AP and lateral views of the thoracolumbar spine should be obtained and the Cobb angle and rib-vertebrae angle difference (RVAD) determined. An RVAD greater than 20 degrees or a rib head overlapping the apical vertebra is an indicator that curve progression will likely occur.[101] The critical number is 20 degrees for the Cobb angle in younger patients (Risser stage 0 and 1 and < 20-degree curve = 22% risk of curve progression and > 20-degree curve = 68% risk).

X-rays are ordered to assess the degree of scoliosis as well as any bony abnormalities, such as butterfly vertebrae or hemivertebrae suggesting a congenital form of the disease. This patient has idiopathic juvenile scoliosis. Eighteen percent to 26% of patients have neural axis abnormalities. Most children are asymptomatic, with right-sided curves being most common. Patients younger than 10 years, boys, curves with an apex to the left, structural abnormalities on plain x-rays, excessive kyphosis, rapid curve progression, or any neurologic signs (absent abdominal reflexes, asymmetric clonus, wide-based gait, weakness) should have an MRI. Chiari I malformations, cervical syrinx, thoracic syrinx, brainstem tumors, dural ectasia, and low-lying conus are commonly seen on MRI.[101] Because this age is atypical for scoliosis, there should be a high index of suspicion for intraspinal pathology.

As far as treatment goes, those with Cobb angles less than 25 degrees and RVADs less than 20 degrees are at low risk for progression and can be followed with serial x-rays every 4 to 6 months, with progression greater than 10 degrees being a trigger for intervention. The key testing point is regarding the crankshaft phenomenon, where anterior growth occurs after isolated posterior spinal fusion. This necessitates a circumferential fusion that will limit development of the thorax and lungs. Most recently, growing rod instrumentation, guided-growth implants, compression-based implants, and a vertical expandable prosthetic titanium rib have been made available to help in treating these young patients with room to grow. Limited data are available for the success of these techniques with potential complications of wound-healing issues, device migration, and rib fracture.[100]

Why Might This Be Tested? It is important to be aware of when a patient is classified as having typical adolescent idiopathic scoliosis vs other causes of scoliosis. Typical adolescent scoliosis usually does not require an MRI or further workup unless neurologic findings are identified. A patient with atypical/infantile scoliosis requires a further workup, and this is important to identify early and quickly.

Here's the Point!

Young patients (Risser 0, 1) with curves greater than 20 degrees need intervention, bracing, or casting because they have a high likelihood of progression (~68%). Plain x-rays are the standard follow-up for idiopathic scoliosis unless there are neurologic findings on physical exam, rapid curve progression, male sex, left-sided curves, or structural abnormalities on x-rays.

Vignette 121: Scapular Winging

A 25-year-old previously healthy male who is an avid backpacker presents with a primary complaint of left shoulder pain and weakness. Symptoms were first noticed approximately 2 months ago when the patient returned home from a 3-week backpacking trip in the Appalachian Mountains. Since that trip, the patient has taken 2 other 1-week backpacking trips and has noted a gradual worsening in symptoms. On physical exam, you notice that the patient has a difficult time raising his left arm. When asked to forward flex and push against a wall, his left shoulder girdle elevates upward, and the inferior border of his scapula migrates medially (Figure 121-1).

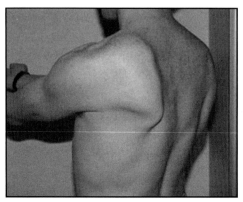

Figure 121-1. Photograph of the patient during his exam.

▶ *What is the diagnosis?*

▶ *What other aspects of the history and physical exam are important?*

▶ *What other tests should be ordered?*

▶ *What is the classification of these injuries?*

▶ *What are the treatment options?*

▶ *When and why would each treatment be used?*

Vignette 121: Answer

The diagnosis is medial scapular winging caused by weakness of the serratus anterior. The patient is an otherwise healthy young man who has a history notable for backpacking long distances. Backpackers, as well as patients with suboptimally healed scapular fractures, often experience compression neuropathies of the long thoracic nerve, resulting in motor deficits of the serratus anterior. On history, these individuals typically present with chief complaints of shoulder weakness, pain, difficulty with overhead activities, and a cosmetic deformity; these symptoms usually owe themselves to the defective biomechanics of the affected shoulder joint. On physical exam, the shoulder girdle will elevate with attempted forward abduction, and the inferior aspect of the scapula will migrate medially. Other mechanisms for long thoracic nerve palsy include traction injuries from sports, such as volleyball and weight lifting, and iatrogenic injuries resulting from an axillary nerve dissection.

Unlike medial scapular winging, lateral scapular winging is caused by weakness of the trapezius muscle. The injury usually results from an iatrogenic event, classically a posterior neck cervical lymph node dissection, which results in injury to the spinal accessory nerve. On history, patients will also note fatigue with abduction, weakness, and cosmetic deformity. However, on exam, the patient's shoulder girdle appears depressed or droopy and the inferior scapular border translates laterally with attempted abduction.

In addition to peripheral nerve injuries that result in medial or lateral scapular winging, the condition is also caused by a number of other conditions. Scapular winging is broadly classified into dystrophic or nondystrophic etiologies. The primary dystrophic condition that leads to scapular winging is fascioscapular humeral dystrophy. Nondystrophic causes include peripheral nerve injuries (long thoracic or spinal accessory nerves), failed tendon transfers, brachial plexus injuries, cerebrovascular disease, medial clavicular insufficiency, painful scapular crepitus, and Sprengel deformity.

When evaluating any patient with scapular winging, it is important to glean the length of time symptoms have been present, family history, and anything else that could point to the etiology (fracture, tumor, recreation). Exam should focus on directionality of scapular winging and shoulder girdle motion during resisted wall push-off and abduction. The examiner may also stabilize the scapula posteriorly to assess for improvement of shoulder function.

X-rays in patients with scapular winging help rule out associated fractures, dislocations, malunion, and deformities but do not provide insight into the cause of the condition. An EMG study may elucidate the cause of the pathology, particularly if a specific peripheral nerve injury pattern is suspected.

In many nondystrophic scapular winging cases, particularly those caused by injury to the long thoracic or spinal accessory nerves, observation for return of function should be attempted first for a minimum of 6 months. Adjunct nonoperative modalities that are frequently useful during this period include serratus anterior or trapezius strengthening as well as bracing.

Operative management of scapular winging is typically managed by tendon transfers or scapulothoracic fusion. Medial scapular winging can be treated with a pectoralis major tendon transfer, whereas lateral scapular winging can be alleviated with the lateralization of the levator scapulae and rhomboids (Eden-Lange transfer). Scapulothoracic fusion is an effective operative alternative and a salvage procedure after failed tendon transfer.

Why Might This Be Tested? Scapular winging is a commonly seen shoulder condition. It is important to differentiate between dystrophic and nondystrophic causes for the condition. When remembering nondystrophic peripheral nerve injuries, bear in mind that medial scapular winging is caused by long thoracic nerve palsy but lateral scapular winging is caused by spinal accessory nerve palsy. Most cases of nondystrophic peripheral nerve injuries often resolve with no specific treatment. Thus, nonoperative management should be attempted first.

Here's the Point!

Identify the diagnosis, classify the type of scapular winging, determine its likely etiology, and choose which treatment(s) is warranted. When operative intervention is required, medial scapular winging can be treated with a pectoralis major tendon transfer, whereas lateral scapular winging can be alleviated with the lateralization of the levator scapulae and rhomboids.

Vignette 122: What Is That Mass on My Daughter's Shoulder?

A 10-year-old female is seen for progressive pain and swelling in her proximal arm. Her parents state that it appeared a week ago after bumping her arm while playing outside. She does not complain of any pain with functional activities. Examination reveals a firm, fixed mass in the proximal humerus. Plain x-rays, MRI, and histology slides of the lesion are obtained (Figures 122-1 to 122-3).

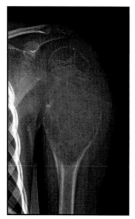

Figure 122-1. AP x-ray of the left shoulder.

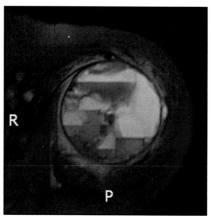

Figure 122-2. Axial cut of a T2-weighted MRI of the left shoulder mass.

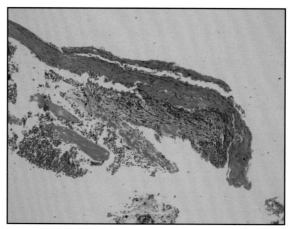

Figure 122-3. Histology section of the mass (200× magnification).

► *What is the diagnosis?*

► *What is the treatment?*

► *What are the risk factors for recurrence?*

Vignette 122: Answer

This is an ABC, a benign reactive entity that can be locally aggressive. Most (~75%) ABCs are diagnosed within the first 2 decades of life. It occurs eccentrically in the metaphyses of long bones, most commonly the femur, tibia, and humerus. Similar to osteoblastoma and osteoid osteoma tumors, ABCs can be found in the posterior elements of the spine. ABCs can be primary or secondary, occurring in conjunction with another lesion, such as GCT, osteoblastoma, chondroblastoma, nonossifying fibroma, fibrous dysplasia, chondromyxoid fibroma, and osteosarcoma. Up to 30% of ABCs are secondary in nature (much like the Red Sox to the Yankees in the 1990s!).

These tumors are staged using the Enneking classification for benign tumors of bone. In this scheme, stage 1 is a latent lesion, demonstrating a well-demarcated radiodense border circumscribing the lesion. There should be no cortical perforation, soft tissue mass, and minimal to no remodeling of the host bone. Stage 2 is an active lesion, radiographically maintaining a geographic pattern and usually demonstrating some changes in the host bone. However, the body is able to effectively contain this lesion, and there is no cortical perforation. Stage 3 lesions are aggressive and defined by perforation of the host bone. ABCs typically are stage 2 or 3 lesions and are located eccentrically, causing an expansile "blow-out" appearance. Plain x-rays will often show internal trabeculation (mnemonic device for internal trabeculations: DCHANG—a shout-out to a former coresident, Dave Chang).

- D = Desmoplastic fibroma
- C = Chondromyxoid fibroma
- H = Hemangioma
- A = ABC
- N = Nonossifying fibroma
- G = GCT

The tumor will often be found as an expansile, lytic, and eccentric area of bone destruction in the metaphyseal region of the affected bone.

The classic MRI and CT findings often found on the Boards/OITE depict fluid-fluid levels in the tumor. However, around 5% are solid with no cystic component. Differential diagnosis includes unicameral bone cysts, cystic fibrous dysplasia, nonossifying fibroma, and telangiectatic osteosarcoma, which can have a similar appearance to aggressive stage 3 lesions.

The histologic appearance is one of blood-filled lakes separated by fibrous septations. The stroma consists mainly of bland fibroblasts and myofibroblasts, occasional giant cells (don't be tricked into believing these are GCTs), and reactive immature bone with rimming osteoblasts. There can be occasional mitotic figures. The appearance differs from telangiectatic osteosarcoma as ABCs lack the cellular pleomorphism, hyperchromatism, and haphazard pattern of osteoid formation (without osteoblastic rimming) indicative of osteosarcoma.

The mainstay of treatment for stage 2 or 3 ABCs is surgical curettage and bone grafting or cementation, with local control rates between 70% and 90%. Adjuvant treatment with phenol, hydrogen peroxide, or argon beam coagulation has been described. Wide excision is reserved for recurrent lesions and expendable bones with local control rates near 100%. Risk factors for recurrence are stage 3 tumors, younger patients, and lesions in close proximity to open growth plates. For inaccessible or extensive lesions, embolization or external beam radiation may be considered.

Why Might This Be Tested? ABCs are often included on standardized exams because they are common tumors that can appear aggressive and malignant in nature. They are also easily confused on histological examination with GCTs, making it a topic the question writers like!

Here's the Point!

ABCs are benign, locally aggressive lesions typically found in patients younger than 20 years. The x-rays show expansile lesions with internal trabeculations. Treatment typically involves curettage and bone grafting with known risk for recurrence, particularly in children with open growth plates.

Vignette 123: Beware Benign Knee Radiographs in a Trauma Patient

A 35-year-old male presents to the emergency department in the trauma bay following a motor vehicle crash. He is complaining of severe pain about his right knee. X-rays from the trauma bay are shown in Figure 123-1. A large joint effusion without obvious fracture is noted. Physical exam reveals global laxity of the knee, including the ACL, PCL, and MCL.

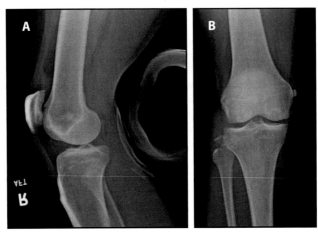

Figure 123-1. (A) Lateral and (B) AP x-rays of the injured right knee.

▶ *What is the diagnosis?*

▶ *What is the most devastating associated injury?*

▶ *What are the indications for immediate surgical intervention?*

▶ *What is the ideal timing for surgical repair/reconstruction?*

Vignette 123: Answer

The diagnosis in this case is a knee dislocation. Spontaneous reduction of a knee dislocation prior to hospital arrival is common. A spontaneously reduced knee can appear deceptively benign, especially in a polytrauma patient with distracting injuries. Although a knee dislocation may reduce spontaneously, there are subtle radiographic findings that may be identified, including mild tibiofemoral subluxation, avulsion fractures, and rim fractures, which act as clues to the injury (pay attention to these clues because they often answer the question). In this case, notice the Segond fracture, which is a small avulsion of the lateral tibial condyle and is pathognomonic for an ACL injury. A thorough physical exam of the knee with neurovascular assessment is required for all victims of high-energy trauma; in particular, a knee dislocation should have a focused assessment of pulses. The presumptive diagnosis of a knee dislocation should be made when there is substantial laxity of 2 or more major ligaments of the knee.[368,369]

Traumatic knee dislocations are uncommon, accounting for an estimated 0.02% of all musculoskeletal injuries.[370,371] Knee dislocations are classified based on the direction of dislocation, which is characterized by the position of tibia relative to the femur (distal bone to the proximal bone), and whether the injury is acute (< 3 weeks) or chronic (> 3 weeks). The most common type of knee dislocation is anterior (40%) as a result of hyperextension. Posterior dislocations comprise 33% of all knee dislocations and typically occur as the result of a so-called dashboard injury, a mechanism whereby the leg strikes the dashboard, resulting in a proximally directed force that causes ligamentous knee injury. Lateral and medial dislocations occur less frequently (18% and 4% incidence, respectively) because they necessitate a direct and violent varus or valgus load. Rotary dislocations are the least common type. Knee dislocations from a twisting injury are usually displaced in 2 directions. Posterolateral dislocation is the most common form; these may be difficult to reduce in a closed manner because the medial femoral condyle often buttonholes through the medial soft tissue structures, including the capsule and/or the MCL.

The most devastating injury associated with a knee dislocation is vascular compromise of the popliteal artery. Popliteal artery injury has been reported in 32% to 45% of knee dislocations. Degree of injury may range from an intimal tear to complete transection of the artery. Vigilance is necessary to identify such an injury because failure to recognize one resulting in delayed revascularization of greater than 6 to 8 hours portends poor outcomes and results in a near 90% amputation rate. Intimal injuries may be subtle and can lead to catastrophic outcomes when missed because this can be a prelude to clotting or aneurysm formation.

A careful and complete neurovascular exam should be documented on initial examination and frequently thereafter. Vascular assessment may include physical examination, use of ABI, or CT angiography. Vascular exam includes palpation of dorsalis pedis and posterior tibialis arteries; a pulse may be present distal to a complete arterial occlusion due to the presence of collateral flow. As such, even with palpable pulses and a normal ABI, many surgeons advocate for CT angiography because the possibility of arterial injury remains despite a normal physical examination. If a patient presents with soft signs of ischemia, including palpable but asymmetric pulses and asymmetric warmth and/or color of the limb, ABIs should be completed. ABIs are determined by dividing the systolic pressure of the affected limb at the level of the ankle (determined by Doppler) by the systolic pressure in the ipsilateral upper extremity with the patient lying flat. An abnormal value, defined as a ratio less than 0.9, should prompt an immediate vascular surgery consult and advanced imaging to investigate arterial integrity. CT angiography is 100% sensitive and specific, and IV contrast may be given through the antecubital fossa. In the setting of hard signs of ischemia, including a cool, pulseless, obviously dysvascular limb, immediate vascular surgeon consultation is warranted.

Neurological damage should be suspected in knee dislocations. The peroneal nerve is injured more frequently than the tibial nerve and occurs in 16% to 40% of cases.

Prompt placement of an AFO in the early postinjury period is necessary to obviate equinus deformity due to Achilles tendon contracture.

Indications for emergent surgery include patients with vascular injury, compartment syndrome, open injury, or an irreducible dislocation. Vascular injuries often require saphenous vein bypass graft and concomitant prophylactic fasciotomies after revascularization. Open injuries and compartment syndromes are treated with aggressive irrigation and debridement and fasciotomies, respectively. External fixation is used to provide stability about the knee while these emergent situations are addressed.

Definitive ligamentous reconstruction should be delayed for several days following knee dislocation to allow resolution of limb swelling and ensure that any vascular repair is adequate. Delay in reconstruction longer than 3 weeks, however, can lead to excessive scar formation and preclude repair of the collateral and posterolateral ligaments. The ideal timing is 10 to 14 days following injury, when partial returns of ROM and quadriceps muscle tone reduce the risk of postoperative arthrofibrosis. Open and/or arthroscopic techniques may be used depending on the integrity of the capsule. Two weeks is typically needed for the capsule to heal sufficiently to prevent extravasation of fluid. Collateral ligaments can be repaired in the acute setting (<3 weeks). The cruciate ligaments are often midsubstance tears and require surgical reconstruction. Knee stiffness is the most common complication after these injuries, and aggressive therapy is important. Rehabilitation focuses on ROM exercises with partial weight bearing for the first 4 weeks, with gradual progression to full weight bearing at 6 to 8 weeks once 90 to 100 degrees of flexion is achieved. Running may resume at 6 months if 80% of quad function has returned, and return to sport averages between 9 and 12 months.

Why Might This Be Tested? Knee dislocations can present with normal x-rays and appear relatively benign, but the consequences of a missed vascular injury are devastating. It is easy to miss this diagnosis on plain x-rays.

Here's the Point!

Suspect a knee dislocation if 2 or more ligaments are substantially unstable on exam. Vascular injury occurs in 40% of patients and must be ruled out with serial exams and arteriography. ABIs of less than 0.9 should prompt an immediate vascular consultation.

Vignette 124: Metabolic Bone Disease

A 70-year-old Black male presents with progressively worsening hip pain. Initial x-rays show severe osteopenia and cystic deformity of the proximal femur. On preoperative evaluation for a THA, the patient is found to have hypocalcemia on laboratory testing and a prolonged QT interval on his EKG. His surgery is cancelled to evaluate these new findings.

▶ *What are the common conditions associated with hypocalcemia?*

▶ *List the physical examination findings classically found with hypocalcemia.*

▶ *Diagram the feedback loop for calcium regulation in hypocalcemia.*

During the medical workup, it is determined that the patient has a history of chronic renal failure, as evidenced by an elevated creatinine.

▶ *What are the metabolic bone disorders associated with renal failure and hypocalcemia?*

▶ *Outline the pathogenesis of bone changes related to this condition.*

▶ *Describe the effect on perioperative management for patients.*

Vignette 124: Answer

Part I

The common conditions associated with hypocalcemia include the following[372]:
- Hypoparathyroidism: Low parathyroid hormone (PTH) levels function to decrease serum calcium levels and increase phosphate levels because the kidney is not stimulated to secrete phosphate and retain calcium (see feedback loop below). Often occurs after thyroid surgery as an iatrogenic condition.

- Pseudohypoparathyroidism (PHP): This is a result of a genetic defect, so we can blame Mom and Dad, at the target cell level. PTH levels are typically normal or high but have no end organ effect due to a receptor defect.
    - Albright hereditary osteodystrophy: A form of PHP with associated findings of shortened metacarpals and metatarsals (often first, fourth, and fifth), shortened extremities, obesity, and poor intelligence.
    - Pseudo-PHP: Has similar clinical findings as PHP but has normal PTH and calcium levels.
- Renal osteodystrophy: Chronic renal disease leads to a disorder in calcium and phosphate regulation. Divided into high- and low-turnover disease.
- Rickets/osteomalacia: This is a failure of mineralization of bone with multiple causes, including the following:
    - Nutritional deficits: Often related to vitamin D deficiency leading to poor calcium absorption, low phosphate, and elevated PTH levels. Treatment is with vitamin D.
    - Hereditary vitamin D–dependent rickets
        - Type I: Defect in renal 25-(OH)-vitamin D-1-α-hydroxylase, AR inheritance, on 12q14 chromosome and inhibits the conversion to the active form of vitamin D
        - Type II: Defect in intracellular receptor for 1,25 (OH)2 vitamin D3
    - Familial hypophosphatemic rickets: The most common form of rickets and inherited as an x-linked disorder, resulting in a decreased tubular reabsorption of phosphate in the kidneys.
    - Others: GI absorption defects, renal tubular defects, renal osteodystrophy, heavy metal intoxication sodium fluoride, medications (anticonvulsants)
- Others: hypoalbuminemia, hypomagnesemia, hyperphosphatemia

The classic findings associated with hypocalcemia include the following:
- Neuromuscular irritability
    - Muscle cramping and tingling sensations
    - Tetany
    - Seizures
    - Chvostek's sign (abnormal reaction of the facial nerve to stimulation)
- Cataracts, dry skin, coarse hair, poor dentition
- Fungal infections of the nails
- EKG changes, prolonged QT interval
- Syncope and CHF

Figure 124-1 outlines the feedback loop for hypocalcemia and its effect on the various sites of regulation in the body.

Part II

Renal osteodystrophy is a pathologic bone condition in the setting of kidney disease. Renal failure is a common condition treated in the United States, with more than 300,000 cases being managed annually. Some factors associated with this condition include Black race (4× more common than in Whites), age (the older we get, the higher the incidence), and sex (males > females). The kidneys are responsible for regulating mineral homeostasis in the body, are a target organ, and excrete PTH (Figure 124-2). The proximal renal tubules are responsible for the hydroxylation and activation of vitamin D (requires 2 hydroxylation reactions

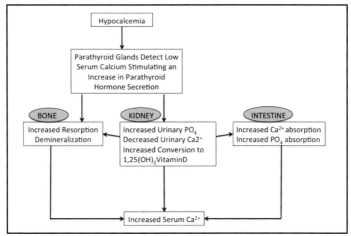

Figure 124-1. Feedback loop for the body's reaction to hypocalcemia. (Adapted from Boden SD, Kaplan FS. Calcium homeostasis. *Orthop Clin North Am.* 1990;21[1]:31-42 and Tejwani NC, Schachter AK, Immerman I, Achan P. Renal osteodystrophy. *J Am Acad Orthop Surg.* 2006;14[5]:303-311.)

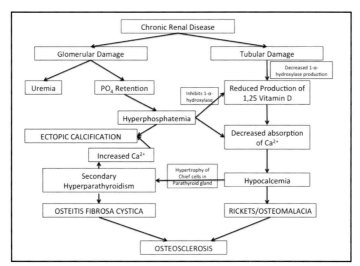

Figure 124-2. The effects of chronic renal disease on calcium homeostasis. (Adapted from Boden SD, Kaplan FS. Calcium homeostasis. *Orthop Clin North Am.* 1990;21[1]:31-42 and Tejwani NC, Schachter AK, Immerman I, Achan P. Renal osteodystrophy. *J Am Acad Orthop Surg.* 2006;14[5]:303-311.)

to become active) as catalyzed by 1-α-hydroxylase, which also feeds back to inhibit PTH synthesis. The following are the 2 forms of renal osteodystrophy (hypocalcemia in setting of renal failure)[372,373]:

1. High-turnover renal bone disease: Classic form of the disease, with chronically elevated levels of PTH, which ultimately leads to hypertrophy of the chief cells of the parathyroid gland. This upregulation leads to continually elevated PTH despite correction of the renal condition, called secondary hyperparathyroidism. Bone turnover remains high and can lead to osteitis fibrosa cystica.
    o   There is a diminished ability to excrete phosphate, causing the heightened production of PTH via the following mechanisms: increased phosphate directly lowers calcium, elevated phosphorus

inhibits activation of the catalyst 1-α-hydroxylase, elevated phosphorus directly increases PTH production.

2. Low-turnover renal osteodystrophy (adynamic lesions): These are patients with renal disease that is well treated and have bone pathology without secondary hyperparathyroidism. The osteoid is not defective in this setting as in osteomalacia, but there is often aluminum overload and secondary bone deposition.
    o   Elevated aluminum levels impair the proliferation and differentiation of cells into mature osteoblasts. PTH release is often impaired, and these adynamic lesions are found in the bones of such patients.

As a side note, chronic dialysis can lead to accumulation of β-2 microglobulin and amyloidosis (often asked about—stains pink with Congo red).

The surgical implications for these patients are substantial and must not be ignored. You cannot chalk this up as a standard joint replacement or fracture case. One must be prepared to treat significant defects in bone stock and poor bone quality as well as a rigorous perioperative assessment of potential sites of infection. Several studies have documented a lower rate of success in this patient population after hip replacement for dislocations, infections, and loosening. Typically, pathologic fractures through these weakened areas of bone occur in the standard locations, wrist, back, ankle, and hip. Careful planning is required because the adjacent bony deformities may be great, making fixation with standard implants more difficult. In certain cases, these fractures may be best treated nonoperatively with large bony deformities in patients who are minimal ambulators. Also, these patients are like walking petri dishes and have a high risk for hematogenous infections due to their renal failure, dialysis, immune deficiency related to medications, and other related comorbidities.[373]

Why Might This Be Tested? There are always some questions that are related to medical conditions and calcium/phosphate regulation. Knowing the calcium feedback loop will allow you to pick up a few questions we often write off as primary care questions.

Here's the Point!

Know the calcium feedback loop and the implications for what happens when something goes awry. Calcium homeostasis is crucial to the bones, and the basics must be understood.

Vignette 125: What's With This Persistent Limp After My Hip Replacement?

A 75-year-old male 3 months status post left THA is doing well but presents to the clinic with a limp. Upon questioning, he states that he was unable to attend many of his postoperative physical therapy visits due to transportation issues. He has a lurch with ambulation and does not want to use a cane. He has questions as to why he continues to have a limp.

▶ *What is a Trendelenburg gait?*

▶ *What causes a Trendelenburg gait?*

The patient follows his physician's recommendations and attends physical therapy regularly, and his gait has normalized after 3 months.

▶ *Based on the free body diagram, how much force must be generated by the abductor musculature to balance the body weight and prevent this gait abnormality?*

▶ *What is the joint reaction force?*

Vignette 125: Answer

A Trendelenburg gait is an abnormal lurch that results from weak abductor musculature, which typically works to keep the pelvis level. When these muscles are weak, the patient compensates by lurching the body to the affected side because the weak muscles cannot hold the body level. This gait is sometimes present following THA, particularly following a direct lateral approach or when sufficient offset of the hip is not restored.[374] A basic understanding of biomechanics is necessary to understand the forces acting on the hip that help keep the pelvis level and prevent this type of gait.

Biomechanics is the study of the biological systems, or in this case the human body, using the laws of physics. Free body diagrams are commonly used to determine forces acting on the tissues under question. To understand these diagrams, some basic laws of physics should be reviewed, starting with Newton's laws, which are as follows. First, velocity of an object remains constant if no force is applied to the object. Second, force equals mass multiplied by acceleration ($F = MA$). Third, when a force is applied to an object, that object applies an equal and opposite force on the first object. A vector is a quantity that has magnitude and direction, and this concept is used to describe forces acting on tissues in the human body. When a vector force causes rotation, as often happens around a joint in the human body, the ability of this force to cause this rotation is called a moment. This is defined as moment = force × distance. This concept is best understood with a real-world example. It is more difficult to hold a 25-lb weight with your arm stretched out then with it close to the body because the distance, and therefore moment, is much greater.

Motion at joints is due to forces acting on the tissues surrounding that joint. The forces come in the form of body weight, objects suspended by the body, or muscular contractions. Joints rotate around their instant COR, which is a point that dynamically changes with joint translation. Joint congruence refers to how well 2 articular surfaces articulate together. A major point to remember is that the greater the contact surface of a joint, the lower the contact forces (the more area touching, the less force is seen on the surface). Joint reaction force is the force acting within a joint that results from the forces acting outside the joint. This can be best understood with a simplified example of the forces acting on a hip joint (Figure 125-1).

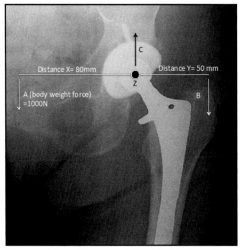

Figure 125-1. AP x-ray of the left hip (used as a diagram to outline the forces around the hip joint).

To solve this free body diagram, consider 2 points rotating around the COR, point Z. This is analyzed as if in a static state because the aim is to keep the pelvis level. Therefore, the forces on one side of the COR must equal the forces on the other side. Another consideration is that the farther away from the COR the force is applied, the less force is needed to produce the same moment, or torque. Therefore, in this case, (A)(X) = (Y)(B), or (80)(1000) = (50)(B). B = 1600. Joint reaction force is the force the joint sees and is a combination of the forces applied on both sides of the COR. Therefore, C = (A) + (B), or C = 1000 + 1600 = 2600. Remember, these diagrams apply to all joints in the body and not just the hip. Overall, the forces in a system must equal out, so when you constrain a joint, the forces must be borne out elsewhere—this goes for all systems.

Some other biomechanic factoids that you should be familiar with include the following:

- In humans, the center of gravity falls just in front of S2.
- Kinetic energy equation: $KE = 1/2mv^2$.
- Electrical charges are created from deforming forces:
    - Compression (concave aspect of a curve) side = electronegative
    - Tension (convex side of a curve) side = electropositive
- Coefficient of friction is the resistance between 2 surfaces gliding over one another. Synovial fluid serves to lubricate the surfaces and provide elastohydrodynamic lubrication.
    - Coefficient of friction is 0.002 to 0.04 for human joints and 0.05 to 0.15 in metal-on-PE articulations.

Why Might This Be Tested? Understanding the concept of a Trendelenburg gait is an easy way to bring in free body diagrams to a test. Biomechanics is the underlying science explaining motion across joints and, therefore, is important for an orthopedic surgeon to understand.

Here's the Point!

For a joint to be held statically in space, the forces across either side of the joint must be equal. If the forces are not equal, the joint will move until the forces equalize. Remember, the greater the contact area, the lower the contact stresses.

Vignette 126: My High-Heeled Shoes Are Unbearable Now

A 69-year-old healthy female and former ballet dancer complains of worsening pain and stiffness of the great toe over many years. Her pain has progressed to the point where she is unable to tolerate high-heeled shoes and can no longer jog for exercise. Physical examination reveals 15 degrees of dorsiflexion of the hallux MTP joint compared with 80 degrees on the contralateral side. X-rays show prominent dorsal osteophyte formation and advanced joint space narrowing of the hallux MTP joint.

▶ *What are the risk factors for DJD of the hallux MTP joint?*

After failing conservative management, the patient has opted to proceed with surgical intervention.

▶ *What treatment options are available for early and endstage disease?*

Vignette 126: Answer

Hallux rigidus is a general term used to describe pain and stiffness of the hallux MTP joint. Other than hallux valgus (bunions), hallux rigidus is the most common condition to affect the first MTP joint and is typically far more disabling than a bunion deformity. Hallux rigidus is typically a local arthritic process but can be associated with systemic arthritides, such as gout, RA, or psoriatic arthritis. The term *hallux rigidus* is often used interchangeably with *hallux limitus*.

Hallux rigidus has been described in the following 2 different age populations: adolescent and adult. The adolescent form occurs predominantly in males and is often bilateral, and a positive family history of great toe problems is common. This condition is relatively common in athletes and is often associated with osteochondritis dissecans or history of a turf toe injury (a forced dorsiflexion compression injury). The adult form may be a continuum of the adolescent condition, but the exact etiology often remains elusive. Hallux rigidus in the adult condition is seen more commonly in active individuals, such as professional athletes, dancers, and runners. It is widely believed to be attributed to repetitive impact stresses on the hallux MTP joint. Although some attribute HR to anatomical considerations (metatarsus primus elevatus, advanced hallux valgus, pes planus, congenital flattening of the metatarsal head, etc), repetitive microtrauma is the most likely cause.

On physical examination, ROM of the hallux MTP joint should be compared with the contralateral side. The classic finding is restricted dorsiflexion, often in the presence of normal or only slightly diminished plantarflexion. Compensatory hyperextension of the hallux interphalangeal joint is another common finding. A gouty flare should always be considered in the setting of significant swelling and with exquisite tenderness to light touch ("Even the weight of the bedsheets on my toe is intolerable"), especially in those fond of cheeseburgers and a few too many glasses of pinot noir (cheese and wine are risk factors for gouty flare).

Staging of hallux rigidus, proposed by Coughlan et al in 2003, is largely based on the radiographic findings and is used to guide treatment. In grade 0, dorsiflexion is restricted in the absence of radiographic findings. Grade 1 hallux rigidus will exhibit a dorsal osteophyte (seen most notably on the lateral foot x-ray) with preservation of the joint space of the hallux MTP. In grade 2, osteophytes may be seen dorsally as well as medially and laterally, while mild to moderate joint space narrowing is now evident. With grade 3, substantial narrowing occurs and subchondral cysts may be present. In grade 4, the joint space is obliterated and the metatarsal head has a flattened appearance.

Nonoperative treatment of hallux rigidus is aimed at reducing the inflammatory process and immobilizing the hallux MTP joint. This will usually involve NSAIDs, activity restrictions (low-impact sports), shoewear modifications (avoidance of heels), and a rigid insert (Morton's extension) to minimize dorsiflexion of the hallux MTP joint. Judicious use of intra-articular corticosteroid can also be considered.

The choice of surgical procedure takes into consideration the patient's age, activity level, and expectations and the severity of the condition. Operative treatment is broadly divided into the following categories: joint debridement, arthroplasty, and arthrodesis. In surgery for grade 1 and 2 hallux rigidus, regardless of age, cheilectomy of the hallux MTP is performed. This procedure, which addresses the dorsal impingement by excising all osteophytes and circumferentially releasing the contracted soft tissues, is the mainstay of surgical treatment of hallux rigidus. Because the pathology in hallux rigidus preferentially affects the dorsal half of the MTP joint, a proximal phalanx closing-wedge dorsiflexion osteotomy (Moberg osteotomy) is often performed in adolescent patients to create additional pseudodorsiflexion, which acts to translate stresses to the plantar aspect of the metatarsal head.

In grade 3 and 4 disease, in order to establish a pain-free joint, joint resection, interpositional arthroplasty, or fusion is preferred. In older and more sedentary patients, a Keller or Mayo resection arthroplasty is the procedure of choice. This allows for effective pain relief and improvement of motion at the expense of weakened plantarflexion (loss of plantar intrinsic insertion), transfer metatarsalgia to the second toe (due to shortening of the hallux), and deformity of the hallux (varus or valgus). In younger and more active patients who favor preservation of motion, a capsular interpositional arthroplasty (Hamilton's technique) is favorable to a pure resection arthroplasty because the extensor hood, extensor hallucis brevis tendon, and capsule are interposed between the phalanx and metatarsal as a soft tissue buffer. Implant arthroplasty procedures, such as a phalanx hemiarthroplasty, metatarsal head resurfacing, or TJA have not been widely endorsed and almost certainly will not be the correct choice on any Board certification examination! However, hallux MTP arthrodesis remains the gold standard surgical treatment for grade 3 or 4 cases of hallux rigidus. Recent literature continues to support the decision to fuse an arthritic MTP joint, which allows for effective pain relief while preserving the relative length of the first ray. This is likely to be the answer that the examiner is looking for. The joint is fused in approximately 10 to 15 degrees of dorsiflexion and 15 to 20 degrees of valgus. Potential issues with fusion include malunion, nonunion, and DJD of the hallux IP joint.

Why Might This Be Tested? Hallux rigidus is the most debilitating condition affecting the great toe. It is often seen in weekend warriors and active individuals later in life as a consequence of repetitive microtrauma but is also seen in younger patients with a positive family history for problems with the hallux.

Here's the Point!

Despite new advances in treatment, the mainstays of treatment for hallux rigidus remain cheilectomy in grade 1 and 2 disease and fusion in grades 3 and 4.

Vignette 127: What Tests Do I Order for This Painful THA?

A first-year resident is called to the emergency room to evaluate an 82-year-old female with a painful left THA performed 4 years ago. The patient is a poor historian but states that a recent fall led to a pelvic fracture that did not require surgery on her right side. She has been sedentary for a couple of weeks and states that her right ankle has started to swell in the past couple of days. In addition, her right TKA has been painful, swollen, and warm for the last 2 weeks. In her confusion, she complains of multiple ailments, and a battery of imaging studies are ordered.

▶ *Describe the following studies and their relevance to this case:*
  - *Technetium bone scan*
  - *WBC-labeled bone scan*
  - *MRI*
  - *CT scan*

Vignette 127: Answer

Multiple tests and their relevance to the patient's complaints are as follows:

- Technetium bone scan: In an elderly patient with multiple vague complaints around joint replacements, a technetium-99m bone scan may allow one to assess for component stability (one has to assume that in the emergency room serial x-rays—the gold standard—are not available), occult fractures (although not as accurate in first 48 hours after fracture), infection, or tumors. There are typically 3 phases to a bone scan, and technetium-99m is used as it is incorporated into metabolically active bone:

  - Phase 1: blood flow (initial or transient phase); basically follows the name and shows the arterial network yielding perfusion images
  - Phase 2: blood pool; allows the labeled cells to equilibrate in the intravascular system for about 30 minutes
  - Phase 3: delayed phase; after about 4 hours, the tracer will accumulate in distant sites with active metabolism of phosphates (bone growth or turnover)

  Scintigraphy using technetium-99m is an easy-to-administer test but may miss acute fractures, multiple myeloma, and can be positive after hardware placement for up to 2 years (89% of tibial and 63% of femoral components remain positive more than 1 year after TKA). Recent studies have questioned the accuracy of bone scans in assessing component stability/loosening and osteolysis. Geerdink et al found a sensitivity and specificity for acetabular loosening of 38% and 73%, respectively, using technetium-99m scintigraphy.[375] Technetium-99mdp is incorporated into metabolically active and immature bone in place of phosphate, creating areas that light up on the scan.

- WBC-labeled bone scan: Indium-111-labeled WBC scan can be used to assess for areas of infection and is a 2-day test.[376] WBCs are harvested from the patient, labeled with indium, and then injected back into the patient. The injected labeled cells are then scanned 24 hours later, with reasonable success for determining periprosthetic infection or osteomyelitis. In this case, although not the first test to come to mind, it could be used to rule out infection in her replacements if more information was needed. Combining a WBC-labeled scan and marrow study (technetium-99m or sulfur colloid scan) improves the accuracy of the test, with reports yielding 100% specificity, 46% sensitivity, 100% positive predictive value, and 89% negative predictive value.[377] Combining the studies helps to account for marrow packing of cells and gives a more accurate assessment for infection. Gallium-67 citrate is another labeled scan that localizes in areas of inflammation and neoplasm. Gallium salts are used and dissolved to create active gallium for which the radioactive isotope is used for these scans. The isotope is injected and will bind to transferrin, leukocyte lactoferrin, bacteria, areas of inflammation, and neutrophils—hence the utility in detecting tumor, inflammation, or infections.

- MRI: MRI is an imaging study that applies a magnetic field with radiofrequency pulses leading to images based on the signal intensity recorded in the tissues. This test has become a mainstay in our imaging portfolio because it does not involve radiation and is good with assessing bone marrow changes, soft tissue injuries, joint effusions, and most human tissues. The protons in each tissue are excited by the magnetic field and then relax into a pattern that gives off various signals, leading to what amounts to a specific signature. Common signatures for various tissues are listed in Table 127-1.

  In this case, an MRI may aid in predicting an infection but is not likely needed. However, in patients with a MOM THA or a persistently painful hip, one may be indicated. Once considered not possible, metal-artifact reduction sequences can be ordered to help with identifying soft tissue injuries adjacent to metallic implants.[378] These sequences involve 2 recently developed 3-dimensional MRI techniques that allow for good peri-implant visualization by correcting for the metal artifact using Slice Encoding for Metal Artifact Correction or Multi-Acquisition Variable-Resonance Image Combination.[378] Both techniques use 3D fast spin-echo readouts and have been shown to be effective in reducing artifact and providing high-resolution images.

- CT scan: CT images are a product of a collimated x-ray beam directed at the patient with a detector that determines how much radiation is absorbed or deflected. This yields a computed map of the x-ray slices, giving a detailed view of the imaging area. Hounsfield units (HU) are used to measure the x-ray densities produced by imaging a specimen. Water is given a 0, whereas fat ranges from -100 to 0 and bone is about 1000 on this HU scale. It remains an excellent means for viewing bone, spinal conditions, rotational

Table 127-1.

COMMON SIGNATURES FOR VARIOUS TISSUES

Tissue Type	T1-Weighted	T2-Weighted
Cortical bone	Dark	Dark
Osteomyelitis	Dark	Bright
Ligaments	Dark	Dark
Fibrocartilage	Dark	Dark
Fluid	Dark	Bright
Fat	Bright	Gray/intermediate
Muscle	Gray/intermediate	Dark
Bone marrow	Bright	Dark
Acute hematoma	Gray	Dark
Chronic hematoma	Bright	Bright

alignment of knee components (internal rotation of components can lead to patellofemoral complications—3 to 8 degrees correlates with patellar subluxation and 7 to 17 degrees correlates with early patellar dislocation and subluxation[379]), acetabular anteversion and femoral, limb lengths, PE, and other medical conditions. Although it is often a worthwhile test to procure, in this case, it is not likely to help as much, unless you are using a contrast CT with vascular imaging to rule out a DVT.

With multiple complaints and concerns, it is reasonable in this case to get a duplex Doppler of both lower extremities to rule out the onset of a DVT, particularly with the description of unilateral ankle swelling. In addition, it is important to x-ray all joints and bones that are exceedingly painful. As it turns out in our case, the patient had a DVT but no evidence of fracture or loosening of the components.

Why Might This Be Tested? Knowing your imaging modalities is critical. Often times you will be given a disease process or injury and you must then select the best possible imaging study to obtain a diagnosis. Also, the MRI signatures of soft tissues are important to remember and just have to be committed to memory.

Here's the Point!

Patients with multiple complaints often require tests to assess what the problem is. Just know what tests can help with certain diagnoses; for total joints, serial x-rays are best, CT scan is good for bone, MRI is great with soft tissues, scintigraphy assesses for infection or areas of bone turnover/growth, and ultrasound is needed to rule out DVT.

Vignette 128: Doc, My Heel Is Killing Me!

A 44-year-old male construction worker complains of 6 months of heel pain. His pain is worse in the morning and gradually improves throughout the course of the day. His symptoms have persisted despite over-the-counter heel inserts, activity modifications, oral NSAIDs, and home stretching exercises.

▶ *What is the differential diagnosis of plantar heel pain?*

▶ *What nerve entrapment conditions are seen in the heel?*

▶ *What systemic or referred sources can be responsible for heel pain?*

Vignette 128: Answer

Plantar heel pain is a very common complaint in patients presenting to the orthopedist. Heel pain is a common reason for lost productivity at work in laborers and time spent on the sidelines by athletes.

The differential diagnosis of plantar heel pain includes plantar fasciitis, plantar fascia rupture, calcaneal stress fracture, tarsal tunnel syndrome, compression of the lateral plantar nerve, fat pad atrophy, L5-S1 radiculopathy, seronegative spondyloarthropathy, and tumor.

A key to proper diagnosis of the source of plantar heel pain is in an understanding of the anatomy. The heel fat pad begins to atrophy after approximately 40 years of age. The decrease in shock absorbency can predispose the patient to plantar fasciitis and calcaneal stress fracture. The plantar fascia is a broad ligament that originates from the anterior and medial calcaneus and inserts distally at the MTP joints. Distal to the tip of the medial malleolus, the tibial nerve branches into the medial and lateral plantar nerves, as well as a medial calcaneal sensory branch.

Plantar fasciitis is more common in females, obese patients, and those who are subjected to repetitive stresses or athletic activities. The central band of the plantar fascia becomes inflamed, and chronic microtears often develop. On exam, the maximal point of tenderness is usually over the medial calcaneal tuberosity. Patients will often exhibit Achilles tendon tightness. Morning pain is the hallmark of this condition, and patients typically demonstrate symptomatic improvement as the day progresses. Lateral x-rays will often reveal a plantar calcaneal heel spur, but it is widely accepted that the spur is a consequence of repetitive microtrauma (traction enthesophyte) and is not a source of pain (and consequently is not removed at the time of surgery). Treatment consists of commitment to a long course of nonsurgical treatment modalities, including prefabricated or custom shoe inserts, activity modifications, stretching exercises, physical therapy, oral NSAIDs, corticosteroid injections, dorsiflexion night splinting, or casting. In patients with significant disability and symptoms beyond 6 months, surgery should be considered. Open and endoscopic plantar fascia release have been recommended; what they have in common is a partial, rather than complete, release of the fascia in order to prevent the potential complication of arch collapse due to loss of the windlass mechanism of the plantar fascia. An open release allows for direct visualization of the thickened portion of the fascia, whereas the endoscopic approach provides less morbidity and an earlier return to work.

Calcaneal stress fractures are a frequent cause of heel pain in military recruits and running athletes. The common clinical presentation is posterior and plantar heel pain with a prodromal period of 7 to 10 days. Swelling is often present (which is rarely seen in plantar fasciitis). Pain is exacerbated by any weight-bearing activities. The classic radiographic finding as seen on the lateral view is a fracture line emanating from the posterosuperior calcaneus and is usually evident 3 to 4 weeks after the onset of symptoms. MRI is also useful in the diagnosis. Weight bearing is allowed during the recovery phase, and most patients return to full activity 8 weeks after diagnosis.

Tarsal tunnel syndrome is an entrapment of the tibial nerve within the tarsal canal just posterior to the medial malleolus. The nerve branches into its 3 terminal branches: the medial plantar nerve, lateral plantar nerve, and medial calcaneal nerve within the tunnel. In 60% of cases, a specific etiology can be identified. Causes include trauma (ankle fracture, dislocation), varicosities, heel deformity (varus, valgus), space-occupying lesion (ganglion, lipoma, exostosis), accessory muscle in canal, and diabetes mellitus. Plantar heel pain is more diffuse and less focal than in other sources of heel pain. One-third of patients report radiation proximally into the medial aspect of the leg. Tinel's sign is often present at the site of entrapment. Definitive diagnosis is confirmed with electrodiagnostic studies. Initial treatment consists of NSAIDs, bracing, orthotics (to address deformity), or corticosteroid injection. Surgical treatment is recommended for space-occupying lesions or with failed conservative treatment.

One of the most commonly overlooked causes of plantar heel pain is entrapment of the first branch of the lateral plantar nerve. This nerve innervates the periosteum of the medial calcaneal tuberosity. The site of compression is between the deep fascia of the abductor hallucis muscle and medial head of the quadratus plantae muscle. Athletes, such as sprinters, figure skaters, and ballet dancers, are prone to this specific entrapment syndrome. Motor weakness of the abductor digiti quinti may be seen. With entrapment of the medial plantar nerve, the point of maximal tenderness is located more distally on the foot (at the level of the navicular tuberosity). In patients who fail nonsurgical treatment for more than 6 months, surgical decompression of the nerve is recommended.

Why Might This Be Tested? Plantar heel pain is a common presenting complaint to the orthopedist and a common cause of lost time from work and from sports.

Here's the Point!

In obese patients with morning pain, think plantar fasciitis; in military recruits and marathoners, think calcaneal stress fracture; with space-occupying lesions, think tarsal tunnel syndrome; in ballet dancers and sprinters, think entrapment of the first branch of the lateral plantar nerve; and when the pain is slightly more distal in the heel in runners, think entrapment of the medial plantar nerve.

Vignette 129: Cut Me Some Slack—My Wrist Hurts!

A 58-year-old retired construction worker presents with gradual-onset right wrist pain over the past 8 months. He hasn't noticed any particular stiffness. He describes it as a deep ache that is worst at the extremes of extension more than flexion. There was no known trauma. His physical exam reveals a lack of 30 degrees of extension and 15 degrees of flexion compared with the unaffected side. He is tender at the radioscaphoid joint dorsally more than volarly and has no ulnar-sided symptoms. Forced extension, especially with radial deviation, reproduces his symptoms. X-rays are shown in Figure 129-1.

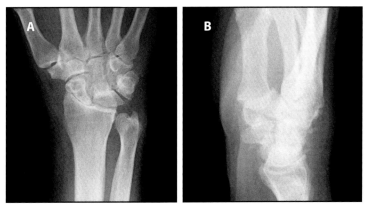

Figure 129-1. (A) AP and (B) lateral x-rays of the wrist.

▶ *What is the patient's underlying diagnosis, and how does it typically progress?*

▶ *What are his primary surgical treatment options?*

▶ *What is the role of arthroscopy in treating this condition?*

▶ *What outcome can be expected from surgery?*

Vignette 129: Answer

The underlying diagnosis in this case is scapholunate advanced collapse (SLAC) arthritis. This arthritis typically develops 15+ years following a complete tear of the scapholunate ligament. Although a complete tear sounds terrible, the patient often cannot recall a specific injury associated with the ligament rupture. SLAC wrist is a common arthritic process found in males who work with their hands heavily during their life. The pathology results in unopposed flexion of the scaphoid, resulting in poor congruency of the radioscaphoid joint and degenerative changes at the styloid first and then the radioscaphoid joint in its entirety. Although the lunate will typically extend due to unopposed pull of the triquetrum, the consistent crescent shape of the lunate in the sagittal plane makes this alteration well tolerated and radiolunate degeneration very rare.[380] As the scaphoid and lunate separate from each other, the capitate begins to descend proximally with resultant midcarpal joint degeneration over time, typically later than the radioscaphoid joint. Patients are often unaware of the fact that they have lost wrist ROM and are bothered instead by the pain. The above has been classified into the following 3 stages: stage I, scaphoid and radial styloid arthritis; stage II, arthritis of the entire scaphoid facet of the radius; and stage III, aforementioned plus capitate and lunate arthritis.

Treatment is based on addressing the arthritic areas. In early stage I disease with arthritis only at the articulation the radial styloid and scaphoid, pain primarily with radial deviation, and well-maintained wrist ROM, arthroscopy with radial styloidectomy can be considered as a less invasive procedure option. This presentation is less common, and the results are not definitively known. When the majority of the radioscaphoid joint is affected (stage II) but the midcarpal joint is spared, proximal row carpectomy (PRC) or partial fusion (typically scaphoid excision and 4-corner fusion) can be considered.[381,382] Both procedures will typically result in approximately 60% of the normal arc of wrist motion and more than 70% return of grip strength, but slightly better radial deviation and grip strength are reported with partial fusion than with PRC.[381] However, partial fusion is technically more challenging, requires more prolonged immobilization, and carries the risk of nonunion. PRC has shown degenerative changes at the radiocapitate articulation in long-term outcome studies but does not appear to correlate with symptoms or the need for further intervention.[380] For stage III disease, the options are scaphoid excision and 4-corner fusion or wrist arthrodesis.

Why Might This Be Tested? SLAC arthritis is the most common form of wrist arthritis and develops in a common pattern of progression based on specific pathomechanics of the wrist. Specific treatments are available and vary depending on stage.

Here's the Point!

SLAC arthritis typically occurs years after a scapholunate ligament tear with a predictable pattern of progression (partial radioscaphoid → entire radioscaphoid → midcarpal joint). Arthroscopic radial styloidectomy can be considered in very early stage I disease. PRC and 4-corner fusion can be considered when the midcarpal joint is unaffected (stage II) with similar results reported. PRC is not an option when the midcarpal joint has degenerated.

Vignette 130: I Am Young and Do Not Want a THA. What Do I Do?

A 22-year-old male presents with endstage DJD from a prior septic arthritis when he was a child. He is a construction worker and is medically healthy with no other specific ailments or conditions. His gait has continued to deteriorate, and he is not able to work a full day without severe pain or oral analgesic agents. THA options have been discussed with several consultants, but the patient is concerned about the need for future surgeries. He inquires about other options of endstage DJD of the hip that do not involve replacement components.

▶ *What other procedures do you have to offer?*

▶ *Describe the surgical techniques.*

▶ *What future outcomes and complications can be expected with these options?*

Vignette 130: Answer

Despite being rarely performed in the United States at this time, hip arthrodesis may be the best alternative to arthroplasty for this patient. He is a young (younger than 40 years) laborer and has unilateral disease, which are the classic indications for hip arthrodesis. Consideration for fusion should also be considered when there are bone deficiencies and neurologic abnormalities leading to abductor dysfunction. Contraindications and relative contraindications for arthrodesis include bilateral hip disease, infection, inflammatory arthropathy, extensive low back pain/disease, ipsilateral knee disease, ON (must check other hip), and psychological instability. Other concerning conditions include obesity, poor health, and advancing age.[383] Girdlestone resection is another nonarthroplasty option but not a particularly good one at this patient's age and activity level. Similarly, arthroscopy and osteotomy have no role in managing this case.

Various techniques have been described to successfully perform an arthrodesis. In the end, the optimal position for hip fusion is between 20 and 30 degrees of flexion, 5 and 7 degrees of adduction, and 5 and 10 degrees of external rotation.[383] Well-described surgical techniques for hip arthrodesis include the following:

- Lateral cobra plating: Abductors are stripped off of the ilium, and the pelvis is osteotomized to increase the contact area of the femur and pelvis. Fusion rates of 94% to 100% have been reported; however, this technique was later modified to bend the plate and avoid the pelvic osteotomy. Furthermore, a trochanteric osteotomy was performed to avoid stripping the abductors in the subsequent modification.[383]

  o Matta et al used an anterior approach through an extended Smith-Petersen approach (remember sartorius and tibiofibular interval). Fixation is placed medial, and the abductors are spared, making later conversion to THA easier.[384]

- Double plating: A lateral approach is used, and one plate is placed laterally, followed by application of an anterior plate.

- Other options:

  o Central dislocation and internal compression
  o Intramedullary arthrodesis
  o Transarticular nailing
  o Extra-articular arthrodesis (with or without subtrochanteric osteotomy)
  o Two-incision: one anteriorly to debride the joint and a second laterally to place a compression hip screw

Early protected weight bearing is suggested, and limited ROM will help avoid overstressing the fixation devices. Older methods occasionally required the use of a hip spica cast to achieve adequate early stability and minimize nonunion.

Overall, for the length of success, arthrodesis results have been favorable, particularly when compared with THA. In 2 well-known studies, Callaghan et al and Sponseller et al reported on hip arthrodesis at an average of 35 and 38 years, respectively. Patients were able to continue working for nearly 30 years after their fusions in these series. Other complications reported included low back pain (~60%), ipsilateral knee pain (~50%), contralateral hip pain (~20% to 25%), and conversion to arthroplasty (~15% to 20%).[385,386] Most of these problems occurred at least 20 years after the arthrodesis, yet up to 65% were unsure if they would undergo the procedure again. Daily activities, such as putting on shoes and socks and sitting in a chair, were difficult, and some reported issues with sexual intercourse.[385,386] Other reports using the anterior technique found an 83% fusion rate, with a high satisfaction rate in 12 patients.[382]

Potential complications with hip arthrodesis include excessive blood loss (1 to 6 L), infection (4% to 8%), nerve injury (rare, initially secondary to prolonged casting), VTE (2% to 9%), nonunion (5% to 15%), femur fracture (1% to 18%), and malunion (up to 17%). Gait efficiency has been found to be approximately 53% of normal after fusion, and adjacent joint pain is common at long-term follow-up (typically 20+ years).[382] The need for reoperation has been reported to be around 20%. The need to convert to a THA is typically related to a painful nonunion, adjacent joint pain (often lower back), or malpositioning of the limb. Success rates are reasonable, but patients have a high risk for complications (~11% to 54%),[387] including aseptic loosening (15%), abductor insufficiency (manifesting as persistent limp or dislocation), nerve injury, and clinically relevant HO. Due to the high risk and complexity of these cases, it is not wise to take down a fusion solely for the purpose of gaining hip motion.

Why Might This Be Tested? Although hip arthrodesis is an uncommon procedure, the indications are narrow, making it a good topic for vignettes. Furthermore, the position of fusion is a common question for multiple joints in the body, including the hip.

Here's the Point!

In patients younger than 40 years, hip arthrodesis is a reasonable option for noninflammatory DJD in a single joint. The position of fusion is 20 to 30 degrees of flexion, 5 to 7 degrees of adduction, and 5 to 10 degrees of external rotation. Conversion to THA after a hip fusion may be compromised by poor bone stock, abductor dysfunction (limp and dislocation), heterotopic bone formation, and aseptic loosening.

Vignette 131: Red Swollen First Toe—Ouch!

A 50-year-old female presents to your office for first-time evaluation of right medial forefoot pain. The pain is described as burning with associated swelling medially that is worse when wearing high heels. On physical exam, there is noted erythema and swelling medial to the first MTP joint. Her first MTP has normal mobility, there is no tenderness to palpation about the joint, and she has no associated deformity.

▶ *What is the most likely diagnosis?*

▶ *What other tests should be ordered?*

▶ *What specific measurements should be assessed?*

▶ *What are the treatment options?*

Vignette 131: Answer

Based on the history, physical exam, and x-rays, the patient has a diagnosis of hallux valgus. In general, this is defined as medial deviation of the distal end of the first metatarsal along with lateral deviation of the proximal phalanx distally. As in our case, the incidence is higher in women and symptoms are aggravated by restrictive shoe wear, specifically high heels with a narrow toe box. There may be a hereditary component; however, increased incidence has been shown in patients with RA and cerebral palsy. On physical exam, one should look for swelling/erythema about the first MTP joint medially. Mobility of the joint (ridged or hypermobile) and deformity is assessed along with tenderness to palpation about the joint. Other concomitant pathology, including hammertoes, pes planus, gastrocnemius contracture, and callus formation, should also be observed.

There are several key aspects to the pathoanatomy that aid in understanding the radiographic interpretation and subsequent surgical management, if necessary. Hallux valgus, as mentioned, consists of valgus deviation of the great toe along with varus angulation of the first MT. This relatively medial position of the first MTP causes the sesamoids to subluxate laterally. The capsule becomes contracted laterally and attenuated medially along with the adductor tendon contributing to the deformity.

X-rays should include weight-bearing AP and lateral views with an optional sesamoid view (Figure 131-1). The key measurements include the hallux valgus angle (HVA),[388] first and second intermetatarsal angle (IMA),[389] distal metatarsal articular angle (DMA),[390] joint congruency, and hallux valgus interphalangeus angle (HVIA),[391] which are demonstrated in Figure 131-2. Joint congruency is observed at the first MTP and should be interpreted in 1 of 3 ways: congruent (DMA or HVIA are abnormal), incongruent (joint is subluxated), or combined deformity. Signs of instability can be seen on the lateral x-ray by plantar widening at the proximal MT along with second TMT joint arthrosis.[392]

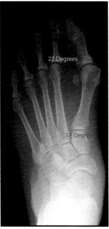

Figure 131-1. Foot radiograph showing a 27-degree HVA and 17-degree IMA.

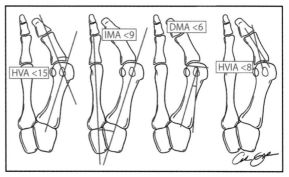

Figure 131-2. Demonstrated from left to right are the normal angles for the measurements of the HVA, first and second IMA, DMA, and HVIA. (Reprinted with permission from Adam B. Yanke, MD.)

The first consideration to be made regarding treatment is whether the patient's deformity is symptomatic. Patients without symptoms and pure cosmetic complaints should, at most, undergo conservative management.[393] Nonoperative treatment includes shoewear with a wide toe box, low heel, and soft leather uppers. Local padding or orthotics to support the medial arch (associated pes planus) or unload symptoms related to transfer metatarsalgia (secondary to failure of the Windlass mechanism) may also be helpful. Several factors will quickly guide the clinician toward the appropriate surgical procedure. Evidence of joint tenderness to palpation, spasticity, or the presence of a rigid deformity are indications for first MTP arthrodesis. Then one should take into consideration the radiographic angles that guide treatment as follows: IMA less than

13 degrees and HV less than 40 degrees=distal MT osteotomy and soft tissue release (possible Akin); IMA greater than 13 degrees OR HV greater than 40 degrees=proximal osteotomy and soft tissue release; and instability of first TMT or joint laxity=first TMT fusion and soft tissue release. Soft tissue or osseous corrections alone are never the answer. Easley et al provides a thorough review of the operative treatment options and their respective level of evidence.[394]

Given our patient's presentation and x-rays, she should be started with a trial of nonoperative management. If this fails, she would be indicated for a proximal opening-wedge osteotomy with soft tissue release.

Why Might This Be Tested? Hallux valgus is commonly encountered, and although there are many different treatment options, one should understand the general principles that guide conservative and surgical treatment.

Here's the Point!

Only operate if painful! If the patient failed conservative management, then evaluate x-rays as follows: fuse rigid/unstable/spastic joints, IMA less than 13 degrees and HV less than 40 degrees=distal MT osteotomy and soft tissue release (possible Akin); IMA greater than 13 degrees OR HV greater than 40 degrees=proximal osteotomy and soft tissue release; and instability of first TMT or joint laxity=first TMT fusion and soft tissue release.

Vignette 132: Pediatric Shoulder Pain

A 3-year-old female was brought into the emergency department because her mother reported that she was having pain and discomfort while taking a bath. The mother stated that she was able to finish the bath, get her dressed, and put to her bed that night. She was later brought in for evaluation due to continued pain, crying, and inability to rest comfortably. There was no reported history of trauma. The child has no medical problems or history of fever or chills and has met all developmental milestones appropriately. Physical examination reveals a swollen left shoulder and pain with any attempted motion. The child refuses to use the left arm at all. Clinical and radiographic images of the shoulder are shown in Figure 132-1.

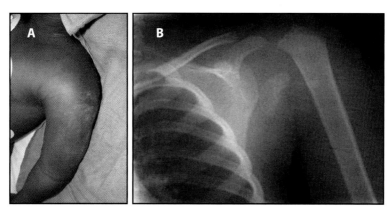

Figure 132-1. (A) Clinical photograph and (B) x-ray of the child's shoulder.

▶ *What studies do you need to obtain?*

▶ *What is the diagnosis? How is this injury classified?*

▶ *After reviewing the studies, what, if anything, is concerning regarding the clinical presentation?*

▶ *What is the appropriate treatment now?*

Vignette 132: Answer

With the reported history, the following differential diagnosis should come to mind: fracture, unreported trauma (abuse), infection, and—less likely but always in the differential—a tumor. With the reported history, several tests should be ordered to determine the appropriate diagnosis, including plain x-rays with AP and axillary views and laboratory tests, such as an ESR, CRP, and CBC. These are good screening tests for infection because a normal CRP has a 95% negative predictive value for infection.[146] Although the aforementioned tests are a good screen for infection, if suspicion is high, consideration for aspirating the shoulder joint should be entertained.

The fracture is classified using the Salter-Harris classification for pediatric fractures. In a type I fracture, there is a separation through the growth plate; in type II, the fracture crosses the physis and exits obliquely across one of the corners of the metaphysis; in type III, the fracture line extends through the growth plate and exits through the epiphysis into the joint; type IV is a vertical fracture that crosses the epiphysis, physis, and metaphysis; and type V is a crush fracture of the growth plate.[20] Our patient has a displaced Salter-Harris I proximal humerus fracture. Proximal humerus fractures in children younger than 5 years are typically Salter-Harris I fractures, as opposed to older children in whom they are typically Salter-Harris II fractures.

These fractures can occur secondary to a direct fall; however, in a child this age and with this degree of displacement, the concern for abuse is extremely high. This fracture would be extremely painful, and the fact that the mother continued to give the child a bath, get her dressed, and put her to bed should be raising a huge red flag in your evaluation. Because of this, Child Protective Services should be called and the concern for child abuse thoroughly investigated (this goes for all fractures in children for whom the history does not fit the injury pattern).

The treatment of this fracture would be a closed reduction and placement of a sling and swath or a shoulder immobilizer for 2 to 3 weeks. The remodeling potential is great in the proximal humerus in this age group, so even if the fracture alignment is not anatomic, the patient will typically have a good result cosmetically and functionally.

Why Might This Be Tested? Knowledge of which fractures are common and their mechanisms is important in order to not only properly treat the fracture, but also to make sure the child is safe in his or her home. Also, it is important to be aware of the remodeling potential in proximal humerus fractures and that it is extremely rare that these require surgery, even in older children.

Here's the Point!

If you suspect abuse (history does not match the injury pattern), you must alert Child Protective Services and evaluate thoroughly. Proximal humerus fractures in children rarely require surgery and are typically Salter-Harris I fractures when the patient is younger than 5 years and Salter-Harris II fractures after that age.

Vignette 133: Shoved in the Mall

A 62-year-old, community-ambulatory female with a medical history of osteoporosis and hypertension comes into clinic after sustaining a fall directly onto her right shoulder. The patient reports no prior injuries and was pushed while walking in the mall, which caused the fall. On physical examination, the patient has severe pain throughout the shoulder region and swelling of the entire arm with ecchymosis. There is no gross evidence of glenohumeral dislocation on exam, but overall exam and ROM testing are limited by pain. The patient has neutral alignment of her shoulder at baseline with notable inability to abduct her right arm. Pulses and capillary refill are symmetric to her upper extremities. Initial x-rays are obtained in the emergency room (Figure 133-1).

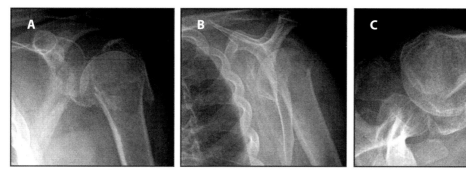

Figure 133-1. (A) AP, (B) scapular Y, and (C) axillary view x-rays of the left shoulder.

▶ *What is the diagnosis?*

▶ *What other aspects of the history and physical exam are important?*

▶ *What other tests should be ordered?*

▶ *What is the classification of these injuries?*

▶ *What are the treatment options?*

Vignette 133: Answer

The diagnosis is a displaced, comminuted 4-part fracture of the right proximal humerus without disloca-tion. Proximal humerus fractures account for 4% to 5% of all fractures in adults, and 75% of these fractures across all age groups occur in females, especially in the older population. These fractures typically result from high-energy injuries in young patients and low-energy falls in older patients. A critical aspect of proximal humerus fractures is the integrity of the vascular supply. The majority of the direct blood supply to the humeral head comes from the anterior circumflex humeral artery via the arcuate artery. The posterior circumflex artery provides blood supply to the posterior portion of the greater tuberosity and a small pos-teroinferior portion of the humeral head. Fracture patterns can help the clinician predict the vascular status of the humeral head and direct appropriate treatment options.[395-400]

It is important to first record the preinjury functional level and any history of previous trauma or disloca-tion. During physical exam, it is important to assess the status of the surrounding neurovascular structures, with particular attention to the axillary nerve because it is commonly injured in fracture-dislocations. Greater tuberosity fracture-dislocations are most frequently associated with an isolated axillary nerve injury. The incidence of associated axillary nerve injuries increases with age, with rates as high as 50% in patients older than 50 years.

Plain x-rays (shoulder trauma series) are most commonly used to diagnose and classify proximal humerus fractures. These views include AP, scapular (Y) lateral, and axillary views of the affected shoulder. Posterior fracture-dislocations and displaced greater tuberosity fractures are most commonly missed because an axil-lary view is not obtained. The axillary view is critical to assess possible dislocation of the glenohumeral joint. CT is not routinely used for proximal humerus fractures unless there is uncertainty regarding the amount of comminution or extent of intra-articular extension. CT can also be used for preoperative planning in dif-ficult cases with severe comminution. MRI can be used concurrently to identify associated rotator cuff injury based on exam findings or clinical suspicion.

Defining and identifying the amount of displacement is the most important aspect of proximal humerus fracture classification. The established Neer classification is based on the anatomic relationship of 4 seg-ments (greater tuberosity, lesser tuberosity, articular surface, and shaft) and states that a fracture is displaced if any major segment is displaced 1 cm or more or is angulated more than 45 degrees. Fracture patterns can be broken down into minimally displaced 2-part, 3-part, 4-part, and articular surface fractures.

Nonsurgical treatment using immobilization with a sling followed by rehabilitation is indicated for minimally displaced or nondisplaced fractures. It is also indicated for minimally displaced fractures in elderly, low-demand patients and patients with multiple medical comorbidities. Most (roughly 85%) proxi-mal humerus fractures are treated nonsurgically. Contraindications include severely displaced fractures in moderate- to high-functioning patients because they may potentially lead to decreased strength and ROM.

There are various surgical treatments available, including closed reduction and percutaneous pinning, ORIF, and hemiarthroplasty. Closed reduction and percutaneous pinning are indicated for displaced surgi-cal neck fractures in patients with good bone quality and, in some cases, with 3-part fractures and valgus-impacted 4-part fractures. A relative contraindication is metaphyseal comminution. ORIF using plate and screws via a deltopectoral or deltoid-splitting approach can be done when bone quality is good and is indi-cated for displaced 2-, 3-, and 4-part fractures. The anterior (Henry) approach follows the interval between the deltoid (axillary nerve) and the pectoralis major (medial and lateral pectoral nerves). With retraction of the cephalic vein, the subscapularis is exposed and divided to enter the joint. Protect the musculocutane-ous nerve (pop quiz—this nerve innervates what muscles? Coracobrachialis, biceps brachii, and brachialis muscles, as well as supplying sensation to the lateral antebrachial cutaneous nerve) as it penetrates the biceps approximately 5 to 8 cm distal to the coracoid (70% of the time). A contraindication is osteoporotic patients with displaced 4-part fractures or severe fracture comminution. Complications of managing proximal humerus fractures include missed dislocation (with nonoperative treatment), adhesive capsulitis, malunion, ON (especially 4-part fractures), nonunion, and rotator cuff injury.

Hemiarthroplasty is the treatment of choice for the case described here because it is indicated for dis-placed, comminuted 4-part fractures, especially in elderly patients with poor bone quality and a history of osteoporosis. Results of hemiarthroplasty vary depending on greater tuberosity healing and rotator cuff function. Humeral head replacement after an acute fracture has been shown to have a better outcome than delaying intervention or choosing nonoperative treatment. TSA is less commonly indicated in cases of an intact rotator cuff, and reverse TSA is an option for elderly patients with nonreconstructable tuberosities but remains controversial.

Why Might This Be Tested? Proximal humerus fractures are common in young and old patients and have important anatomy associated with each fracture pattern. There are a variety of treatment options and indications, making it a commonly tested topic.

Here's the Point!

Hemiarthroplasty is indicated for elderly patients with displaced 4-part fractures or fracture-dislocations, and the majority of proximal humerus fractures can be treated non-surgically with acceptable long-term functional outcomes. Also, the vascular supply of the humeral head and the various fracture patterns can disrupt the surrounding vascular and nervous structures.

Vignette 134: Doc, I Have Atraumatic Knee Pain and Swelling... Hope It's Not a Tumor

A 28-year-old female presents to your clinic with a 5-month history of increasing knee pain and swelling. She has some mild rest and night pain, but the majority is activity associated. On examination, she has fullness of her distal thigh and tenderness to palpation laterally. A plain x-ray is shown in Figure 134-1, and a sagittal MRI cut is shown in Figure 134-2. A histologic specimen after biopsy is represented in Figure 134-3.

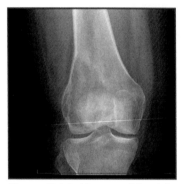

Figure 134-1. AP x-ray of the right knee.

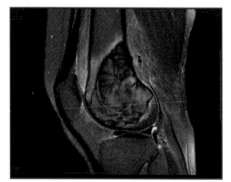

Figure 134-2. Sagittal MRI cut of the right knee.

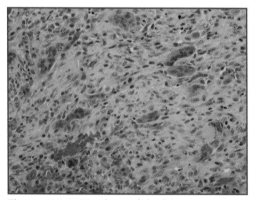

Figure 134-3. Histology of the biopsy specimen (400× magnification).

▶ *What is the likely diagnosis?*

▶ *How would you manage this patient?*

Vignette 134: Answer

GCT is a benign, aggressive process that occurs in the epiphyses or apophyses of long bones in young adults. This typically affects individuals in early adulthood, ages 25 to 40, when many other diagnoses are uncommon. It is more commonly found in women and is rare in children with open growth plates. It must be distinguished from chondroblastoma, a benign tumor typically seen in a younger age group, and clear cell CHS, a rare epiphyseal malignancy. The most common sites of involvement are the distal femur, proximal tibia, and distal radius, although nearly any bone can be affected.

Radiographic features typically show an eccentrically based epiphyseal-metaphyseal lesion with variable amounts of cortical destruction. The lesions tend to be predominantly radiolucent, but they occasionally have septations and areas reminiscent of an ABC. GCT is a likely entity in an epiphyseal lesion in a skeletally mature patient (closed growth plates). In a skeletally immature patient, a similar-appearing epiphyseal lesion is more likely to be chondroblastoma.

Histologically, GCT contains very large multinucleated giant cells, often containing more than 50 nuclei. There is a proliferation of uniform, ovoid mononuclear cells with numerous, evenly dispersed osteoclast-like giant cells. Characteristically, the nuclei of the individual monocytes in the stroma are identical to the nuclei that make up the giant cells. Mitotic figures are usually present.

Staging is done radiographically as described by Campanacci. Stage 1 is latent, with a well-defined margin and no cortical involvement. Stage 2 is active, with a thinned cortex but no frank perforation. Stage 3 is aggressive, with cortical perforation and soft tissue extension. MRI or CT scan can further assess the extent of the lesion.

Benign pulmonary metastasis can occur in 2% to 3% of patients. The clinical course of pulmonary metastasis is variable; some remain stable without treatment and others can progress and be lethal. Multiple sites of osseous disease are rare but possible. Malignant degeneration can occur but is rare.

Treatment consists of curettage of the lesion for stage 1, stage 2, and some stage 3 tumors. It is imperative to open a large enough bone window to visualize and remove the entire tumor, using a high-speed burr at the margins. Most advocate some type of adjuvant treatment at the time of surgery to decrease local recurrence. These include phenol, cryoablation with liquid nitrogen, argon beam coagulation, and high-intensity cauterization. The defect can be filled with bone graft or polymethylmethacrylate. Polymethylmethacrylate has an added benefit of being exothermic and expansive as it cures, theoretically extending the margin of excision and reducing recurrence. Without adjuvant treatment, the recurrence rates can be as high as 50%. With adjuvants, the rates are closer to 10% to 25%, depending on the bone and stage (distal radius and stage 3 lesions have the highest recurrence). The recurrence rate after en bloc excision is much lower and is often implemented in advanced stage 3 disease or after local recurrence.

Chemotherapy and radiation may be used in metastatic disease or unresectable lesions. Adjuvant chemical treatments attempt to exploit the role of osteoclastic-mediated destruction in GCT. Under normal conditions, monocytes express receptor activator of nuclear factor kappa B (RANK), the stimulation of which induces osteoclastic differentiation and subsequent bone resorption. The stromal cells in GCT, thought to be of osteoblastic lineage, secrete pathologic amounts of RANK ligand (RANKL), which stimulates this osteoclastic pathway. New treatments using denosumab, a monoclonal antibody to RANKL, and zoledronic acid, a potent bisphosphonate, are under investigation.

Why Might This Be Tested? This is a common tumor to encounter, so it is frequently tested. There are also many tumors that have giant cells within them but are not GCTs. It is important to be able to distinguish these tumors and have the correct diagnosis.

Here's the Point!

GCT is a benign but aggressive tumor in younger females with closed physes. These lytic lesions typically have a tremendous number of giant cells on histological evaluation. Treatment consists of local excision and some adjunctive modality (argon, phenol, cryotherapy). Recurrence is not uncommon, with 10% to 25% recurring even after resection and adjuvant management.

Vignette 135: Osteoporosis

A female patient's DEXA report noted a T-score of -3.6 at the femoral neck and a T-score of -3.3 at the lumbar spine, further confirming the diagnosis of osteoporosis. Also, her CBC, calcium, vitamin D, and chemistry laboratory tests were all within normal limits, and a detailed history and physical exam were relatively unremarkable, ruling out common secondary causes of osteoporosis. Given her overall concern about future fracture risk and after further discussion with her family, she is now interested in starting pharmacologic treatment for her osteoporosis.

▶ *In which patient populations should pharmacologic treatment be considered?*

▶ *What is the basic mechanism of bisphosphonate treatment?*

▶ *What are the common side effects of bisphosphonates?*

Vignette 135: Answer

Males and females older than 50 years with a known fracture of the hip or spine or osteoporosis diagnosed by bone density testing should consider taking medication. Patients with low bone mass or osteopenia should be considered for treatment if risk factors are present or a history of fractures makes the 10-year probability of hip fracture greater than or equal to 3% or any osteoporosis-related fracture that is greater than or equal to 20%. The WHO algorithm or FRAX tool is a clinical tool to help determine a patient's absolute risk of fracture based on bone mineral density and 10 specific risk factors. By estimating the likelihood of a person to break a bone in the upcoming 10 years, those most appropriate for treatment can more easily be identified. Of note, appropriate daily calcium and vitamin D intake is recommended for all patients in addition to any other pharmacologic therapy.[401,402]

Bisphosphonates have generally been considered first-line medications for the treatment of osteoporosis to reduce future fracture risk. These antiresorptive drugs specifically slow the bone loss that occurs in the breakdown part of the remodeling cycle by attaching to hydroxyapatite binding sites on bony surfaces and inhibiting osteoclast resorption activity, osteoclast progenitor development, and promoting osteoclast apoptosis. Although osteoblast activity is also affected, bone homeostasis is overall tipped toward bone formation and overall bone loss is decreased.[401,402]

Common side effects may include abdominal pain, nausea, diarrhea, and heartburn with a risk for esophageal ulceration if strict administration guidelines are not followed. More serious yet rare conditions associated with bisphosphonate therapy include atrial fibrillation, ON of the jaw, and atypical hip or diaphyseal femur fractures.[402]

Why Might This Be Tested? Bone health is an extremely common yet generally underaddressed issue throughout the health care system. During the past 10 to 20 years, postmenopausal osteoporosis, and to a lesser extent male osteoporosis, have been recognized as important diseases that have a great effect on physical function, quality of life, disability, and mortality, through increasing the risk of fractures.

Here's the Point!

Although a range of effective and well-tolerated therapies that can halve the rate of fractures are now available, even the most basic of treatments are often not implemented. A multidisciplinary and proactive approach to bone health and osteoporosis should be included as part of routine fracture care.

Vignette 136: My Hip Hurts

A 76-year-old male presents to the clinic with right hip pain. As he walks into the clinic room, you note that he has an antalgic gait and that he is leaning over a cane held in his right hand. Subsequent AP and lateral hip x-rays demonstrate moderate hip OA. You have a discussion with him about various potential nonoperative and operative treatment options, including THA, but he wishes to pursue conservative treatment at this time. You have some recommendations for him, including some modifications in his cane use.

▶ *What recommendations would you make about his cane use?*

▶ *Biomechanically describe why he would benefit from your modifications.*

Vignette 136: Answer

Hip OA is extremely common and often quite disabling for patients. Several treatment options exist for patients depending on their pain level, degree of arthritis, and desire to pursue operative or nonoperative treatment. The use of an assistive device, such as a cane, can be part of a conservative treatment plan for hip, knee, and ankle arthritis. Although any weight that can be unloaded from the affected joint is likely to reduce pain, it is biomechanically beneficial to have the cane in the opposite hand of the affected hip. To understand why this is, one needs to be comfortable with several biomechanical concepts and be able to use free body diagrams (Table 136-1).

Table 136-1.	
BIOMECHANIC TERMS AND DEFINITIONS	
Term	*Definition*
Kinematics	The part of biomechanics that describes motion without regard for the forces required to produce motion.
Kinetics	The part of biomechanics that concerns studying the forces causing movement or maintaining equilibrium.
Scalar	Quantities that are specified by a single number that describes magnitude (eg, time, mass, volume, speed).
Vector	Composed of magnitude, direction, sense, and position (eg, force, stress, strain, velocity, torque, displacement).
Force	A push or pull upon an object resulting from the object's interaction with another object. It is measured in Newtons (N). Force = mass × acceleration
Velocity	The rate of change in the position of an object with respect to time (aka speed). Velocity = rate/time
Acceleration	The rate of change in velocity with respect to time. Acceleration = $\Delta v/\Delta t$
Moment	The product of a force and the perpendicular distance between the line of action of force and the axis of rotation of the motion that the force produces. Moment = force (perpendicular) × distance
Rigid body	A rigid body assumes no deformation of the body despite the magnitude of the forces acting upon it.
Static equilibrium	When the sum of all forces acting upon a rigid body is zero. The body at static equilibrium is at rest or at constant velocity.
Free body diagram	When analyzing the forces acting upon a rigid body, the body part/joint is isolated from the environment and replaced with forces acting on the system. Forces and moments are both vectors, and their sum must equal zero at equilibrium.
Joint reaction force	The force generated within a joint by the forces acting upon the joint.

Biomechanics is the study of the mechanical forces acting on the musculoskeletal system. Newton's laws of mechanics are the basis for understanding biomechanics and the effects of various forces on the human body (Table 136-2).[403] By applying Newton's laws to a free body diagram, one can analyze and determine how various forces act upon a body and how alterations can be made to benefit the patient. A free body diagram is a drawing or pictorial that is used to analyze all of the forces and moments acting upon a body.[404] It can help determine the unknown forces or moments that are applied to the body and thus help to analyze problems in static or dynamic forces.

Table 136-2. NEWTON'S THREE LAWS	
Term	Definition
Newton's first law	An object in motion moves at a constant velocity unless another force acts upon it.
Newton's second law	The acceleration of a body is proportional to the magnitude and direction to the force applied to it and is inversely proportional to its mass. Force = mass × acceleration ($F = m \times a$)
Newton's third law	When a body exerts a force on a second body, the second body exerts an equal force on the first body, but in the opposite direction.
Mechanics	The study of conditions of rest or motion of bodies under the action of forces.

To understand the joint reaction forces that occur during single-leg stance, one needs to grasp the forces involved in bilateral stance. When both feet are on the ground, it is estimated that the weight of the head, arms, and trunk (HAT) is distributed evenly between each hip joint. The HAT is two-thirds of the entire body weight, with the remaining one-third of body weight being distributed evenly between each lower limb (one-sixth per limb). During unilateral stance, as occurs with normal gait when the contralateral limb is elevated, five-sixths of the entire body's weight must be supported by the ipsilateral hip joint. To maintain a balanced and level pelvis, the forces acting around the hip joint need to be in equilibrium. The forces of gravity acting on the body weight must be balanced by the contraction of hip abductor muscles. These 2 forces must be equal in magnitude but opposite in direction to maintain balance. The joint reaction force of the hip due to body weight alone is calculated with the following equation: joint reaction force = five-sixths × body weight.

Assuming an individual weighs 150 lb, the joint reaction force in the hip during single-leg stance is 125 lb (or five-sixths of 150 lb). This is the force of compression from the body weight of the head, arms, trunk, and contralateral leg alone. In this setting, the hip is being compressed not only by body weight, but also by the muscular compressive forces required to keep the pelvis level. The force of gravity acting upon the body's center of gravity will create an adduction torque around the hip joint that is the weight of the body (125 lb) multiplied by the distance from the COR (center of hip joint) to the center of gravity. Assuming this distance is 4 inches, the resulting torque will be 125 lb × 4 in = 500 in-lb.

To counterbalance this and maintain the pelvis in equilibrium, we know that the hip abductors will need to create a torque that is equal but in the opposite direction. Working backward from 500 in-lb and assuming that the hip abductor moment arm is 2 in, we can determine the force that the hip abductors must generate:

$$\text{Torque} = 500 \text{ in-lb} = 2 \text{ in} \times \text{Fabd}$$
$$\text{Fabd} = 500 \text{ in-lb}/2 \text{ in} = 250 \text{ lb}$$

So, the hip joint not only feels the 150 lb from the individual's body weight, but also the 250 lb of compressive force generated by the hip abductor muscles, for a total of 400 lb of force. A good estimation of forces across the joint is 3 times that of body weight.

As can be seen from the calculations above, the majority of hip joint reaction force comes from the muscle contraction of the hip abductors as opposed to just one's body weight (250 lb vs 150 lb). While patients' efforts to lose weight are helpful in decreasing the joint reaction force and relieving pain, finding a way to decrease the force that the hip abductors need to generate to maintain equilibrium will have a larger effect on decreasing to compressive forces across the joint. One intrinsic compensatory method is to decrease the distance of the center of gravity from the COR. This is accomplished by a compensatory trunk lean toward the affected hip. This effectively decreases the moment arm for the body weight.

Assuming again that an individual weighs 150 lb, 5/6 × BW = 125 lbs. By moving the moment arm at the hip closer to the COR, the rotational torque and the compressive forces across the hip are decreased. Just by leaning toward the affected hip, it will decrease the compressive forces of body weight (Fbw) from 500 in-lb to 250 in-lb. As a result, this will also decrease the forces that need to be generated by the hip abductors to maintain a level pelvis. If the force that the abductors needs to balance is now only 250 in-lb, the compressive forces can be again calculated as follows:

$$0 = ([[(5/6 \times 150 \text{ lb}]0 \times 2 \text{ in}]) - (2 \text{ in} \times \text{Fabd})$$
$$0 = (125 \text{ lb} \times 2 \text{ in}) - (2 \text{ Fabd})$$
$$0 = 250 \text{ in-lb} - 2 \text{ Fabd}$$
$$2 \text{ Fabd} = 250 \text{ in-lb}$$
$$\text{Fabd} = 125 \text{ lb}$$
$$250 \text{ in-lb} = 2 \text{ in} \times \text{F}$$
$$\text{F} = 250 \text{ in-lb}/2 \text{ in} = 125 \text{ lb}$$

So, the net joint reaction force from the pull of the hip abductors and the compressive force of body weight is now 375 lb, which is decreased from 500 lb just by leaning toward the affected hip. Now, what about using a cane? Using the cane in the ipsilateral hand will decrease the joint reaction force, but only by the amount of weight that can be transmitted up the arm instead of through the hip. It has been estimated that an average individual can push down on a cane with approximately 15% of their body weight. In this case, 22.5 lb will travel through the cane in a 150-lb individual. This will reduce the weight of his head, arms, trunk and contralateral leg to 127.5 lb. We can then use this number in the above equations to calculate the joint reaction force:

$$150 - 22.5 = 127.5$$
$$127.5 \times (5/6 \text{ BW}) = 106.25$$
$$\text{Fbw} = 106.25 \times 4 \text{ in}$$
$$\text{F bw} = 425 \text{ in-lb}$$
$$0 = (425 \text{ in-lb}) - (2 \text{ in} \times \text{Fabd})$$
$$2 \text{ in} \times \text{Fab} = 425 \text{ in-lb}$$
$$\text{Fab} = 212.5$$

The total joint reaction force with the cane on the ipsilateral side is as follows:

$$\text{F} = \text{Fbw} + \text{Fabd}$$
$$\text{F} = 127.5 + 212.5$$
$$\text{F} = 340 \text{ lb}$$

This is decreased from the 375 lb without the cane.

Now, with the cane in the contralateral hand, we not only decrease the body weight by the force of the hand pushing down on the cane, but we also have a force providing a counter-torque to the hip abductors. To calculate this, we have the patient's body weight and subtract the force provided by pushing through the cane, which we are assuming to be 15% of his or her body weight.

This is 127.5 lb, and five-sixths of this is 106.25.

This will create a torque at the COR of the following:

$$106.25 \text{ lb} \times 4 \text{ in} = 425 \text{ lb-in}$$

The cane in the contralateral hand produces a counter-torque centered around the latissimus dorsi muscle, which is developing the downward force. Assuming the COR for the counter-torque is 8 inches, the counter-torque is as follows:

$$\text{F} = 22.5 \text{ lb} \times 8 \text{ in}$$
$$\text{F} = 180 \text{ in-lb}$$

The torque produced by body weight is 425 in-lb and the counter-torque provided by the latissimus dorsi muscle is 180 in-lb, which leaves 245 in-lb. To balance the pelvis, the torque generated by the hip abductors must equal this. So the force generated can be calculated as follows:

$$245 \text{ in-lb} = 2 \text{ in} \times \text{Fabd}$$
$$245 \text{ in-lb}/2 \text{ in} = \text{Fabd}$$
$$\text{Fabd} = 122.5$$
$$\text{Total joint compression} = 122.5 + 106.25 = 228.75$$

Placing the cane in the opposite hand decreases compression forces across the hip from 340 lb with the cane in the ipsilateral hand to 228.75 lb in the contralateral hand. This is a reduction in force across the hip of approximately 33% compared with using the cane in the ipsilateral hand.

Why Might This Be Tested? A basic understanding of biomechanics and how it relates to joint structure, function, and movement is essential for all aspects of orthopedic surgery. An orthopedic surgeon needs to be able to analyze a joint structure and the forces that are acting upon it and see how alterations that are made can affect movement and joint reaction forces.

Here's the Point!

Through the use of biomechanical principles and free body diagrams, you can manipulate the forces acting upon a joint to improve your patient's function and pain. Moving the cane to the opposite hand decreases the adduction torque produced by body weight, but more importantly, it decreases the force required by the hip abductors to maintain a level pelvis.

Vignette 137: Adolescent Foot Pain and Stiffness

A 12-year-old female with no significant medical history and a normal developmental history comes into the clinic with her parents with a 6-month history of pain in the calf and hindfoot and difficulty walking on uneven ground. The patient has no history of past or recent trauma. On exam, the patient has notable pes planus deformity, limited subtalar motion, and pain in the tarsal sinus and longitudinal arch. The patient has neutral alignment of her foot and is neurovascularly intact. The initial x-ray obtained is shown in Figure 137-1.

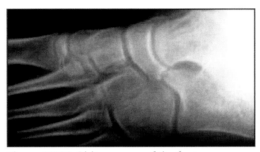

Figure 137-1. Oblique x-ray of the foot.

▶ *What is the diagnosis?*

▶ *What are the demographics and typical findings of this disorder?*

▶ *What other tests should be ordered?*

▶ *What are the treatment options?*

Vignette 137: Answer

The diagnosis is a tarsal coalition of the calcaneus and navicular bones (calcaneonavicular coalition). Tarsal coalition is an abnormal connection (bony, cartilaginous, or fibrous) between bones of the midfoot and hindfoot that occurs in approximately 1% to 10% of the population. Approximately half of all cases are bilateral, and most coalitions are asymptomatic and found incidentally during the workup of other disorders. Calcaneonavicular coalitions are the most common type and generally occur in patients aged 10 to 12 years, and talocalcaneal are the next most frequent, with an age of onset at 12 to 14 years. Talocalcaneal coalitions can occur at any of the 3 facets and most commonly occur at the middle facet. Calcaneonavicular coalitions on x-rays show an elongated dorsal process of the calcaneus ("anteater's nose"), and talocalcaneal coalitions show a C-shaped line that extends from the talar dome to the sustentaculum tali (C-sign of Lefleur).[405-409]

X-rays to be obtained during workup include AP, lateral oblique, and Harris heel views. A bridge between the affected bones will often be visible on x-ray with accompanying dorsal talar beaking. Harris heel views are prone to false-positive reads for tarsal coalition. A CT scan is helpful in showing the coalition, bar size, and the presence of multiple coalitions. Multiple coalitions are often present in Apert's syndrome and fibular deficiency. MRI can be useful to visualize cartilaginous or fibrous coalitions.

No treatment is needed for asymptomatic coalitions, and symptomatic coalitions with pain can be treated with NSAIDs, decreased physical activity, shoe orthotics, and cast immobilization. Roughly 30% of symptomatic coalitions can be successfully treated with immobilization. Surgical intervention involves coalition resection and interposition of tendon (extensor digitorum brevis) or fat where the coalition was previously located. Contraindications to simple excision include advanced degenerative changes or multiple coalitions that require triple arthrodesis or subtalar fusion.

Why Might This Be Tested? Tarsal coalition can be easily confused with other soft tissue and tendon disorders of the foot, especially if x-rays are not carefully examined.

Here's the Point!

Multiple coalitions can be present, and there are limited indications for surgical intervention. Asymptomatic coalitions do not require treatment, and most patients with painful coalitions do well with nonoperative treatment. Also, calcaneonavicular and then talocalcaneal coalitions are the most common in frequency.

Vignette 138: Ouch! A Slip on Ice Leads to Pain Between My THA and TKA

A 73-year-old female presents with pain, swelling, and deformity around a previously well-functioning TKA after falling on ice. The skin around the knee demonstrates a mild abrasion without frank laceration. There is gross crepitus with any ROM of the knee or entire leg. She is neurovascularly intact distally to motor and sensory function. The patient also has no significant medical history except for generalized OA with a well-functioning THA on the same side. Plain x-rays are shown in Figure 138-1.

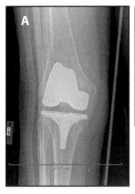
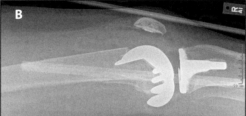
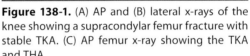
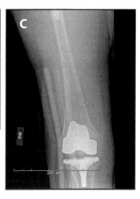

Figure 138-1. (A) AP and (B) lateral x-rays of the knee showing a supracondylar femur fracture with stable TKA. (C) AP femur x-ray showing the TKA and THA.

▶ *What is the diagnosis?*

▶ *What are the treatment options?*

▶ *What are the goals of surgical intervention?*

▶ *What findings would necessitate revision surgery?*

Vignette 138: Answer

The patient has a periprosthetic fracture just proximal to the femoral component of her TKA in the supracondylar region and between the hip stem above. Periprosthetic fractures after TKA have a reported incidence of 0.3% to 5.5% after primary surgery and up to 30% after revision procedures.[186,410] Supracondylar femur fractures are the most common type, with an incidence of 0.3% to 2.5% for primary TKA and 1.6% to 38% for revision TKA.[186,410] A modified Vancouver classification system has been described to highlight the critical points of the fracture and help guide treatment options.[187]

- Type I fracture: distal to the hip stem and proximal to the knee stem
- Type II fracture: adjacent to either the hip or knee components
- Type III fracture: adjacent to both prostheses
- Each type is further categorized with an A, B, or C modifier as follows:
    - A: Both components are stable
    - B: One component is loose (B1: hip is loose, B2: knee is loose)
    - C: Both components are loose

Nonsurgical management requires prolonged immobilization of the knee, has an unacceptable rate of malunion, and could place the skin at risk for breakdown and ultimately lead to an infection. Other options include ORIF with a plate and screws (with or without bone graft), IM rod fixation, or component revision and fracture stabilization. The short-term goal of operative intervention is to provide the patient with a stable knee/femur to allow for ROM and early mobilization. The long-term goal is to provide a well-functioning, pain-free TKA. In the setting of an unstable interprosthetic fracture, operative intervention will be dictated by several factors. ORIF with retention of the components should be performed if the following conditions are present:

1. The TKA was well functioning prior to the fracture.
2. The TKA components have a good long-term track record.
3. There is no evidence of acute or chronic infection.
4. The component/cement/bone interfaces are intact without evidence of loosening of the component from the distal fracture fragment.
5. There is sufficient bone stock to obtain acceptable distal fixation.
6. The resulting construct is stable enough to allow for near immediate ROM.

More specifically for interprosthetic fractures, the zone between the 2 prostheses must be adequately spanned, leaving no stress risers for future fracture (never end components or fixation devices at the end of one another; always span so there is no increased fracture risk). If the hip or knee components are loose, it is imperative that revision surgery be performed because fractures will not heal in the setting of a loose implant, and loose implants can be a source of pain and disability (most important part of looking at the x-rays is making sure the components are stable). Although an interprosthetic fracture is rare and more challenging than even a periprosthetic fracture, when treated appropriately, good results can be achieved. Locked lateral plating techniques have become the most popular method for treating these fractures and are successful when long plates are used, periosteal and muscle stripping are minimized, a large span of fixation is achieved, and a good reduction is performed. Despite reasonable clinical results (73% return to preinjury level of function), nonunion, malunion, delayed union, and hardware complications are common adverse events.[187]

Why Might This Be Tested? Interprosthetic and periprosthetic fractures are treated similarly and together are not an infrequent cause of reoperation in hip and knee patients. Fracture classification systems are available and help guide management.

Here's the Point!

Interprosthetic fractures are difficult to manage, and the first step in the treatment algorithm is determining component stability. If the THA or TKA is loose, then revision surgery is necessary. If components are stable, then locked lateral plating (with overlap of the components of at least 50%) is the treatment of choice, with high rates of union and perioperative complications.

Vignette 139: Metabolic Bone Disease

A 32-year-old female in her postpartum period of her pregnancy complains of increasing left hip pain. She has had difficulty ambulating due to the incapacitating groin pain. She denies a history of trauma, prior hip pain, or other difficulties during the pregnancy. The child developed normally during the intrauterine pregnancy, and the delivery was uncomplicated.

▶ *List the differential diagnosis.*

▶ *What tests would you obtain to confirm the diagnosis?*

▶ *What are the appropriate treatment options?*

Vignette 139: Answer

The differential diagnosis for this case is bone marrow edema, transient osteoporosis of the hip, regional migratory osteoporosis (typically affects men and is a migratory polyarticular arthralgia), femoral neck fracture, pelvic fracture (diastasis of ring), ON (assess for risk factors, alcohol, steroid use, etc), neoplasia (metastatic carcinoma, multiple myeloma, and lymphoma), inflammatory arthritis (infectious, RA, gout, multifocal osteomyelitis, and tuberculosis), osteitis pubis, hernia, or intrapelvic source of pain. The history was picked on purpose to distract you from the underlying diagnosis and would have been more clear if this was a middle-aged man without atraumatic pain.[411]

Regardless, with this history in the postpartum setting, the best test to make the correct diagnosis is a plain x-ray. In this case, the plain x-ray is normal without evidence of fracture, pelvic ring diastasis, neoplasia, or osteitis pubis. This will rule out many of the diagnoses listed above but would have been more helpful if it showed periarticular osseous demineralization or the phantom appearance of the femoral head. Have you picked up on the diagnosis yet?

More advanced imaging options to confirm the diagnosis are the following[411]:

- Bone scintigraphy: May not be specific for our diagnosis but will often show an increased uptake within a few days of the onset of symptoms. For this case, let's presume that we obtained a bone scan and it showed a homogenous, diffuse increased uptake to the entire femoral head. This again rules out ON, fracture, and most neoplastic lesions.

- CT scan: Not recommended for diagnosis of our disorder.

- MRI: Because we expect some bone marrow abnormality or are just still shooting in the dark, an MRI is the examination of choice. In our case, the T1-weighted images show a low signal intensity and the T2-weighted images show high signal intensity in the entire femoral head uniformly. Coupled with our history, this confirms the diagnosis of transient osteoporosis of the hip, although to be 100% sure of the diagnosis, we would ultimately need to see this signal pattern return to normal in the future.

Transient osteoporosis typically affects healthy middle-aged men or women in the third trimester of pregnancy or postpartum. The hip pain is often disabling; however, it usually runs a short course and will certainly resolve within 6 to 8 months (shorter than a hockey season!). Typically, x-rays will show extensive bone loss in the femoral head within 3 to 6 weeks of the onset of symptoms. Spontaneous clinical and radiographic resolution typically occurs. Treatment involves focusing on the clinical symptoms present and often involves partial weight bearing, analgesics, NSAIDs, and rest. Protecting the weight bearing is important so that collapse of the femoral head does not occur and should continue until clinical and radiographic resolution of findings are seen. There is some evidence that bisphosphonates can be used to treat transient osteoporosis.[411]

Why Might This Be Tested? Hip pain is a great test question because it can go down the fracture, arthritis, metabolic bone disease, ON, etc, pathway. This will be the lead-in for several questions on most standardized orthopedic tests.

Here's the Point!

Transient osteoporosis is self-limited and usually occurs in women during or just after pregnancy and in late-middle-aged men. An MRI is the diagnostic imaging of choice, and treatment is conservative, with protected weight bearing and time.

Vignette 140: What Do You Mean My Blood Is Too Thin for Surgery?

A 75-year-old female presents to the emergency department after sustaining a fall from standing at her home. She was washing some dishes when she slipped on the floor and fell onto her right hip. She was not able to get up secondary to pain and had to call her daughter to bring her to the hospital. She has a medical history significant for atrial fibrillation, for which she takes warfarin. She has no past surgical history. Physical exam reveals a frail-appearing woman in no acute distress. Vital signs are within normal limits. She has pain with any motion of her right hip, but you do not notice any gross deformity. X-rays reveal mild right hip OA and a displaced right femoral neck fracture. Your plan is to take her to the operating room for a right hemiarthroplasty, but you notice that her INR comes back at 3.0.

▶ *What is the mechanism of action behind her elevated INR?*

▶ *What is the mechanism of action for the commonly used anticoagulants?*

▶ *How long before surgery should routine anticoagulation be stopped?*

Vignette 140: Answer

The diagnosis is a femoral neck fracture requiring a hemiarthroplasty given the patient's age and functional status. She is taking warfarin and therefore has an elevated INR (with a likely goal of 2 to 3 given her history of atrial fibrillation). The vignette asks several relevant questions, even to an orthopedist! First, what is the mechanism of action behind her elevated INR? Warfarin acts to inhibit vitamin K epoxide reductase (functions to add carboxyl groups to the vitamin K–dependent clotting factors [II, VII, IX, X], thereby activating them), leading to inhibition of fibrin clot formation. The INR or prothrombin time (PT) is used to measure the effects of warfarin on the clotting cascade. The INR and PT specifically measure the extrinsic pathway (while the PTT measures the intrinsic pathway [Figure 140-1]) and tell the clinician the clotting tendency of blood, with higher values correlating to decreased ability to form a stable clot.

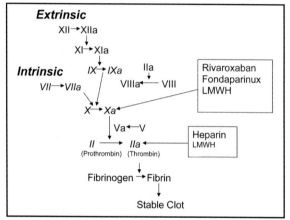

Figure 140-1. Clotting cascade with mechanism of action of common anticoagulants: italic Factors (II, VII, IX, X) are acted on by warfarin. The intrinsic and extrinsic pathways converge at Factor X; from this point on the pathway is known as the common pathway. LMWH = low-molecular-weight heparin.

The effects of warfarin can be reversed over a rapid or relatively longer period of time. In order to reverse it in a short period of time, the patient is given fresh-frozen plasma (and in some countries, prothrombin complex concentrate), which acts to replete the clotting factors. Vitamin K, oral or IV, has a slower onset and can take 24 hours or more to have a significant effect.[412]

As the flowchart demonstrates, warfarin works on Factors II, VII, IX, and X. Heparin and LMWH act on Factor IIa via antithrombin III. This is the primary place in the clotting cascade in which heparin works, while it is a secondary site of action for LMWH. Rivaroxaban, fondaparinux, and LMWH all work on Factor Xa. LMWHs inhibit clot formation via binding antithrombin and accelerating its inactivation of Factor Xa. Rivaroxaban is an oral direct inhibitor of Factor Xa and selectively blocks this molecule in the cascade. The downside to heparin and warfarin is that these must be monitored with the PTT and INR, respectively, whereas the other agents do not have to be monitored. For coumadin, there are specific drug-drug interactions to avoid, such as increased bleeding with NSAIDs or aspirin-like drugs; decreased action with inducers of CYP2C9, 1A2, or 3A4 (eg, rifampin, phenobarbital, phenytoin, montelukast, and carbamazepine); increased action with inhibitors of CYP2C9, 1A2, or 3A4 (eg, amiodarone, fluconazole, metronidazole, tigecycline, acyclovir, allopurinol, caffeine, cimetidine, ciprofloxacin, oral contraceptives, calcium channel blockers, anti-retrovirals, and ketoconazole); and increased bleeding with serotonin reuptake inhibitors (eg, paroxetine, sertraline, venlafaxine, duloxetine, and citalopram). Furthermore, there are specific foods that are high in vitamin K that need to be avoided or eaten consistently so as to not throw off the monitored blood levels, including kale, spinach, broccoli, cabbage, lettuce, Brussels sprouts, parsley, collard greens, mustard greens, chard, green tea, and dietary supplements. Alternatively, alcohol and cranberry juice consumption can potentiate the effects of warfarin.

A common problem orthopedic surgeons face is deciding when to stop anticoagulation prior to elective surgery. For the majority of patients, Table 140-1 is a good rule of thumb for when to stop anticoagulation. Of note, patients with metal stents should not have their anticoagulation stopped in the 4 to 6 weeks after stent placement, and if they have a drug-eluding stent, it should not be stopped earlier than 12 months.

Table 140-1.
COMMON ANTICOAGULANTS, THEIR HALF-LIVES, AND WHEN THEY SHOULD BE STOPPED PREOPERATIVELY TO REDUCE THE RISK OF INTRAOPERATIVE BLEEDING

Anticoagulant	Average Half-Life	When to Stop Preoperatively	Reversal Agent
Coumadin	40 h	5 d	Vitamin K, FFP
Fondaparinux	19 h	12 to 24 h	FFP/factor VII (partial effect)
Heparin	30 to 60 min	30 to 60 min	Protamine sulfate
LMWH	12 h	12 to 24 h	Protamine sulfate (partial effect)
Rivaroxaban	7 h	24 to 36 h in elderly	PCC, APCC, or factor VII
Aspirin	20 min to 6 h	7 to 10 d	Platelets
Clopidogrel	6 to 8 h	7 to 10 d	Platelets

APCC = activated prothrombin complex concentrate; FFP = fresh-frozen plasma; PCC = prothrombin complex concentrate.

Adapted from Horlocker TT, Wedel DJ, Rowlingson JC, et al. Regional anesthesia in the patient receiving antithrombotic or thrombolytic therapy: American Society of Regional Anesthesia and Pain Medicine Evidence-Based Guidelines (Third Edition). *Reg Anesth Pain Med.* 2010;35(1):64-101 and White RH, McKittrick T, Hutchinson R, Twitchell J. Temporary discontinuation of warfarin therapy: changes in the international normalized ratio. *Ann Intern Med.* 1995;122(1):40-42.

Aspirin is notably absent from Figure 140-1 because it does not affect the clotting cascade. The mechanism of action of aspirin is to irreversibly inhibit thromboxane and prostaglandin synthesis via inhibition of cyclooxygenase (enzyme required for thromboxane and prostaglandin synthesis). Thromboxane A2 is necessary for platelet aggregation to form the platelet plug, and aspirin works to inhibit that. Clopidogrel is also an inhibitor of platelet aggregation and is a prodrug, activated by the liver (CYP450 enzymes). The drug irreversibly binds the platelet receptor, rendering platelets ineffective for their 7- to 10-day lifespan.

Why Might This Be Tested? Many orthopedic patients are on some form of anticoagulation either prior to or for prophylaxis after surgery. It is vital to the success of the orthopedic surgeon to completely understand this cascade so he or she can ensure patients are properly anticoagulated before and after surgery.

Here's the Point!

The clotting cascade is a unique interplay of several clotting factors activating and inhibiting one another to achieve a stable clot. Warfarin inhibits factors II, VII, IX, and X (extrinsic pathway). The INR is used to monitor warfarin efficacy. The effects of warfarin can be reversed acutely with fresh-frozen plasma or more slowly by administering vitamin K.

Vignette 141: Something Is Wrong With My Son's Knee!

A 13-year-old male presents to the emergency department with knee pain and a general feeling of malaise. He has a fever of 39°C. He reports no trauma. He has limited ROM secondary to pain but a minimal effusion. A plain x-ray is seen in Figure 141-1.

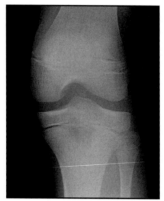

Figure 141-1. AP x-ray of the left knee.

▶ *What are the potential diagnoses?*

▶ *What additional tests would you order?*

An MRI and biopsy specimen are shown in Figures 141-2 and 141-3.

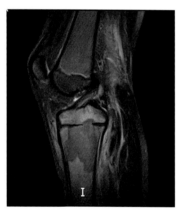

Figure 141-2. Sagittal fat-suppressed T2-weighted MRI of the left knee.

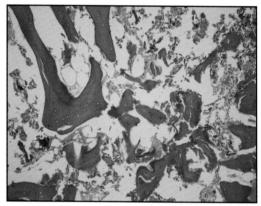

Figure 141-3. Biopsy specimen from the left knee (100× magnification).

▶ *What is the definitive treatment?*

Vignette 141: Answer

Acute osteomyelitis can have a clinical presentation and radiographic analysis that overlap with malignancy. Although patients will often have helpful clinical findings, such as fever, a history of penetrating trauma, or a recent illness, many times the diagnosis remains uncertain until a tissue biopsy. Because of the variability in presentation and array of radiographic findings, infection should be considered when diagnosing bone or soft tissue lesions.

On examination, the presence of a fever should be documented. In the area of concern, the overlaying skin should be assessed for pain and warmth. A soft tissue abscess, alone or from cortical perforation of a bone infection, may be fluctuant and painful. The patient may appear systemically ill, or the symptoms may be localized to the affected extremity.

Initial x-rays of the site should be obtained. Osteomyelitis can have a very aggressive appearance on imaging that could potentially represent a neoplastic process. Acute osteomyelitis can have an associated periosteal reaction with or without osseous erosions. Chronic osteomyelitis can show a sequestrum (nidus of infection) with a surrounding sclerotic involucrum. In children, infection routinely will cross the physis (common description for test taking purposes). An open growth plate can act as a barrier to tumor extension, although this is not universally true. MRI can further define the inflammatory reaction (substantial in acute osteomyelitis), cortical perforation, and soft tissue extension.

If infection is suspected, laboratory values (CBC, ESR, CRP) should be obtained to look for signs of inflammation. Again, this can overlap with a neoplastic presentation.

Whether the process is expected to be a malignancy or infection, a tissue diagnosis is typically required. When the clinical picture is consistent with infection, it is reasonable to be prepared to treat it if the intraoperative findings and frozen section show acute inflammation without signs of tumor. It is important to send tissue for culture and permanent sectioning because tumors may be quite inflammatory and necrotic. Fragments of bony trabeculae with numerous intervening inflammatory cells and necrotic debris are seen on histological examination of infection. The finding of neutrophils invading bone is necessary for a diagnosis of acute osteomyelitis. It is important to have cultures and a diagnosis prior to initiating antibiotic therapy.

The treatment of acute osteomyelitis is irrigation and debridement, with or without antibiotic beads, and systemic antibiotics. The treatment of chronic osteomyelitis is more complex, requiring removal of all necrotic bone and possibly a staged reconstruction. Other forms of osteomyelitis include the following:

- Chronic sclerosing osteomyelitis: Affects the diaphysis of adolescents, insidious onset, often anaerobic bacteria, periosteal proliferation, must rule out tumor

- Chronic multifocal osteomyelitis: Commonly appears in children without systemic symptoms, multiple metaphyseal lytic lesions seen on x-ray (often clavicle, distal tibia, distal femur), resolves spontaneously

Why Might This Be Tested? This is a common problem, and osteomyelitis is a classic imitator of many conditions. Due to the confusion it can cause on presentation, it is a favorite topic for question writers. Make sure you understand how to make the diagnosis.

Here's the Point!

Osteomyelitis is a very common condition that must be worked up and a diagnosis confirmed (cultures and histology section showing neutrophils invading bone) before antibiotic treatment is initiated. Chronic multifocal osteomyelitis is a self-limiting condition.

Vignette 142: Case of My Legs Feeling Too Heavy

A 60-year-old female reports symptoms of leg heaviness bilaterally when she is walking. She states that she feels better when she flexes forward, which provides her with substantial relief of these symptoms. She also describes pain in her mid to lower back that is worse at the end of the day. She has tried a course of physical therapy, which consisted of back-strengthening exercises with minimal relief. She is referred to you after seeing a pain doctor who provided her with transforaminal injections for the past year, which initially provided benefit but now are decreasing in efficacy. On exam, patient has 4/5 dorsiflexion of her ankle and extensor hallucis longus bilaterally. She has no focal sensory deficits. In describing her deformity, her head is over her pelvis and is well balanced in the sagittal plane with no significant hip or knee flexion contractures. She has a slight fullness in her lower back but coronally is well balanced, too. Her only medical problem is hypertension and diet-controlled diabetes mellitus. She is looking for definitive management for her pain and restoration of her functional activities.

▶ *What is the most likely diagnosis?*

▶ *What do you recommend for her?*

Vignette 142: Answer

This patient is suffering from 2 processes. The first and main issue is spinal stenosis. Spinal stenosis is defined as narrowing or stricture of the spinal canal. In some patients, this compression becomes symptomatic. The classical presentation, which this patient has, is that of bilateral neurogenic claudication, defined as intermittent pain radiating to the buttocks/thigh and/or leg that is worse with prolonged standing, walking, or lumbar extension. When patients suffer from lumbar stenosis, various studies have demonstrated favorable surgical outcomes.[413-415] The most recent study analyzing outcomes of spinal stenosis in patients without scoliosis or spondylolisthesis found in an as-treated analysis, all primary outcomes benefited surgery over nonoperative management.[413] In another study looking at patients with degenerative spondylolisthesis in an as-treated analysis, surgical treatment substantially demonstrated greater improvement in pain and function at 2 years.[416] Because this patient has tried nonoperative management and it has failed, she should be offered the option of surgical correction, namely decompression at the level of her spinal stenosis.

Secondly, this patient suffers from an element of degenerative scoliosis of her lumbar spine. Unlike idiopathic adolescent scoliosis, in which the pathogenesis is still elusive, the scoliosis that this patient has is the result of a progressive degenerative process, subluxation of the facet joints, asymmetric disk height loss, and ultimately scoliosis. Another difference between adult and adolescent idiopathic scoliosis is that adult curves are more rigid. Predictors of progression are curves greater than 50 degrees, lateral and rotatory listhesis, and large apical rotation. In this patient, the description depicts a decent amount of lateral and rotatory listhesis at the apex of the curve.

Third, this patient's leg and buttock pain is likely from her stenosis. However, her back pain may also stem from muscle fatigue. Fourth, the issue of deformity correction is not critical in these patients. The main deformity principle is coronal and sagittal balance, sagittal having a little more precedence. In a study by Glassman et al of 298 patients with adult scoliosis, positive sagittal balance was the most reliable predictor of clinical symptoms. Thoracolumbar and lumbar curves generated less favorable scores than thoracic curves. Magnitude of coronal deformity and extent of coronal correction are less critical parameters.[417]

Finally, the treatment algorithm for patients with degenerative scoliosis is similar to that of other deformity cases. Conservative treatment is indicated for nonprogressive curves causing localized back pain as well as for spinal stenosis. If the patient fails nonoperative treatment or the curve demonstrates progression, then surgical treatment is warranted. If fusion is necessary, the decision is made on a case-by-case basis. Because many of these patients have other comorbidities, they may be too feeble to undergo an extensive fusion procedure. The focus of these patients should be neurological decompression. In addition, patients may demonstrate autofusion of their functional spinal motion segments and thus be relatively stable. Therefore, these patients may benefit from selective fusion rather than fusing all involved segments. Principles in fusing spondylolisthesis levels (anterior, rotatory, and lateral) should be followed as well as not stopping a fusion at the apex of a curve. It is not wise to end a fusion at the thoracolumbar junction because there may be a tendency for kyphosis to occur at this level; similarly, the issue of stopping at S1 or extending to the ilium for long constructs has been heavily debated.

Why Might This Be Tested? Adult scoliosis is a different disease in many aspects compared with adolescent scoliosis. Many of these patients have other comorbid conditions precluding extensive surgery and making surgery technically challenging due to previous surgeries or osteoporosis. This disease is reasonably common and involves the convergence of deformity and degenerative principles of the spine, making this a commonly tested entity.

Here's the Point!

One must determine what the predominant problem is for these patients and manage the adult scoliosis appropriately. A distinction between the symptoms of neurogenic claudication, back pain, or progressing deformity must be made in order to formulate a treatment strategy. For adult scoliosis, predictors of progression are curves greater than 50 degrees, lateral and rotatory listhesis, and large apical rotation.

Vignette 143: Doc, I Can't Bench My Weight Anymore!

A 30-year-old male football lineman complains of vague shoulder pain. He has no history of acute trauma or prior dislocations. When asked to describe his pain, he has difficulty locating it but says if he has to pick the front or back of his shoulder, it is more posterior. Playing football (blocking) and bench press cause him the most discomfort. On physical exam, his ROM, strength, and sulcus exam are all normal. An MRI of the patient's shoulder is shown in Figure 143-1.

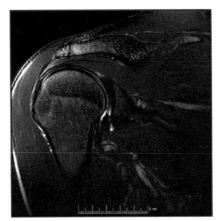

Figure 143-1. Axial T2-weighted MRI of the shoulder.

▶ *What is the most likely diagnosis?*

▶ *What specific physical exam will help elucidate this pathology?*

▶ *What other tests should be considered?*

▶ *What are the treatment options?*

Vignette 143: Answer

The history and imaging are concerning for posterior shoulder instability with associated attritional labral damage. Although only in 5% of instability cases, posterior shoulder instability should be high on your differential in patients who partake in activities with the arm in front of the body and internally rotated and complain of vague, deep shoulder pain (lineman, pushing activities).[418] The main restraints to posterior subluxation are the posterior inferior band of the glenohumeral ligament (static) and the subscapularis (dynamic). Suspicion is highest for football linemen, weight lifters, pitchers, golfers, and swimmers. With the latter three, the injury tends to be secondary to dynamic stabilizer fatigue and scapulothoracic muscle imbalance along with contributions of glenohumeral internal rotation deficit in pitchers. The most sensitive exam finding is a positive Kim and jerk test.[419] The Kim test involves positioning the arm with 90 degrees of abduction and while holding the elbow pressing posteroinferior on the humerus, which will reproduce the patient's pain. To perform the jerk test, have the patient stand with the arm in front of the body and internally rotated with a posteriorly directed force and feel for relocation when bringing the arm into a position of straight abduction.

Plain x-rays and possibly a CT scan are important in these patients to rule out osseous contributions to their instability. These include glenoid retroversion, erosion, or a reverse osseous Bankart or Hill-Sachs lesion. The axillary x-ray is important in the acute setting to determine a diagnosis of dislocation, and chronically it can elucidate bone loss. The West Point view can also demonstrate the glenoid rim clearly. CT scans provide the most detailed information and should be obtained if there is suspicion for bone loss. MRI or MRA should be obtained to evaluate the glenoid labrum, posterior glenohumeral ligament, and rotator cuff. The labrum can demonstrate a reverse Bankart or a Kim lesion, which is an attritional injury causing fissuring of the labrum from multiple microtraumatic events (Figure 143-2).

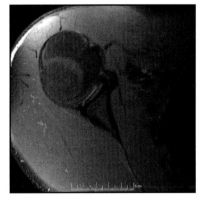

Figure 143-2. Coronal T2-weighted MRI of the shoulder.

Treatment should always begin with physical therapy focusing on the rotator cuff (subscapularis) and scapulothoracic stabilization. That said, 90% of patients with acute traumatic etiology or frank posterior labral tears will fail nonoperative management.[420] Indication for open stabilization is patients who require bony stabilization. Arthroscopic stabilization can be performed for recurrent, posttraumatic, unidirectional posterior subluxation, multidirectional instability with symptoms in the posteroinferior direction, and a symptomatic posterior labral tear. Patients with syndromic laxity or voluntary instability should be treated nonoperatively.

Why Might This Be Tested? Posterior shoulder instability represents 5% of cases of shoulder instability but should be high on your differential in patients who partake in activities with the arm in front of the body and internally rotated and complain of vague, deep shoulder pain.

Here's the Point!

Keep posterior shoulder instability on your radar as a cause of posterior shoulder pain, and remember that attritional injuries usually respond to therapy, whereas acute injuries can be treated arthroscopically.

Vignette 144: Restrained Driver in a Motor Vehicle Accident With Multiple Injuries

A 22-year-old male is brought to the emergency department by emergency medical services following an interstate motor vehicle collision in which he was the restrained driver. In the trauma bay, he is noted to have gross deformity and swelling of his left thigh and shortening of the left lower extremity compared with the right. Initial trauma evaluation reveals multiple associated injuries, including multiple rib fractures, pneumothorax, and a large hepatic hematoma consistent with a liver laceration. On further physical examination, he is noted to have palpable pedal pulses and normal distal motor and sensory function. AP and lateral x-rays of the femur are shown in Figure 144-1.

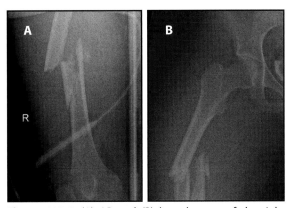

Figure 144-1. (A) AP and (B) lateral x-rays of the right femur.

▶ *What is the diagnosis?*

▶ *What injuries are commonly associated with this diagnosis?*

▶ *What are the key elements of the history and physical examination?*

After operative management of the fracture, the following questions were discussed at monthly trauma grand rounds:

▶ *What should be checked in a patient who had an IM nail prior to leaving the operating room?*

▶ *What are the indications for retrograde femoral nailing?*

▶ *What are the disadvantages of a piriformis-entry IM nail?*

▶ *What are the fixation options for concurrent femoral diaphysis and neck fractures?*

▶ *What are the advantages of early operative fixation of femoral diaphyseal fractures?*

▶ *What are the deforming forces on the proximal femur following diaphyseal fracture?*

▶ *What is the incidence of femoral neck fracture in association with femoral diaphyseal fracture?*

▶ *What are the indications for obtaining a CT scan in femoral diaphyseal fractures?*

▶ *What is the age and sex distribution of the incidence of femur fractures?*

▶ *What are the commonly associated orthopedic injuries associated with femur fracture?*

Vignette 144: Answer

The x-rays show a diaphyseal femur fracture. The mechanism of injury is an important aspect of the history, especially the energy of the injury, which provides an indication of degree of soft tissue injury and presence of other associated injuries. It is critical to obtain a detailed examination, which should include inspection and palpation of all extremities, the pelvis, and the spine, as well as a detailed neurovascular exam, including palpation and/or Doppler examination of the pedal pulses and assessment of the ABI if indicated. Commonly associated injuries include abdominal, thoracic, and/or head trauma; it is important to be aware of these injuries because they will influence the timing and method of treatment. Commonly associated orthopedic injuries include spine, pelvic, and acetabular fractures; hip fractures and/or dislocations; distal femur, patella, and tibial plateau fractures; and ligamentous and/or meniscal injuries of the knee.[370,371]

Femur fractures occur in individuals of all ages and are the result of multiple mechanisms of injury. There is a tendency toward a bimodal distribution, with a greater proportion of fractures occurring in young males secondary to high-energy mechanisms and elderly females secondary to lower levels of trauma. High-energy mechanisms include automobile and motorcycle crashes, falls from a height, and gunshot wounds. Radiographic evaluation should include AP pelvis and AP/lateral views of the femur and knee; dedicated x-rays of the hip should be obtained in every patient with a femoral shaft fracture. If there is suspicion of occult femoral neck fracture or distal intra-articular extension into the knee, then a CT scan may be indicated (Figure 144-2). Do not miss these diagnoses!

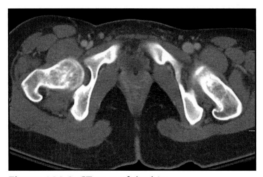

Figure 144-2. CT scan of the hip.

It is useful to be aware of the deforming forces acting on the fracture because this knowledge may aid in treatment. Shortening occurs due to the pull of the hamstrings and quadriceps. The abductors—gluteus medius and minimus—abduct, the iliopsoas flexes, and the short hip external rotators externally rotate the proximal segment. The adductors—adduct longus, brevis, magnus, and gracilis—medialize the distal fragment and pull it into varus. The gastrocnemius flexes the distal fragment in more distal fractures.

Initial management consists of skin or skeletal traction. Skeletal traction can be placed either in the distal femur (pin goes in medial to lateral) or proximal tibia (pin goes in lateral to medial). Traction functions to maintain femoral length, lessen soft tissue injury and blood loss, and increase patient comfort until operative fixation is possible. If proximal tibial traction is chosen, the knee must be carefully examined to exclude ligamentous injury.

Nonsurgical treatment is rarely chosen as a means of definitive management and is only indicated in patients in whom medical comorbidities contraindicate surgery. The prolonged immobility required for nonsurgical management carries its own set of morbidities and complications. Nonsurgical options consist of skeletal traction, spica casting, and cast bracing.

Research has shown that early stabilization of femur fractures (within the first 24 hours) minimizes the complication rates and can decrease the length of hospital stay. Surgical options include anterograde IM nail, retrograde IM nail, plate and screw fixation, or external fixation. The standard of care for femoral diaphyseal fractures is a statically locked, reamed IM nail.

Options for anterograde nailing include piriformis and trochanteric entry nails. The advantage of the piriformis entry nail is that the piriformis fossa lies in line with the mechanical axis of the femur, thereby minimizing the risk of iatrogenic fracture comminution and varus malalignment vs trochanteric entry nailing. Disadvantages include the difficulty of obtaining the starting point, more muscle and tendon damage, and possible damage to the blood supply of the femoral head (more commonly an issue in pediatric vs adult patients) compared with trochanteric entry nails. Too anterior of a starting point may result in iatrogenic femoral neck fracture due to increased hoop stresses in the proximal femur. The trochanteric entry nail starting point is more lateral, which is an easier starting point to obtain and results in less abductor muscle damage. There is also a lower likelihood of damage to the blood supply of the femoral head. Modifications in nail design have drastically reduced the incidence of varus malalignment and fracture comminution seen with earlier trochanteric entry nails.

Indications for retrograde femoral nailing include factors that make proximal access for anterograde nailing difficult or undesirable (pregnancy, bilateral femur fractures, morbid obesity, and ipsilateral femoral neck and acetabular fractures) or that make distal access desirable (patellar or tibial fractures). Retrograde nailing also has the advantage of decreased operating time and blood loss, making it more desirable in polytrauma patients. Data also show that in distal metadiaphyseal fractures, alignment is improved with retrograde nailing.

Reaming leads to greater fracture stability due to improved cortical nail fit, provides osteoinductive and conductive factors to the site of the fracture, and, despite damaging the endosteal circulation, has been shown to produce a periosteal vascular response that increases local blood flow. For these reasons, reaming is recommended as standard practice. Despite these advantages, there are some concerns with reaming, such as aggressive reaming at the fracture site, which can lead to malreduction; forceful reaming, which can lead to thermal necrosis; and reaming multiple canals, which can lead to marrow emboli (certainly a concern if considering nail fixation of multiple long bones in a single patient).

Indications for plate and screw fixation include fractures involving the distal metadiaphyseal region of the femur, a very narrow medullary canal, fractures around or adjacent to a previous malunion, extension of the fracture into the peritrochanteric or metaphyseal regions, associated vascular injury requiring repair, adjacent hip or knee prostheses, and ipsilateral femoral neck fracture.

External fixation is used as a temporizing measure until definitive fixation can be performed in severely injured patients; patients with severe soft tissue injury or contamination, which prohibits initial fixation; and patients with an arterial injury requiring repair.

Ipsilateral femoral neck fracture occurs in 3% to 10% of patients with femoral shaft fractures. These fractures are often nondisplaced or minimally displaced and often have a vertical orientation (more difficult to manage). Treatment options include cephalomedullary nail or retrograde nail with cannulated screws or a sliding hip screw.

Nonunion is uncommon in femoral diaphyseal fractures. The most common form of malunion after femoral diaphyseal fracture fixation is rotational malalignment. In most patients, rotational deformities of greater than 15 degrees are not well tolerated and require operative correction. Angular malunion is more common in proximal and distal fractures where the interference fit of the nail in the isthmus does not function to align the fracture.

Why Might This Be Tested? Diaphyseal femur fractures are high-energy injuries that should prompt evaluation of potential associated injuries, including femoral neck fracture, acetabular fractures, and knee injury (ligamentous and osseous). Damage control orthopedics is used in the setting of polytrauma and aims to minimize a "second hit" resulting in further pulmonary compromise by providing rapid temporizing stabilization with external fixation or traction.

Here's the Point!

The diagnosis of femur fracture will be apparent. Less obvious are the associated injuries, which require proper evaluation. Antegrade, reamed IM nail placement is the standard of treatment for diaphyseal femur fracture.

Vignette 145: Doc, My Hip Feels Unstable When I Stand Up. What Do I Do?

A 28-year-old female presents with a 2-year history of hip pain and instability. She does not recall an acute injury. The discomfort is more pronounced with prolonged weight bearing and is mainly located in her groin and laterally at times.

Functional abductor strength tested with the Trendelenburg test and side-lying abduction strength testing is negative and similar to the other hip. The anterior apprehension test consists of passive hip extension, adduction, and external rotation and is found to be positive. Groin pain with flexion, internal rotation, and adduction is indicative of a positive impingement test, also found with our patient.

On further physical examination, the patient's right hip extension is 0 degrees, flexion to 135 degrees, external rotation of 40 degrees, and internal rotation to 15 degrees. The patient has 5/5 strength with hip flexion, abduction, and adduction. The patient has positive impingement, positive psoas impingement, positive anterior apprehension, negative posterior impingement, negative lateral rim impingement, negative trochanteric pain sign, negative ischiofemoral impingement, negative straight-leg raise, and negative circumduction clunk. The patient has a painful arc from 12 to 4 o'clock.

▶ *What are the relevant radiographic studies that need to be obtained?*

▶ *What is the diagnosis?*

▶ *What nonoperative treatments are available?*

▶ *What are potential surgical options?*

Vignette 145: Answer

Typical radiographic views for assessing hip dysplasia include standing AP pelvis and false profile (described by Lequesne as a standing x-ray at an angle of 65 degrees between the pelvis and the film), frog-leg lateral, Dunn lateral, and cross-table lateral. A standing AP pelvis view is good for assessing if the femoral head is centered in the acetabulum. It also allows for measuring the acetabular lateral center-edge angle (vertical line through the center of the femoral head and a line to the lateral roof of the acetabulum), alpha angle (best on MRI; angle measured from line along femoral neck to the center of the head and line from center of the head to the head-neck junction), acetabular inclination, and joint center position. The femoral head-neck morphology can be evaluated and the greater trochanter position assessed (looking for coxa vara, lateral greater trochanters, and femoral neck morphology). The crossover sign is diagnostic of acetabular retroversion (can see on AP x-rays, with the anterior wall and posterior wall crossing often near the center of the femoral head). Prominent ischial spines are also indicative of acetabular and pelvic retroversion. Coxa profunda or protrusio acetabula is defined as a relatively medial and deep acetabulum.

The frog-leg, Dunn, and cross-table lateral views allow for particular assessment of the proximal femoral head-neck junction, particularly the alpha angle (normal, < 55 degrees). MRI and MRA help to assess intra-articular pathologies, particularly cartilage and labral defects. CT and 3D reconstruction can assist to delineate abnormalities of the femoral head and acetabulum with regard to location and extent and acetabular version.

Acetabular dysplasia is assessed by measuring the lateral center-edge angle (normal, ≥ 25 degrees) on an AP x-ray and the anterior center-edge angle (normal, ≥ 20 degrees) on a false-profile x-ray. The Tönnis angle of inclination of the acetabulum weight-bearing zone can be measured on the AP x-ray (normal, 0 to 10 degrees; angle measured from horizontal line and line to the lateral edge of the sourcil). A broken Shenton line indicates hip subluxation (follow the curve of the obturator foramen to the femoral neck). Hip joint lateralization is quantified by measuring the distance between the medial border of the femoral head and the ilioischial line (normal, < 10 mm). Acetabular version is assessed on the AP pelvic x-ray. There has been shown to be a correlation between retroversion in patients with symptomatic acetabular dysplasia. Anterolateral femoral head morphology, which is often abnormal in hip dysplasia due to an offset deficiency, is assessed on the frog-leg or Dunn view.

The x-rays in our case demonstrate that the patient has a lateral center-edge angle of 20 degrees (Figure 145-1), an alpha angle of 65 degrees (Figure 145-2), and an associated labral tear (Figure 145-3).

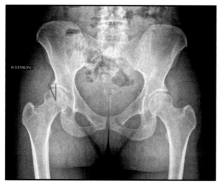

Figure 145-1. AP pelvis x-ray showing how to measure the center-edge angle. In this case, the angle is 20 degrees, which indicates hip dysplasia.

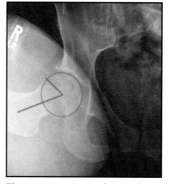

Figure 145-2. Lateral x-ray showing a 65-degree alpha angle.

The patient's symptoms of groin pain and instability, in combination with her radiographic findings, are consistent with painful hip dysplasia. Insufficient acetabular coverage leads to the anterior instability and subsequent pain. The differential for atraumatic hip instability includes hip dysplasia, FAI, congenital

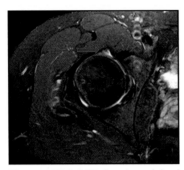

Figure 145-3. MRI showing a labral tear at the red arrow.

ligamentous laxity, Down syndrome, Ehlers-Danlos syndrome, Marfan syndrome, arthrochalasis multiplex congenita, and other forms of ligamentous laxity (acquired, idiopathic, iatrogenic).[421]

Nonoperative modalities include physical therapy for improving ROM and strength. NSAIDs also help to control symptoms. An intra-articular injection with a local anesthetic and corticosteroid can serve diagnostic purposes to confirm intra-articular contribution to symptoms but may also provide relief. However, since this is largely a mechanical problem, the progression of symptoms is likely, and there is an increased risk of developing OA.

The surgical options include the 2 broad categories of joint-preserving techniques and joint replacement. Patients with hip dysplasia often present at a young age when hip replacement should be avoided. Joint-preserving techniques strive at a minimum to delay or even prevent the onset of OA requiring hip replacement by aiming to restore stability, reduce pathologic stress, and reduce impingement. Hip preservation surgeries typically consist of an acetabular redirectional osteotomy, sometimes in combination with a proximal femoral osteotomy. In the presence of severe coxa valga, a varus-producing intertrochanteric femoral osteotomy is performed concomitantly to improve lateral femoral head coverage. It is generally accepted that when bony dysplasia is present, the role of arthroscopic procedures is unclear and osteotomy is more likely the procedure of choice.

For the skeletally mature patient, the Bernese periacetabular osteotomy (PAO) and other rotational acetabular osteotomies (eg, Wagner, Schramm, or Nakamura) are being used. The Bernese PAO is the most commonly used acetabular redirectional procedure for management of symptomatic hip instability secondary to primary acetabular hip dysplasia. Symptomatic management of acetabular hip dysplasia with Bernese PAO is indicated in patients with pain and/or progressive limp. Patients should ideally have no advanced radiographic signs of OA. Adequate and relatively painless passive ROM (flexion, ≥ 90 degrees; abduction, ≥ 30 degrees) should be present on physical examination.

The Bernese PAO involves the following 4 osteotomies: the anterior ischium below the acetabulum, through the superior pubic ramus, the supra-acetabular ilium, and the posterior column, connecting the initial cut. Typically, this is performed via an abductor-sparing procedure using a modified Smith-Petersen approach. ROM is tested intraoperatively, and osteotomy is fixed with 3 to 4 cortical screws. The capsule should be opened to address any labral pathology, and an osteochondroplasty should be performed as necessary.[422]

Why Might This Be Tested? Hip dysplasia and femoroacetabular impingement have increasingly been recognized over the past decade as a source of hip pain and a risk factor for developing degenerative changes in the hip. Familiarity with the concepts of these clinical entities is becoming more important.

Here's the Point!

Hip dysplasia refers to abnormal acetabular and femoral anatomy and can lead to hip instability, pain, and degenerative changes. Reorientation osteotomies are aimed at recreating normal anatomy and delaying or stopping the progression of degenerative changes and symptoms.

Vignette 146: My Knee Has a Fever!

A 72-year-old morbidly obese female with a history of peripheral vascular disease and type 2 diabetes mellitus presents with knee pain and stiffness 18 months after a TKA. Her initial postoperative course was complicated by persistent drainage 2 weeks out from surgery that "was cured" with a course of oral antibiotics and dressing changes. She has been off of antibiotics for over 1 year and denies systemic symptoms of fevers or chills. The patient reports near constant pain and swelling that is unrelated to specific activities. Despite NSAIDs, oral narcotics, and a short course of physical therapy, nothing has been reported to help for any extended period of time. On examination, the surgical scar is well healed and without erythema. There is a moderate effusion with a passive ROM from 15 to 90 degrees of flexion. X-rays demonstrate well-positioned and fixed components without evidence of loosening or failure.

▶ *What is the differential diagnosis?*

▶ *What serological studies should be ordered?*

▶ *What is the role of a joint aspiration?*

▶ *What preoperative strategies exist to prevent this complication?*

Serologic testing is elevated, and the cell count and positive cultures are consistent with periprosthetic infection. Assuming this is the confirmed diagnosis, answer the following questions:

▶ *What is the treatment of choice?*

▶ *What are the advantages/disadvantages of articulating antibiotic spacers?*

▶ *What other options exist, and how successful are they in management of this condition?*

Vignette 146: Answer

The patient's history of a chronic draining wound and a course of oral antibiotics is a red flag for PJI. Her medical history of morbid obesity, type 2 diabetes mellitus, and peripheral vascular disease also place her at risk, particularly if she had open foot ulcers at the time of surgery. Other risk factors associated with an increased risk for infection include malnutrition (albumin <3.5 g/dL or total lymphocyte count <1500 cells/mm^3), smoking, alcoholism, prior open surgical procedures, multiple blood transfusions, steroid use, RA, immunosuppression, and urinary tract infections.[423] Systemic symptoms are often not present, and their absence should not be used in ruling out PJI (often meant to lead you astray). The remainder of the differential for a painless, stiff TKA includes arthrofibrosis, instability, malrotation, loosening, complex regional pain syndrome, and joint stuffing (too tight in flexion and/or extension).

The AAOS has outlined a diagnostic and treatment strategy for patients with suspected PJI.[424] All patients should have a serum ESR and CRP drawn. If these results are elevated (ESR, >30 mm/h; CRP, >10 mg/L; must be taken in context of the normal for that particular laboratory; will be indicated in a question) or if there is a high index of suspicion, the knee should be aspirated and the fluid sent for WBC count/ differential and culture. A Gram stain should not be performed. A WBC count greater than 3000 and/or a differential greater than 67% segmental neutrophils is highly sensitive for chronic PJI.[425] Indium/sulfur colloid scans, leukocyte esterase strips, synovial and serum IL-6, synovial CRP, and synovial biomarker assays are other options that are being explored to rule out PJI.

Prevention is now paramount for TJA, and several strategies have recently been used in this regard. Preoperative modalities that have been initiated include the use of advance cutaneous disinfection protocols (chlorhexidine baths) and preoperative screening for colonization of MRSA (nasal swabs and ointment for positive cultures).[426,427] Optimization of preoperative medical conditions should be part of the clearance process for surgery. In addition, prophylactic antibiotics should be initiated within 1 hour of the surgical incision and continued for 24 hours postoperatively. Routine prophylaxis typically consists of second-generation cephalosporin medications, with clindamycin being reserved for those with beta-lactam allergies and vancomycin for those who have been identified with preoperative screening to be colonized with MRSA. Recent thinking is that vancomycin should be used in conjunction with a more broad-spectrum antibiotic for adequate prophylaxis. Furthermore, many patients will be undertreated with a simple 1-g dose of vancomycin, which should be weight based, even for prophylaxis dosing.

Given the chronic nature of this infection, a 2-stage procedure is the most successful option in the United States. All components should be removed, the knee thoroughly debrided and irrigated, and an antibiotic (typically vancomycin and an aminoglycoside; 3:1-g ratio as a minimum, per batch of cement; with typically 2 to 3 batches being needed for the spacer depending on the size of the bone defects) impregnated cement spacer placed. A course of IV antibiotics (usually 6 weeks) is then administered, with reimplantation performed between 8 and 12 weeks post resection arthroplasty. At this point, the infection should be eradicated or a repeat spacer may be necessary. Articulating spacers allow the patient some continued motion during this period, with a theoretical benefit of maintaining tissue plains and an easier exposure at time of reimplantation.[428,429] Static spacers provide the theoretical benefit of allowing for less stress on the injured/ healing soft tissues and a lower risk of spacer dislocation and/or fracture. Irrigation and debridement with polyethylene articular surface exchange is an option only in acute (<4 weeks, but <2 weeks is ideal) PJIs.[430] Resistant bacteria have a much lower success rate with component retention (MRSA, methicillin-sensitive *S aureus*, gram-negative bacteria, and atypical bugs). Furthermore, recent data suggest that a failed liner exchange leads to worse results and greater rates of recurrent infection after a subsequent 2-stage procedure. Single-stage exchange of components has been shown to be significantly less effective in curing PJI compared with a 2-stage procedure in the current US literature.[431]

Why Might This Be Tested? Infections and total joint complications are frequently tested. There are AAOS clinical practice guidelines regarding this topic, so make sure you know them!

Here's the Point!

For cases in which infection is suspected, start with laboratory tests (ESR and CRP) and proceed to aspiration if the results are elevated. Cell counts that are greater than 3000 WBCs with greater than 65% PMNs are concerning for infection. Early infections up to 4 weeks can be treated with a modular component exchange, and later infections are best treated with a 2-stage exchange procedure.

Vignette 147: Case of the "Pussed Out" Finger

A 42-year-old male IV drug user presents to the emergency room with a painful, swollen, erythematous finger that has an area of fluctuance. The affected finger is incised and drained, cultures are obtained, and the patient is started on empiric antibiotics. Cultures demonstrate growth of MRSA, and the patient's IV antibiotics are optimized to cover this organism. After sufficient IV antibiotics, the patient is transitioned to an outpatient regimen of oral antibiotics.

▶ *What is a reasonable antibiotic regimen for this patient?*

▶ *What are the mechanisms of action and side effects of the most commonly used antibiotics in orthopedic surgery?*

Vignette 147: Answer

An initial treatment regimen in an IV drug user with a subcutaneous abscess would start with broad coverage. One example is using vancomycin to cover MRSA and other gram-positive organisms, with the addition of piperacillin/tazobactam to cover gram-negative and anaerobic organisms. Once cultures grow MRSA, more narrow coverage using a single antibiotic, such as IV vancomycin, daptomycin, tigecycline, or clindamycin, would be appropriate. Various antibiotics can be taken orally to cover MRSA and may include trimethoprim/sulfamethoxazole, clindamycin, linezolid, tetracyclines, and quinolones.[432]

Other commonly tested antibiotics are listed in Table 147-1.

A final point regarding antibiotics is their recommended use with open fractures. The Gustilo and Anderson system[433] is used to classify the type of injury, and choice of antibiotics is based on this classification. Type I and II open fractures are treated with first-generation cephalosporins. Type III open fractures are treated with a first-generation cephalosporin plus an aminoglycoside. Farm injuries, or those that are grossly contaminated, require penicillin as well as prophylaxis against clostridia organisms.[434]

Why Might This Be Tested? Orthopedic surgeons of all subspecialties treat infections of native and post-surgical tissues. Therefore, it is important to have the knowledge necessary to optimize a treatment regimen using antimicrobial agents. In addition, mechanisms of action for antibiotics are favorite test questions.

Here's the Point!

For the purposes of orthopedic standardized testing, learn the basics of common antibiotics with regard to spectrum of organism coverage, side effects, and mechanism of action (Table 147-1).

Table 147-1.

COMMONLY TESTED ANTIBIOTICS AND THEIR INDICATIONS, SIDE EFFECTS, AND MECHANISMS OF ACTION

Drug	Indication	Side Effects	Mechanism of Action
Penicillin	Gm Pos, mostly strep, weak broad coverage, open fracture if farm injury (*Clostridium*)	Rashes/ hypersensitivity	Cell wall inhibitor
Amoxicillin	Gm Pos, mostly strep with some Gm Neg	5% to 10% cross-sensitivity with PCN	Cell wall inhibitor
First-generation cephalosporin	Gm Pos, weak Gm Neg	Possible cross-sensitivity with PCN	Cell wall inhibitor
Second-generation cephalosporin	Gm Pos, better Gm Neg coverage than first generation	Possible cross-sensitivity with PCN	Cell wall inhibitor
Third-generation cephalosporin	Gm Pos, Gm Neg, *Pseudomonas*	Possible cross-sensitivity with PCN	Cell wall inhibitor
Vancomycin	MRSA, Gm Pos in PCN-allergic patients	Red man syndrome	Cell wall inhibitor
Carbapenem	Very broad coverage, except MRSA (typically)	Asymptomatic LFT elevation	Cell wall inhibitor
Polymyxin	Gm Neg, used topically	Local reaction	Cell wall inhibitor
Bacitracin	Gm Pos, used topically	Local reaction	Cell wall inhibitor
Piperacillin/ tazobactam	Gm Neg, anaerobes, some Gm Pos	Diarrhea	Cell wall inhibitor
Tetracycline	Lyme disease, rickettsia (Rocky Mountain spotted fever)	Discolored teeth in children	Inhibit 30S subunit
Gentamycin	Aerobic Gm Neg, add for grade III open injury	Nephrotoxicity, ototoxicity	Inhibit 30S subunit
Erythromycin	Strep, *Haemophilus influenzae*	Interact with Coumadin	Inhibit 50s subunit
Clindamycin	Oral MRSA coverage, Gm Pos, anaerobes, prophylaxis in PCN-allergic patients	*Clostridium difficile*, pseudomembranous colitis	Inhibit 50s subunit
Levofloxacin	*Pseudomonas*, aerobic Gm Pos	Tendon rupture, impaired fracture healing	Inhibit DNA gyrase
Trimethoprim/ sulfamethoxazole	Oral community-acquired MRSA coverage, UTIs	Kernicterus in new-borns (late pregnancy), thrombocytopenia	Inhibit folic acid synthesis
Rifampin	*Mycobacterium*	Discolored body fluids, hepatotoxic	Inhibit RNA synthesis
Isoniazid	*Mycobacterium*	Neuropathy without vitamin B6 supplements	Inhibit mycolic acid synthesis

Gm Neg=gram-negative; Gm Pos=gram-positive; LFT=liver function test; MRSA=methicillin-resistant *Staphylococcus aureus*; PCN=penicillin; Strep=*Streptococcus*; UTIs=urinary tract infections.

Vignette 148: When It Rains, It Pours: Complications After TKA

Patient A

A 54-year-old male with a history of a multiligamentous knee injury and reconstruction undergoes TKA for advanced DJD. The surgery is uncomplicated, and the tourniquet is let down after the dressing is on. In the postanesthesia care unit, the patient's drain has a recorded output of more than 1 L in the first hour under suction. Despite releasing the suction, the drain continues to collect bloody drainage. The nurses note that the foot is cold, there are no palpable pulses, and there is decreased capillary refill.

▶ *What is the likely diagnosis?*

▶ *What is the next step in management?*

Patient B

The patient in the adjacent bed in the recovery room is a 73-year-old female status post TKA for advanced RA, valgus deformity, and a flexion contracture. The regional anesthesia is no longer working, and she is unable to actively dorsiflex her ankle in the postanesthesia care unit.

▶ *What is the likely diagnosis?*

▶ *What is the next step in management?*

Patient C

Your office calls with a patient reporting increasing calf pain and swelling after forgetting to take his blood thinner medication for 3 days. This 75-year-old male complains of insidious onset of pain and swelling localized to his calf 12 days after TKA. He has a medical history of hypertension and hyperlipidemia, which are well controlled with oral medications. His knee has a moderate effusion and there are symmetrical pulses palpated in the foot.

▶ *What is a likely diagnosis?*

▶ *What are the next steps in management?*

Patient D

A 76-year-old female complains of dyspnea and mild chest pain on postoperative day 3 after a TKA. Routine VTE prophylaxis was initiated within the first 24 hours of surgery with warfarin, and the patient was mobilized on the evening after surgery.

▶ *What is the most likely diagnosis?*

▶ *What is the next step in management?*

Vignette 148: Answer

Patient A

The patient has likely sustained an injury to his popliteal artery during surgery. The patient's prior surgery, which may have included a PCL reconstruction, has likely led to scarring of the vessels to the posterior capsule. This patient requires emergent vascular surgery consultation for exploration with possible repair or bypass of the injured vessel. Overall, these are uncommon but serious complications occurring in less than 0.25% of cases. Typically, the popliteal artery lies anterior to the vein in knee flexion and is more prone to injury with surgical dissection or use of the saw. Common sequelae of popliteal artery injury include hemorrhage, thrombus formation, pseudoaneurysm, and/or AV fistula formation. Prompt recognition and treatment is crucial, and prophylactic fasciotomies may need to be performed with revascularization attempts.

Patient B

Correction of the patient's valgus and flexion deformity has likely resulted in a stretch injury to her peroneal nerve. The patient's dressing should be loosened and the knee flexed immediately. (This is always the answer on the test, so don't get it wrong!) The peroneal nerve is tethered at the fibula head and is susceptible to a stretch injury when correcting a valgus deformity. Peroneal nerve exploration and decompression is becoming popular for those injuries without return of function. Risk factors for injury include a prior HTO, history of lumbar laminectomy, tourniquet time greater than 2 hours, dressing applied too tightly, and epidural anesthesia.

Patient C

In a patient with calf pain after TKA, a DVT must be ruled out. The diagnostic study of choice is a duplex Doppler scan of both lower extremities. Most practitioners believe symptomatic DVT should be treated with therapeutic doses of anticoagulation. The length of treatment is controversial, with the American College of Chest Physicians recommending at least 3 months of treatment dose anticoagulation.[435] Recent data suggest that elevated preoperative D-dimer values and/or a history of hyperlipidemia may place one at risk for DVT after a TJA.[436] Alternatively, data conflict on using D-dimer in the diagnosis of DVT, and this test may serve to rule out clots.

Patient D

Many physicians have been trained to immediately think of pulmonary embolism in this situation. Although a PE can cause the aforementioned symptoms, cardiac etiologies are more common, and MI and arrhythmia have been shown to be more prevalent and have a higher rate of mortality after TKA than PE. Workup of this patient must include a 12-lead EKG and a set of cardiac enzymes.[325] Although in-hospital mortality has been shown to be declining, there has been a trend toward an increasing incidence of PE after TKA in the United States.[326] In diagnosing a PE, one can expect to find tachypnea, tachycardia, and chest pain with lower oxygen saturations that typically do not completely reconstitute with adjunctive oxygen therapy. Diagnosis can be made using CT scans with PE protocols, ventilation perfusion scans, or pulmonary angiography. Some have suggested that elevated D-dimer and leukocyte elastase levels may be used early on as markers for VTE events. Despite appropriate prophylaxis, no specific regimen has been shown to lower the rates of fatal PE after TJA procedures.

Why Might This Be Tested? Complications are always testable items. In TJA, neurovascular injuries often dominate the question material regarding complications. These injuries are rare but devastating functionally and clinically to the patient.

Here's the Point!

Know where the neurovascular structures are about the knee, and protect all vital structures during the surgical procedure. Prompt recognition and management is crucial for popliteal artery injury (vascular consult, STAT!), peroneal nerve injury (flex knee and loosen bandage), and VTE (diagnosis early and anticoagulate).

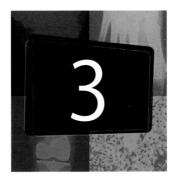

BOARD REVIEW
CRITICAL FACTS AND FIGURES

They key to answering many questions hinges upon one's knowledge of critical facts and figures. These may be numerical values, short clinical factoids, or important anatomical/clinical correlations. For example, what is the translocation associated with Ewing's sarcoma? Or, in an adult, what degree of scoliotic deformity is required to indicate surgical management? Although this involves a certain amount of memorization, many of these points hold the key to unlocking many of the tough vignettes you will encounter. What follows is a "one-stop shop" for all of the critical facts and figures one will need to ace the Boards.

0.1 mm/year = The approximate wear rate below which osteolysis is not commonly seen.

0.9, 6 hours = Ankle-brachial index less than this indicates a likely arterial injury; repairs should be performed within 6 hours, and distal fasciotomies may be required for reperfusion-associated compartment syndrome.

1% = Approximate risk of developing an ileus after a total joint arthroplasty. Risk factors include THA > total knee arthroplasty (TKA), older age, males, history of abdominal surgery, and aggressive narcotic use.

1% = Ligament of Struthers is found in 1% of the population and extends between the shaft of the humerus and the medial epicondyle and can cause median nerve and brachial artery compression (supracondylar process syndrome).

1% to 9% = Percentage of ipsilateral femoral neck fractures seen with traumatic femoral shaft fractures; 20% to 50% of these are missed initially.

1 in 500 = Number of births in which polydactyly occurs: postaxial (small finger), preaxial (thumb), or central (ring, long, and index). Postaxial polydactyly is commonly found in Black children (1.2%) with an AD transmission mode. Also found more commonly in males.

1.5 to 2 cm = The distance above the fibular head where the joint line should be located at the time of revision or primary TKA. During revision TKA, success is contingent on restoring the anatomic joint line and achieving the best balance with the least constraining implants.

2:1 = The ratio of glenohumeral-to-scapulothoracic motion during shoulder abduction.

>4 or 6 mm = Widening seen with stress x-ray of the medial clear space and tibiofibular clear space, respectively, with external rotation in a syndesmotic injury.

Levine BR. *Acing the Orthopedic Board Exam:*
The Ultimate Crunch-Time Resource (pp 407-423).
© 2016 SLACK Incorporated.

5 L = Typical blood volume for a 70-kg adult.

5% to 10% = The incidence of full-thickness rotator cuff tears in patients undergoing TSA for osteoarthritis.

5% to 25% = Number of patients who can develop an inhibitor for factor replenishment with hemophilia (factor VIII deficiency). The inhibitor is an immunoglobulin antibody to the clotting factor protein (makes replenishment unsuccessful), and its presence is a relative contraindication to any elective surgical procedure.

6 to 12 days = Period of time in which flexor tendon repairs are at the weakest. Tendons have more collagen and remain less viscoelastic compared with ligaments. The tendon-healing phases include inflammatory (neoangiogenesis, days 0 to 5), fibroblastic (disorganized collagen, days 5 to 28), and remodeling (collagen cross-linking, > 28 days).

6 to 12 weeks = Time period in which a radial nerve injury associated with a type 3 supracondylar humerus fracture can be expected to spontaneously recover after closed reduction and pinning. Complete recovery is by 3 to 6 months after injury.

6.5 mm = The average transverse diameter of the L1 pedicles; smaller than T1 (7.5 mm), T12 (7.5 mm), and L3 (9.2 mm).

> 7 mm = With lateral mass displacement greater than 7 mm, injury to the transverse ligament can be inferred, making it an unstable injury. Therefore, a C1 fracture with this displacement should be managed with a posterior arthrodesis with lateral mass screws.

< 8 = Glasgow Coma Scale score significant for major head injury (eye opening: 1 to 4; motor response: 1 to 6; verbal response: 1 to 5).

8 cm = Distance proximal to elbow in which the arcade of Struthers can be found and where it can be responsible for ulnar nerve impingement.

8× = In placement of a reverse shoulder arthroplasty, the height of implantation of the glenosphere has an 8× greater influence on scapular notching (associated with poor clinical outcomes) compared with the prosthesis-neck angle.

≤ 9 degrees = Normal intermetatarsal angle.

9 mm = The length change (greatest from flexion to extension of elbow) of the posterior bundle of the MCL when moving from 60 to 120 degrees of flexion. The lateral ulnar collateral changes approximately 3 mm, and the anterior bundle of the MCL has a small length change.

9 mm/year = The growth rate of the distal femoral physis. Growth stops around 14 years for women and around 16 years for men. Others include 6 mm in the proximal tibia and 3 mm in the proximal femur.

9 weeks = Length of time it takes after open reduction and internal fixation of the ankle to resume normal total braking times when driving.

10% = The death rate associated with a scapulothoracic dissociation. There is also a vascular injury or nerve injury in 88% and 94%, respectively.

≤ 10 degrees = Normal distal metatarsal articular angle.

10 years old = Children aged 10 years or younger with a slipped capital femoral epiphysis should receive an endocrine workup. It is typically recommended that patients younger than 10 years or those with an endocrinopathy should have the contralateral side prophylactically pinned.

10 years old and 10 cm = Pathologic genu varum; can be associated with renal osteodystrophy (if bilateral), tumors, infections, or trauma. Surgery is considered for those older than 10 years and with 10 cm between the medial malleoli or greater than 15 to 20 degrees of valgus. Can staple the opposite side of the growth plate if the physis is still open.

12 cm = The optimal bone length of the femur above the knee joint for an above-knee amputation. The adductor myodesis is critical to the outcome and solves the problem of adductor roll.

14.7 mm = The mean distance of the transverse dimension of the rotator cuff insertion at the midportion of the supraspinatus. The cuff inserts near the articular surface along the anterior 2.1 cm of the greater tuberosity.

< 15 degrees = Normal metatarsophalangeal angle, hallux valgus angle.

>15 mm Hg = Chronic exertional compartment syndrome, pressures greater than 15 mm Hg 15 minutes after exercise, an absolute value greater than 15 mm Hg while at rest or greater than 30 mm Hg after exercise. The anterior and deep posterior compartments of the leg are most commonly affected.

15% to 30% = Anatomic variation of the sciatic nerve in the literature. Approximately 80% of the nerve exits below the piriformis muscle (lies anterior to the muscle); 14.3% of the nerve separates into 2 divisions above the piriformis (one branch passes through and the other below the muscle); 2.2% of the nerve undivided passes through the muscle; 4.4% of the nerve splits above the piriformis, with one branch exiting above and one below the muscle.

> 18 = Injury Severity Score = the sum of the squares for the highest Abbreviated Injury Score in the 3 most severely injured body regions (> 18 represents a multiply injured patient)

< 25 mm = Tip-apex distance less than 25 mm will optimize outcomes in fixation of hip fractures and will improve upon the reported 8% to 13% failure rates.

25% = The percent gain with a 30-degree z-plasty; 50% with 45-degree and 75% with 60-degree.

30% = Percent of cases in which trauma is attributed to an insufficiency fracture of the pelvis after at THA. Beware: x-rays may be normal and a CT may be needed to make the diagnosis. Risk factors include rheumatoid arthritis, steroid use, and mechanical constraint. Beware the question with severe groin pain and normal x-rays (look for subtle osteolysis).

30% to 50% = The incidence of vascular injury with anterior dislocation of the knee. Dislocation is based on the direction of the tibia.

36 months = Time point in which physiologic bowing of the lower extremities should spontaneously correct (usually corrects by 2 years, but for sure by 36 months). Typically, an x-ray is ordered at 2 years of age with persistent lower extremity bowing.

43% = Greater stiffness of fixation if central vs eccentric placement in the proximal fragment is achieved in fixing a scaphoid waist fracture. Greater loads to failure are reported with this pattern of optimal fixation.

43% = Greater stiffness with fixation of a scaphoid fracture in the central axis of the proximal and distal fragments. There was a 39% greater load to failure when biomechanical testing evaluated central fixation vs eccentric positioning. The failure mode was screw migration and fracture at the screw-bone interface with dorsal wedge opening.

48% = The amputation rate associated with injection injury into a digit. This requires emergent irrigation and debridement. Outcomes depend on the material injected, quantity injected, injection pressure, and interval to removal of the foreign material.

50 to 150 μ = A common answer for THA; this is the optimal pore size for a porous surface; 50 is the limit for gaps between an implant and the bone; 150 is the limit for micromotion between an implant and bone, as well as the limit for radial clearance in alternative bearings; 50 is the optimal thickness for hydroxyapatite coating.

53% to 60% = The contribution of the medial patellofemoral ligament to patella stability, namely restraint to lateral placement. The joint typically must withstand forces greater than 3× body weight.

< 60% = Tendon lacerations less than 60% should be treated without repair (trim frayed edges to avoid triggering) and early motion.

60/40 = Stance occupies 60% of the gait cycle starting with initial contact through preswing. Swing phase is 40% of the cycle, beginning with toe-off to limb deceleration at terminal swing. Initial swing is marked by hip and knee flexion and ankle dorsiflexion.

70% = By age 70 years, 70% will have degenerative joint disease on plain x-rays, and by age 40 years, 25% will have MRI findings of herniated nucleus pulposus or stenosis without symptoms.

> 70% = The percentage of crystalline structure of polyethylene that is associated with higher failure rates. The goal is to keep the crystalline phase to 50% to 56%. Beware: remelting of polyethylene can increase the percentage of the crystalline phase.

73% = More than 73% of patients with spina bifida develop a latex allergy.

77.3% = Survivorship of Charnley all-polyethylene cups at 20 years; equates to a revision rate of 15% to 20%, up from the early 5% failure rate at 10 years.

85% = Approximate percentage of metatarsus adductus cases that will resolve spontaneously. Often associated with hip dysplasia (10% to 15%), this process often responds to minimal treatment and stretching when flexible. If osteotomy is required, it is best to wait until after age 5 years.

97% = Percentage of cases of achondroplasia caused by a mutation in the fibroblast growth receptor gene 3: active receptor leads to shortened bones.

100% = With advancing age, this is the percentage of patients older than 70 years with a rotator cuff tear and a prior shoulder dislocation. Older patient + shoulder dislocation = likely rotator cuff tear.

300 mg = The amount of calcium found in an 8-oz cup of milk.

1300 mg = The amount of calcium intake recommended for women and men between ages 9 and 18 years as well as pregnant or nursing women aged 14 to 18 years. Men and women aged 19 to 50 years should have 1000 mg; for patients aged 51 years and older, 1200 mg is recommended.

2200 to 2500 N = The tensile strength of a young ACL. A 10-mm patella tendon graft has 2900 N and will be 30% stronger if it's rotated 90 degrees. The posterior collateral ligament and medial collateral ligament (MCL) (2×) have greater tensile strength than the ACL, whereas the lateral collateral ligament is only about 750 N.

3000 = Synovial fluid WBC counts greater than this number are the most sensitive (100%), specific (98%), and accurate (99%) in detecting a prosthetic joint infection.

Accuracy = True-positive + true-negatives/all cases.

AD = The following disorders are inherited via an AD pattern: achondroplasia, osteogenesis imperfecta (IA, IB, IV), postaxial polydactyly, osteopetrosis (mild form), spondyloepiphyseal dysplasia (congenital), Kniest dysplasia, multiple epiphyseal dysplasia, malformations of cortical development (Schmid and Jansen types), malignant hyperthermia, Marfan syndrome, Ehlers-Danlos syndrome, osteochondromatosis, cleidocranial dysostosis, and Apert's syndrome.

Adamantinoma = Rare tumor that typically affects the tibia (rarely can affect the fibula, femur, ulna, or radius) in young patients. Typically presents with chronic pain and has multiple sharply circumscribed lucent lesions (giving it a soap bubble appearance). On histology, there are fibrous and nests of epithelial tissue in a gland-like pattern. Wide surgical excision is the appropriated treatment. Do not confuse with osteofibrous dysplasia.

Age at presentation and hip range of motion = The 2 most significant predictors of long-term outcomes with Legg-Calvé-Perthes disease. Chronologic age younger than 8 years or bone age of 6 years or less are associated with better outcomes.

AM and PL = The ACL is made up of the anteromedial bundle (AM), which is more involved in AP instability, and the posterolateral (PL) bundle, which is tight in extension and internal rotation and helps with rotary instability (such as preventing the pivot shift test).

Aminoterminal residues 1-34 = This is the portion of human parathyroid (total molecule is 84 amino acids) that is found in teriparatide, a common treatment for osteoporosis. More popular now with the concern for abnormal subtrochanteric fractures associated with long-term bisphosphonate use.

Anterior-posterior compression fractures = Often associated with hemorrhage (venous bleeding, superior gluteal vein, or internal pudendal vein), so assess the patient. If he or she is unstable, resuscitate with fluids and stabilize the pelvis emergently with a pelvic binder, bed sheets, c-clamps, pneumatic anti-shock garments, or external fixation. If still unstable, then head to the angiography suite. If the patient stabilizes, you can follow up with a CT scan.

Apprehension sign = Tests for anterior instability and Bankhart lesions, tested with arm at 90 degrees abduction and external rotation; patients feel apprehension about potential dislocation.

Arthrodesis positions =

- Ankle: Neutral dorsiflexion, 5 to 10 degrees of external rotation, and 5 degrees of hindfoot valgus.

- Elbow: Unilateral is 90 degrees of flexion; bilateral includes one at 110 and the other at 65 degrees of flexion.

- Hip: 25 to 30 degrees of flexion, 0 degrees of abduction and rotation (err on side of external rotation).

- Knee: 0 to 7 degrees of valgus and 10 to 15 degrees of flexion.

- Shoulder: 15 to 20 degrees of abduction, 20 to 25 degrees of forward flexion, and 40 to 50 degrees of internal rotation.

Autonomic dysreflexia = An extreme hypertensive reaction caused by an obstructed urinary catheter or fecal impaction in patients with an injury above T5.

Autosomal recessive (AR) = The following disorders are inherited via an AR pattern: Morquio's syndrome, osteopetrosis (severe type), osteogenesis imperfect (II and III), Sanfilippo's syndrome, Hurler's syndrome, malformations of cortical development (McKusick type), diastrophic dysplasia, Laron's dysplasia, sickle cell anemia, hypophosphatasia, hereditary vitamin D–dependent rickets, and homocystinuria.

Baker's cyst = Located between the semimembranosus and the medial head of the gastrocnemius (just an anatomy question you need to know).

Baxter's nerve = The first branch of the lateral plantar nerve and the most common pain generator in the heel. Can be confused with plantar fasciitis in athletes.

Bennett lesion = Mineralization of the posterior inferior glenoid (can see on CT or plain films). This lesion is often seen in overhead-throwing athletes (found in ~22% of asymptomatic professional pitchers).

Bisphosphonates = Inhibit the ruffled border from forming on osteoclasts, inhibiting their ability to produce acid hydrolase enzymes and resorb bone. On the molecular level, they inhibit protein prenylation by blocking farnesyl diphosphate synthase and GTPase formation (geranylgeranyl diphospate). This blocks proteins (Ras, Rho, Rac, Cdc 42, and Rab families) associated with signaling osteoclasts to function.

Blue sclerae = Type IA, IB, and II osteogenesis imperfecta. Type I is autosomal dominant (AD) with A and B designating teeth involvement or not. Type II is autosomal recessive and is lethal. Type III is autosomal recessive, and there are multiple fractures at birth with a short stature. Type IVA and B have normal sclerae with normal healing and an overall milder form.

Body-powered prosthetics = The terminal end of the device is activated by shoulder flexion and abduction, whereas elbow flexion/extension are managed with shoulder extension and depression. The figure-8 harness must be positioned at the level of the C7 spinous process and slightly toward the contralateral side. Hybrid prosthetic systems provide the best function at the lightest weight.

C5, C7, and L3 = Critical levels of spinal cord injury.

- C5: Elbow flexors are working, but motor function below the elbow motor is out. Transfers are assisted at this level, and patients can use an electric wheelchair with mouth-driven accessories.

- C7: Elbow extensors work, and grasp is out. Patients can cut meat, groom themselves, and transfer independently. They can manually manage a wheelchair.

- L3: Quadriceps are functioning but ankle muscles are not. With an ankle-foot orthosis, patients can be community ambulatory.

Calcium phosphate cement = A better alternative than allograft, autograft, bone morphogenic protein, and polymethylmethacrylate for managing defects associated with a tibial plateau fracture. Found to have a higher level of mechanical strength than these other options.

Capacitive coupling stimulation = Functions to stimulate bone healing by upregulating appropriate factors such as transforming growth factor-beta and prostaglandin E. This occurs via calmodulin activation, which results from calcium translocation across voltage-gated channels.

Cerebral palsy (CP) classification = Nonprogressive upper motor neuron disease.

- Physiologic:
    - O   Ataxia: Hard-to-treat form of CP; patients have a wide-based gait and have trouble coordinating muscle movements.
    - O   Athetosis: Less common and very hard-to-treat form of CP. Slow, involuntary movements occur, appears like patient is constantly writhing.
    - O   Mixed: Often a combination of spastic and athetosis involving the whole body.
    - O   Spastic: Most common form. Struggle between agonist and antagonist (velocity dependent) muscle groups stemming from increased muscle tone and hyperreflexia.
- Anatomic:
    - O   Diplegia: Lower extremities are much more involved than upper extremities. Often, patients have strabismus and normal intelligence and can walk.
    - O   Hemiplegia: Involves one side of the body, both upper and lower extremities, and patients can typically walk (most reliable predictor to walk is independent sitting by age 2 years).
    - O   Total body (quadriplegic): Unable to walk, high early mortality rate, low intelligence.

Child abuse = Suspect in fractures in children associated with long bone fracture in nonambulatory patients, multiple fractures in various stages of healing, and midshaft spiral fractures. True physeal fractures are rare in child abuse except the transphyseal fractures of the distal humerus in children younger than 1 year. Check the skeletal survey and note that a forearm fracture in a child younger than 1 year old has a greater than 50% chance of abuse.

Chordoma = A slow-growing tumor that presents as a lytic lesion in the midline of the sacrum (50%) or base of the skull (35%) and has a 3:1 male predominance. Patients are typically older than 50 years and have abdominal pain and a presacral mass. Originates from malignant transformation of residual notochordal cells. Radiation and wide surgical excision are favored for surgery; however, local recurrence is common (50%). On histology, the tumor has foamy physaliferous cells, and they are keratin positive (differentiates it from a chondrosarcoma).

Chromosomal disorders =

- Beckwith-Wiedemann syndrome: Triad of organomegaly, omphalocele, and large tongue is found. Often find spastic cerebral palsy (may be related to hypoglycemia from hypertrophic pancreatic islet cells) and hemihypertrophy. Must be screened regularly for a Wilms' tumor.

- Down syndrome: Trisomy 21, typically find ligamentous laxity, hypotonia, mental retardation, heart disease (50%), endocrine disorders (hypothyroid and diabetes), and premature aging. Hip subluxation/dislocation, scoliosis, atlantoaxial instability, primus varus, pes planus, and slipped capital femoral epiphysis are often found in these patients.

- Menkes syndrome: Copper transport defect that leads to kinky hair

- Prader-Willi syndrome: Found with a partial deletion of chromosome 15, leaving the child to be obese, floppy/hypotonic, and intellectually impaired and to maintain an insatiable appetite. Will commonly see hip dysplasia, scoliosis, and growth disturbances.

- Rett syndrome: Infants develop normally until a progressive and rapid impairment and developmental delay occurs in girls aged 6 to 18 months. MECP2 gene mutation on the male copy of the X chromosome. Typically see ataxia, hypotonia, C-shaped unresponsive scoliosis, spasticity, and joint contractures.

- Turner syndrome: 45 XO females with short stature, web neck, cubitus valgus, sexual infantilism, osteoporosis, and scoliosis. Beware that malignant hyperthermia is common with anesthesia.

Classic tendon transfers =

- Radial nerve palsy: Wrist extension = pronator teres → extensor carpi radialis brevis
- Low ulnar palsy: Thumb extension = flexor digitorum superficialis → radial lateral band
- High median and ulnar palsy: thumb interphalangeal flexion = brachioradialis → flexor pollicis longus; thumb abduction = extensor indicis proprius → abductor pollicis brevis; finger flexion = extensor carpi radialis longus → flexor digitorum profundus

Cobalt alloys = Consist of cobalt, chromium, and molybdenum vs stainless steel (iron-carbon, cobalt, and silicon).

Common translocations =

- T(11;22): Ewing's sarcoma
- T(12;16): Myxoid liposarcoma (q13;p11)
- T(12;22): Clear cell sarcoma
- T(17;22): Dermatofibrosarcoma protuberans
- T(2;13): Rhabdomyosarcoma
- T(9;22): Philadelphia chromosome (chronic myelogenous leukemia, acute lymphoblastic leukemia, chondrosarcoma)
- T(X;18): Synovial sarcoma (p11.2;q11.2)

Concussion syndrome =

- Grade I: No loss of consciousness or retrograde amnesia. Can return to play as soon as symptoms resolve (3 grade I concussions = long-term suspension).
- Grade II: Loss of consciousness, but less than 5 minutes, plus retrograde amnesia, confusion, and disorientation. After first one can return to play 1 week after symptoms resolve. Any repeat episode = long-term suspension.
- Grade III: Prolonged period of unconsciousness, permanent amnesia, and persistent confusion and disorientation. Automatic long-term suspension of play.

Constrained THA liners = Avoid using unless abductor insufficiency exists (never use in malpositioned implants); usually not the correct answer when associated with an acute acetabular reconstruction. The increased stress at the component-bone interface will lead to early failure and component pullout.

Cord syndromes =

- Anterior: The second most common injury; associated with a flexion-compression injury. The anterior two-thirds of the cord are injured, leaving the posterior columns intact (proprioception and vibratory sensation). Incomplete motor and sensory loss is found with greater loss in the legs than the arms. This syndrome carries the worst prognosis for recovery.
- Brown-Séquard: Half of the cord is injured, usually from a penetrating trauma. Will find a loss of ipsilateral motor function and contralateral pain and temperature sensation. Has the best prognosis of the cord injuries.
- Central: Most common; often seen with preexisting cervical spondylosis with a hyperextension injury. Central cord matter is injured, leading to a greater deficit to the motor function of the upper extremities compared with the lower extremities with some sensory loss. The prognosis for recovery is fair.
- Complete: Often related to a burst fracture or canal-occupying lesions/injuries. No function is found below the level for injury. Recovery prognosis is poor.
- Root: Related to foramina compression or a herniated disk. Weakness is related to the level of injury. Prognosis is generally good with these injuries.

Corona mortis = An anomalous connection between the obturator artery and the external iliac artery, found in 10% to 15% of patients during the ilioinguinal approach to the acetabulum.

Cozen fracture = This is a proximal tibial metaphyseal fracture associated with a high incidence of post-traumatic genu valgum deformity. The deformity typically resolves spontaneously and does not need surgery.

Direct compression molding of polyethylene = Gives the best wear rates compared with other techniques for component fabrication (hot isostatic pressing with machining, ram bar extrusion with machining, or compression molding into bars and machining).

Doxycycline = Low dose of this antibiotic can be used to treat rheumatoid arthritis in conjunction with methotrexate. Doxycycline appears to have an anti-metalloproteinase effect in this setting.

Elbow stability = Relies on the coronoid, lateral collateral ligament (aka lateral ulnar collateral ligament [UCL]), and anterior band of the MCL. The anterior oblique fibers of the MCL are the most important for elbow stability, whereas the radial head is the most important secondary stabilizer of the elbow (particularly up to 30 degrees of flexion and pronation).

Estrogen receptor = Tamoxifen is an antagonist to estrogen receptors and can be used to treat desmoid tumors (50% success) in poor candidates for surgery or chemotherapy (methotrexate). These are benign, locally aggressive neoplasms found in 15- to 40-year-olds. Typically a hard, fixed, deep, painless mass with a histology consistent with sweeping bundles of collagen. Can be surgically removed or managed with chemotherapy/hormonal therapy or radiation.

EXT 1 = Genotype of hereditary exostoses that is more commonly associated with a worse condition/phenotype and at higher risk for sarcoma development compared with EXT 2 mutations.

EXT1, EXT2, and EXT3 = Gene mutations associated with multiple hereditary exostosis, which is inherited via an AD pattern. Multiple osteochondromas are found in the distal femur (70%), proximal tibia (70%), proximal humerus (50%), scapula (40%), ribs, distal radius, hands, and proximal fibula. There is a 1% to 2% risk for malignant transformation to a chondrosarcoma.

Extensor carpi radialis brevis = The site of tendinopathy associated with lateral epicondylitis. Pain on resisted wrist extension is a common physical exam finding.

Femoral fracture = The most common cause for malpractice (> failure to diagnose > infection > death) suits secondary to malrotation, compartment syndrome, foot drop, and poor surgical technique.

Fibrillin = Defect in collagen synthesis associated with cardiac abnormalities; long, slender fingers (arachnodactyly); scoliosis (50%); superior lens dislocation (60%); and pectus deformities. Joint laxity is common, and orthopedic conditions found include recurrent dislocations, scoliosis, pes planovalgus, and acetabulum protrusio. The mutation is found on chromosome 15 (CH 15q21).

Four types of flexor digitorum longus avulsion (Jersey finger) =

- Bone and tendon avulsion: early fixation of bone and tendon back to bone
- Large bony avulsion fracture, typically catches on A4 pulley: open reduction and internal fixation of fracture
- Tendon retraction to palm, vincula ruptured: repair within 7 to 10 days
- Tendon retracts to PIP held in place by vincula: repair within 6 weeks

Freiberg's infraction = Osteonecrosis of the second metatarsal head, seen in female athletes aged 13 to 18 years. Patients often have a long second metatarsal. There are 5 stages as classified by Smillie: 1, subchondral fracture on MRI only; 2, dorsal collapse on plain films; 3, dorsal metatarsal head collapse with intact plantar portion; 4, collapse of entire metatarsal head; and 5, severe arthritic changes. Treatment involves removal of loose bodies, dorsiflexion closing, and shortening osteotomy or partial metatarsal head resection (DuVries arthroplasty).

G protein = Somatic mutation in the gene coding for the alpha subunit of Gs, which is the protein that stimulates cAMP formation, leading to fibrous dysplasia.

Gene defects =

- Connexin: Oculodentodigital dysplasia
- Dystrophin: Muscular dystrophy (Duchenne's and Becker's)
- Frataxin: Friedreich's ataxia, wide-based gait, cavus foot, cardiomyopathy
- Myotonin: Myotonic dystrophy
- Neurofibromin: Neurofibromatosis 1, 17q11.2 chromosomal defect, find cervical kyphosis (treat with circumferential fusion), scoliosis, pseudarthrosis of clavicle and extremities, and congenital anterolateral bowing of the tibia
- Periaxin: Charcot-Marie-Tooth type 4F, AR inheritance (normal reflexes)
- Peripheral myelin protein 22: Charcot-Marie-Tooth type I, DNA testing for duplication in portion of chromosome 17 (absent reflexes)

- Sarcoglycan: Limb girdle muscular dystrophy (AR, 10 to 30 years old)
- Schwannomin: Neurofibromatosis 2, mutated in NF2 (see acoustic neuromas)

Groove of Ranvier = A place of appositional bone growth that is found on the periphery of the growth plate that bridges the epiphysis to the diaphysis. It serves to strengthen the physis and grows around and not in length.

Hard-on-hard bearing terms =

- Equatorial contact: Associated with a femoral head that is larger than the cup, leads to high frictional torque on the component (almost like seizing).
- Polar contact: Associated with a femoral head that is smaller than the cup; high-contact stress over a small area = increased wear.
- Radial clearance: The difference between the radius of the head and the cup.
- Run-in wear: In the first million cycles, there is a higher wear rate until the larger surface asperities are polished out.
- Surface roughness: Need surfaces to be smooth; metal alloys have a surface roughness of 0.05 µ, ceramic = 0.02 µ and polyethylene = > 200 µ.

High-grade tumors = Osteosarcoma, postradiation sarcoma, Paget's sarcoma, fibrosarcoma, malignant fibrous histiocytoma, pleomorphic liposarcoma, synovial sarcoma, rhabdomyosarcoma, and alveolar cell sarcoma.

High tibial osteotomy contraindications = Lateral compartment disease, lateral tibial subluxation greater than 1 cm, medial compartment bone loss greater than 2 to 3 mm, greater than 15-degree flexion contracture, less than 90 degrees of knee flexion, greater than 20 degrees of correction needed, inflammatory arthritis, and a varus thrust on exam.

Hilgenreiner's epiphyseal angle = This is the angle from Hilgenreiner's line to a line drawn across the femoral head physis. Used to determine management for congenital coxa vara: less than 45 degrees will resolve spontaneously; 45 to 60 degrees requires close observation; and greater than 60 degrees will usually require surgery, particularly with a neck shaft angle less than 110 degrees.

Hip approaches = Posterior (Kocher) approach for interval split gluteus maximus; direct lateral (modified Hardinge) approach for interval transgluteus medius; anterolateral (Watson-Jones) approach for interval gluteus medius and tensor fascia lata.

Hypocalcemia = Table 3-1.

Immune responses = Type I (IgE mediated), type II (antibody mediated), type III (immune complex mediated), type IV (delayed hypersensitivity reaction), type V (IgM mediated).

Incidence = The number of new cases of the studied variable over a specified time period.

Increased ESR, WBC > 12,000/mm³, fever > 38.5°C, unable to bear weight = In a child, the next step is to aspirate to rule septic arthritis vs toxic synovitis.

Internal rotation = Always the wrong answer with positioning TKA implants; optimally, femoral and tibial components should be externally rotated and central or lateralized to minimize the Q angle in TKA. Similarly, the patella should be medialized.

Intrinsic minus = Claw hand is often associated with a median/ulnar nerve palsy or Volkmann's ischemic contracture. The metacarpophalangeal joints are in hyperextension (focus of surgical management) and the interphalangeal joints are in flexion.

IT band syndrome = Look for vignettes with runners (lots of hills) or cyclists with localized lateral knee pain. Pain is worse with the knee flexed 30 degrees. Check Ober test (hip extension and abduction will tighten IT band). Usually treated with therapy.

Jerk test = Tests for posterior instability and reverse Bankart lesions; down at 90 degrees abduction, internal rotation, and loading of the humerus.

Keratan sulfate = Accumulation is associated with a rare form of dwarfism called Morquio's syndrome and often presents clinically with odontoid hypoplasia.

Table 3-1.

HYPOCALCEMIA

Disease	Pathophysiology	Clinical Symptoms	X-Ray Findings
Hypoparathyroidism	Not enough PTH, often due to ablation of thyroid • Decreased Ca, PTH • Increased Phos	Neuromuscular irritability (tetany, seizures, Chvostek's sign), cataracts, EKG changes (prolonged QT interval), hair loss, nail infections	Calcified basal ganglia
Pseudohypo-parathyroidism (Albright's disease)	PTH receptor abnormality • Decreased Ca • Increased phos, PTH (can be normal)	Short first, fourth, and fifth metacarpals/metatarsals, obesity, diminished intelligence	Brachydactyly, exostosis
Renal osteodystrophy • High turnover: chief cell hyperplasia • Low turnover: no secondary hyperparathyroidism, aluminum toxicity	Chronic renal failure leads to reduced phosphate excretion • Decreased Ca • Increased phos (very high), PTH, alk phos	Hypocalcemia symptoms as above, with secondary hyperparathyroidism in high-turnover disease; amyloidosis can lead to carpal tunnel syndrome, arthropathy, fractures	Rugger jersey spine, osteitis fibrosa, amyloidosis
Rickets (osteomalacia) • Vitamin D deficient	• Low vit D in diet or malabsorption; low Ca, phos, and vit D; and high alk phos and PTH	• Osteomalacia, hypotonia, muscle weakness, dental disease, bowing of bones, waddling gait	• Rachitic rosary, wide growth plates, codfish vertebrae, physeal cupping, Looser's zones, fractures
• Vitamin D dependent	• Normal vit D, inc alk phos and PTH 　o Type I: defect in 25-OH-Vit D1αhydroxylase on 12q14 chromosome 　o Type II: defect in 1,25 (OH)-Vitamin D receptor	• Same as above	• Poor mineralization
• Vitamin D resistant	• Decreased phos resorption in kidneys; low phos and high alk phos and very high 1,25 vit D; x-linked disease	• Same, without changes of secondary hyperparathyroidism (PTH works by activating adenylyl cyclase and phospholipase C)	• Poor mineralization

Alk phos=alkaline phosphatase; Ca=calcium; EKG=electrocardiogram; Phos=phosphate; PTH=parathyroid hormone; vit=vitamin.

Klippel-Feil syndrome = Triad (1). Low posterior hairline (2). Web neck (3). Limited C-spine ROM found in 50% of cases. Basis of disease is failure of normal segmentation of formation of cervical vertebrae. Often associated with Sprengel's deformity, heart disease, renal disease, congenital scoliosis, and synkinesis.

L4, L5, S1, S2, S3 = Nerve roots that lead to the sciatic nerve and innervate the lateral rotators, biceps femoris, semitendinosus, semimembranosus, and adductor magnus.

Lateral talocalcaneal and anterior talofibular ligaments = Both attach to the lateral process of the talus, which is often injured in snowboarders. The lateral process articulates with the calcaneus and lateral malleolus. Structures that attach to the rest of talus are as follows:

- Os trigonum: Trigonocalcaneal ligament (posterior talocalcaneal), posterior talofibular, fibulotalocalcaneal ligaments
- Posterolateral tubercle: Posterior talocalcaneal, posterior talofibular, and fibulotalocalcaneal ligaments
- Posteromedial tubercle: Medial talocalcaneal, medial band of posterior talocalcaneal, superficial posterior talotibial, and deep posterior talotibial ligaments

Lift-off test = Tests for subscapularis injuries; inability to lift arm off of back.

Little League shoulder = Proximal humerus epiphyseolysis is an overuse injury in the skeletally immature overhead-throwing athlete. Early management is cessation of throwing for 6 to 8 weeks, followed by a progressive return to sporting activity.

Low-grade tumors = Parosteal osteosarcoma, chondrosarcoma, hemangioendothelioma, chordoma, adamantinoma, myxoid liposarcoma, angiomatoid malignant fibrous histiocytoma.

Lyme disease = Contracted via a tick bite (deer tick: Ixodes scapularis) and is endemic to the northeastern US and northern California regions. The bug is Borrelia burgdorferi spirochete, and the target-like rash is characteristic (erythema migrans) of stage 1 disease. Stage 2 occurs weeks to months later, and neurologic sequelae and migratory polyarthritis are common. Stage 3 is chronic, and arthritis is common, as is acrodermatitis chronica atrophicans. Treatment is a 4-week course of oral amoxicillin or doxycycline.

Malpositioned tunnels = The most common cause of anterior cruciate ligament (ACL) reconstruction failure! Beware vertical tunnel placement as well as anteroposterior tunnel positions.

Marjolin ulcer = A carcinoma (most often squamous cell) that develops from a chronically irritated, traumatized, or draining area of skin. This is commonly aggressive and occurs in the setting of a deep tissue burn. Other cancers to occur in such an ulcer include basal cell carcinoma, melanoma, and sarcoma.

Match the imaging sign with the correct diagnosis = Table 3-2.

Table 3-2.	
MATCH IMAGING SIGN WITH CORRECT DIAGNOSIS	
A. Segond/lateral capsule sign	1. PCL injury
B. Pellegrini-Stieda lesion	2. Early DJD
C. Square lateral condyle	3. Chronic MCL injury
D. Fairbanks changes	4. ACL tear
E. Lateral stress view: ant stress to tibia with knee flexed 70 degrees	5. Discoid meniscus
ACL=anterior cruciate ligament; ant=anterior; DJD=degenerative joint disease; MCL=medial collateral ligament; PCL=posterior cruciate ligament.	
Answers: A-4; B-3; C-5; D-2; E-1	

Mayfield classification for perilunate instability =

- I: Scapholunate dissociation
- II, VII, IX, X = Clotting factors affected by the inhibition of vitamin K 2,3-epoxide reductase by warfarin (prevents gamma carboxylation of these factors and decreased activation of prothrombin).
- II: Lunocapitate disruption
- III: Lunotriquetral disruption
- IV: Lunate dislocation
- Treatments: Early management consists of open ligament repair and late consists of fusion or proximal row carpectomy

McCune-Albright syndrome = Triad of polyostotic fibrous dysplasia, cutaneous café-au-lait spots (coast of Maine), and endocrine dysfunction (precocious puberty). Found in 30% to 50% of cases of polyostotic fibrous dysplasia resulting from a mutation in the Gs G protein.

Medial epicondyle = The most common fracture associated with a pediatric elbow dislocation. Coronoid and radial neck fractures are common as well, whereas medial humeral condyle and olecranon fractures are infrequently found.

Meet the dactylys! =

- Camptodactyly: Congenital digital flexion; occurs at the PIP of the small finger; 3 types (all often treated nonoperatively); Kirner's deformity is an apex dorsal and ulnar curvature of the distal phalanx.
- Clinodactyly: Congenital curvature of the digit in the radioulnar plane; 3 types (type I, minor angulation and normal length; type II, minor angulation and short phalanx; type III, severe angulation, delta phalanx).
- Macrodactyly: Congenital digital enlargement, often unilateral and 70% affect more than one digit.
- Polydactyly: Duplication of digits; preaxial: thumb duplication; postaxial: small finger duplication.
- Syndactyly: Most common congenital hand deformity; based on the presence or absence of bony connections between digits; 5-15-50-30 → thumb-index 5%, index-middle 15%, middle-ring 50%, ring-small 30%.

Modulus of elasticity = (Highest to lowest) Ceramic > cobalt-chromium alloy > stainless steel > titanium > cortical bone > polymethylmethacrylate > polyethylene > cancellous bone > tendon/ligament > cartilage.

Most common osteochondroses = Table 3-3.

Table 3-3.		
MOST COMMON OSTEOCHONDROSES		
Disorder	**Location**	**Age of Onset**
Legg-Calvé-Perthes disease	Femoral head	4 to 8 years
Osgood-Schlatter disease	Tibial tuberosity	11 to 15 years
Sinding-Larsen-Johansson syndrome	Inferior patella	10 to 14 years
Blount disease	Epiphysis: proximal tibia	Infantile: 1 to 3 years / Adolescent: 8 to 15 years
Sever's disease	Calcaneus	9 to 11 years
Panner's disease	Capitellum: distal humerus	5 to 10 years
Kienböck's disease	Lunate: wrist	20 to 40 years
Köhler's disease	Navicular bone: tarsal	3 to 7 years

Most common tumors of the hand =

- Bony malignancy: chondrosarcoma
- Metastatic lesion: lung cancer (distal phalanx)
- Primary malignancy: squamous cell carcinoma
- Primary sarcoma: epithelioid sarcoma

Mucopolysaccharidosis = Proportionate dwarfisms based on sugars found in the urine.

- Hunter's syndrome: Sex-linked recessive; mental retardation; clear eyes; production of dermatan/heparin sulfate in the urine.
- Hurler's syndrome: Autosomal recessive; most severe form; produces dermatan/heparin sulfate in the urine. Cloudy corneas and mental retardation are common.
- Morquio's syndrome: Autosomal recessive; most common one; presents by age 2 years with waddling gait, kyphosis, cloudy eyes, and normal intelligence. Produces keratan sulfate in the urine.
- Sanfilippo's syndrome: Autosomal recessive; heparin sulfate excretion in the urine; mental retardation; normal until 2 years old; clear eyes.

Multidirectional instability = Typically treated with physical therapy for 6 months. If this fails, an inferior capsular shift procedure is recommended.

Myofibroblast = The offending cell in Dupuytren's contracture. Commonly found in the fifth to seventh decades of life; 2:1 male:female ratio. Pathologic cords form, and surgery is indicated when metacarpophalangeal flexion contractures are greater than 30 degrees and proximal interphalangeal joint (PIP) flexion contractures are greater than 30 degrees. Recurrence rate is approximately 50%.

Negative predictive value = True-negatives/(false-negatives + true-negatives).

Neutrophils = The first cell to appear after muscle injury, followed by an increase in macrophages.

Nicotine = Can delay fracture healing times, increase the risk of nonunion, and reduce the strength of fracture callus. Also associated with an increased risk of pseudoarthrosis after lumbar fusion and infection after a total joint arthroplasty.

Nonrotatory, concave scoliosis = A same-side scoliosis related to an osteoid osteoma that is typically painful. The scoliosis develops due to spasm from the ipsilateral lesion. Often found in the second decade in males more often than females. Pain is relieved by NSAID administration. It is typically managed with medication or marginal excision; radiofrequency ablation may injure neural elements.

Normal values for wrist x-rays =

- Capitolunate angle: 0 to 15 degrees
- Radiolunate angle: -25 to +10 degrees
- SL angle: 30 to 60 degrees
- SL gap: < 3 mm

Odds ratio = This describes the odds of being exposed to a condition or disease in those who have the disease or condition compared with the odds in those without the disease or condition.

Open-chain = Exercises in which the hand or foot is free to move. Differs from closed-chain, in which the foot or hand is in contact with the ground or equipment. Examples are chest press, biceps curls, leg extensions, and leg curls. Closed-chain examples include pushups, pull-ups, squats, lunges, and squats.

PAD/DAB = Stands for Palmar = ADduction and Dorsal = ABbduction. Interosseous muscles of the hand: palmar 3, adduct the fingers and dorsal 4, abduct the fingers.

Parsonage-Turner syndrome = Bilateral anterior interosseous nerve palsy secondary to viral brachial neuritis. Results in motor loss (radial 2 flexor digitorum profundus, flexor pollicis longus, pronator quadratus) with no accompanying sensory deficit.

Physeal growth contributions =

- Femur: 30% proximal and 70% distal
- Fibula: 60% proximal and 40% distal

- Humerus: 80% proximal and 20% distal
- Radius: 25% proximal and 75% distal
- Tibia: 55% proximal and 45% distal
- Ulna: 80% proximal and 20% distal

Plyometric exercises = The most efficient means for improving power during conditioning training. The muscle stretch (stores elastic energy) is followed by an immediate rapid contraction (increased force of concentric muscle contraction).

Positive predictive value = True-positives/(true-positives + false-positives).

Posterior lateral corner = Made up of the popliteus tendon, popliteofibular ligament, arcuate ligament, fabellofibular ligament, biceps femoris tendon, iliotibial (IT) band, and lateral gastroc tendon. Its function is to stabilize the knee against external rotation and posterior translation. Varus alignment is the greatest predictor of failure in posterior lateral corner reconstructions.

Preserved disk space = Commonly found with Pott's disease or tuberculosis of the spine, compared with pyogenic infections, which cross the disk space. Pott's disease can occur in the thoracic and lumbar spine and can lead to a kyphotic deformity.

Prevalence = This is the total number of people who are affected by the variable being studied at a single time point over the total number of individuals at risk in a population.

Prevalence = True-positive + false-negative/all cases.

Proximal femoral focal deficiency = A congenital defect leading to a short, bulky thigh, often associated with coxa vara or fibular hemimelia. Treatment consists of amputation, femoral-pelvic fusion, Van Ness rotationplasty, and limb lengthening.

Punnett square = Diagram.

Quadriceps avoidance gait = Often found in the ACL-deficient knee and characterized by a weaker quadriceps moment during midstance.

Radial club hand = Associated with Holt-Oram syndrome; thrombocytopenia-absent radius; Fanconi's anemia; and vertebral anomalies, anal atresia, cardiac defects, tracheoesophageal fistula/atresia, renal and radial anomalies and limb defects (VACTERL). The ulna is often short too, and elbow stiffness is a contraindication to surgery. Centralization procedures start at age 6 to 12 months. Often found bilaterally, with the following 4 stages of the deformity noted:

- Stage I: Deficient distal radial epiphysis
- Stage II: Hypoplastic radius
- Stage III: Partial aplasia (present proximally, absent distally)
- Stage IV: Total aplasia (most common form)

Radial tunnel syndrome = Pain only; no motor or sensory deficits noted with the posterior interosseous nerve being involved. The long finger extension test and the resisted supination test can help with diagnosis, while electromyography/nerve conduction velocity is relatively useless for such a determination. Tender 2 to 3 cm distal to the radial head over the radial tunnel. Treat nonoperatively for a long time because only 50% to 80% good-to-excellent results are found with surgery.

Relative risk = Incidence of exposed group/incidence of unexposed group. As this number reaches 1, the incidence rates of both groups reach equality. Greater than 1, there is a positive correlation between the risk and the variable being studied; less than 1 affords a protective effect on the population that has been exposed.

Replantation operative sequence = Bone, extensor tendons, flexor tendons, arteries, nerves, veins, and skin. In order, the priority for reimplantation is thumb, long, ring, small, and then index finger. Do not replant if warm ischemia time is longer than 6 hours for proximal to carpus and longer than 12 hours for a digit vs less than 12 and less than 24 hours for cool ischemia time, respectively.

Rheumatoid spine =

- Atlantoaxial subluxation: The most common issue is that pannus destroys the transverse ligament, dens of both. Instability is defined as motion on flexion-extension films greater than 3.5 mm. A difference greater than 7 mm implies a disruption of the alar ligaments, and a difference greater than 9 mm of space available for the cord greater than 14 mm is related to an increased risk of neurovascular injury. Treated with posterior C1-C2 fusion.

- Basilar invagination: Seen as superior migration of the odontoid into the cranium (dens tip is above the foramen magnum). Found in 40% of cases. Treated with C2 to occiput fusion. Know the following lines:
  - O McGregor's line: From the base of the occiput to hard palate; settling is noted when the tip of the dens is more than 4.5 mm above this line.
  - O Chamberlain's line: From the hard palate to the edge of the occiput posteriorly; abnormal if more than 5 mm above this line with tip of dens.
  - O McRae's line: From the anterior to posterior margin of the foramen magnum; if above this line, be suspicious for basilar invagination.

- Subaxial subluxation: Only found in about 20% of cases and can occur at multiple levels. Subluxation of more than 4 mm or more than 20% of the vertebral body typically correlates with cord compression. The cervical body height-to-width ratio of less than 2 is almost always predictive of neurological injury. Treat with posterior fusion if necessary.

Risk and incidence of scoliosis curve progression =

- Curves greater than 20 degrees, age younger than 12 years, and skeletal immaturity (Risser 0, 1).

- Right-sided thoracic curves are common, whereas left-sided curves are rare and must be worked up with early MRI.

- Risser stages 0 and 1 have a 22% and 68% incidence of progression when presenting with a 5- to 19-degree curve or a 20- to 29-degree curve, respectively.

- Risser stages 2, 3, and 4 have a 1.6% and 23% incidence of progression when presenting with a 5- to 19-degree curve or a 20- to 29-degree curve, respectively.

Salmonella = A common cause of osteomyelitis in patients with sickle cell disease. Staphylococcus aureus is still the most common; this is just the classic answer.

Sarcomeres = Muscle units composed of thick (myosin) and thin (actin) filaments strategically arranged in bands and lines. The A band contains actin and myosin, I band contains actin only, H band contains only myosin, M line is an interconnection site of thick filaments, and Z line anchors the thin filaments and is the boundary for a sarcomere on each side.

Sensation and muscle receptor types =

- Flutter: Pacini's corpuscle and hair down

- Limb proprioception: Muscle spindle primary and secondary, Golgi tendon organ, and joint capsule mechanoreceptor

- Steady skin indentation: Merkel's receptor

- Touch: Meissner's corpuscle

- Vibration: Ruffini's corpuscle

Sensitivity = True-positives/(false-negative + true-positives).

Slip angle = The measurement that predicts the likelihood of progression with spondylolisthesis in children, most commonly seen at L5-S1.

Specificity = True-negatives/(false-positives + true-negatives).

Spine facet orientation = The inferior facets of the more proximal vertebra are always more posterior.

- C-spine: 45 degrees to the transverse plane and parallel to the frontal plane

- T-spine: 60 degrees to the transverse plane and 20 degrees to the frontal plane

- L-spine: 90 degrees to the transverse plane and 45 degrees to the frontal plane

Spinal nerves, trunks, divisions, cords, and branches of the brachial plexus =

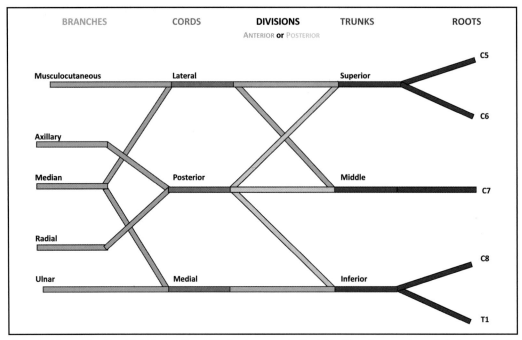

(Adapted from The Brachial Plexus. TeachMeAnatomy website. http://teachmeanatomy.info/upper-limb/ nerves/brachial-plexus/.)

Stener lesion = Interposition of adductor aponeurosis with a gamekeeper's thumb (ulnar collateral ligament injury). A sprain will not open up more than 35 to 45 degrees with stress testing.

Superior border of the pectoralis major = The most reliable anatomic landmark to determine humeral length (anatomic height) and version in a 4-part proximal humerus fracture treated with an arthroplasty procedure.

Supraorbital nerve = The most common nerve injury with the application of a halo, resulting in pain and numbness over the medial one-third of the eyebrow.

Tarsal coalition = Calf pain, peroneal spasticity, flatfoot, and repeated ankle sprains. X-rays are good but CT scan is better at detecting coalition and ruling out that both types exist.

- Calcaneonavicular: 10- to 12-year-olds; surgical resection in persistently painful cases is often successful.
- Subtalar: 12- to 14-year-olds; resect if less than 50% of the middle facet of talus is involved; arthrodesis is preferred if greater than 50% is involved.

Third power = The bending stiffness of a plate is proportional to the plate thickness to the third power. Plates are load-bearing devices and ideally should be placed on the tension side of the bone.

Titanium alloys = Typically consists of varying amounts of aluminum, titanium, and vanadium or niobium.

Toughness = Amount of energy per volume that a material can absorb prior to failure.

Tumor necrosis factor-α = A cytokine that stimulates an acute phase reaction. It is involved in apoptotic cell death, inflammation, and the inhibition of tumorigenesis.

Tumors that metastasize to bone = Breast, prostate, lung, kidney, and thyroid.

Type III tibial tubercle fracture = Fracture extends posteriorly and across the primary ossification center, proximal tibial physis. This injury has a high incidence of compartment syndrome (anterior tibial recurrent artery injury) and meniscal injuries. Delayed complications include recurvatum deformity and refracture.

Types of studies =

- Case control: Begins with a group of subjects with a known disease or injury who are analyzed to identify clinically relevant data.

- Meta-analysis: Combines many smaller studies into a single large cohort review to examine for outcome and management variables.

- Prospective cohort study: A group of normal subjects are followed over time to identify the onset of an injury or disease. Can be used to determine relative risk.

Unilateral unsegmented bar and a contralateral, fully segmented hemivertebra = Has the worst prognosis with congenital scoliosis. Rapidly progressive and should be treated with surgery (posterior spinal fusion with combined anterior for girls younger than 10 years and boys younger than 12 years).

Vertebral squaring = The hallmark radiological sign of ankylosing spondylitis on lateral x-rays. Sacroiliac joint involvement delineates ankylosing spondylitis from diffuse idiopathic skeletal hyperostosis (nonmarginal syndesmophytes at 3 vertebral levels).

X-linked dominant = Hypophosphatemic rickets, Léri-Weill dyschondrosteosis (Madelung's deformity)

X-linked recessive = Spondyloepiphyseal dysplasia (tarda form), Hunter's syndrome, hemophilia, and Duchenne's muscular dystrophy

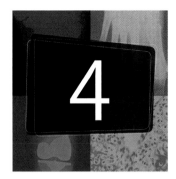

"CRUNCH-TIME" SELF-TEST
TIME TO GET YOUR GAME ON

The following is a high-yield rapid-fire series of review questions. These questions are related to common facts that are often found on orthopedic standardized examinations. They are meant to supplement the vignettes, so know these answers well. Typically, Board questions are more detailed; however, knowing the answers to this self-test serves as a good start to determining the crux of more difficult vignettes. This will test your knowledge of the "tough stuff" that might show up on the Boards or OITE.

Many of these questions will relate to a prior vignette and should reaffirm your knowledge of these commonly tested topics. There are also some stand-alone questions that do not correspond to a prior vignette, but they will bolster your ability to ace your exam. Upon completion of the test, which may take several sessions, check the answer key. To determine how prepared you are for your upcoming examination, use the key to interpret your results to the self-test. Cheating will cloud your results and make the interpretation page irrelevant. During crunch time, correlate your wrong answers with the appropriate vignettes and topics to focus your last-minute studying where you need help.

1. What is the diagnosis and treatment for a shoulder with limited active and passive range of motion with normal x-rays and good rotator cuff strength?
2. What are the most common sites for posttraumatic physeal arrest?
3. List the insertion of structures on the fibula from anterior to posterior.
4. What muscles in the hand originate and insert on a tendon?
5. True or false: The anterolateral portion of the posterior cruciate ligament is tight in extension.
6. In what position should a Monteggia-type fracture be immobilized?
7. What are the fundamental differences between effects of aging on cartilage vs osteoarthritis?
8. What are the most common sites for fractures associated with child abuse?
9. What should preoperative management of a metastatic renal cell carcinoma include?
10. What is the most common type of Monteggia fracture?
11. Describe a swan neck deformity.
12. What are the common locations of ulnar nerve compression about the elbow?
13. What is the most important fluoroscopic view required for inserting iliosacral screws in the proper orientation?
14. What conditions are associated with protrusio acetabulum?

Levine BR. *Acing the Orthopedic Board Exam:*
The Ultimate Crunch-Time Resource (pp 425-429).
© 2016 SLACK Incorporated.

15. What is an acceptable reduction for a Colles' fracture?
16. What is the most common malignant bone tumor in children?
17. What are the borders of the quadrilateral space?
18. What are the levels of evidence for published literature?
19. What structure is typically injured in a Boutonnière deformity?
20. When releasing lateral structures during the balancing of a TKA in flexion and extension, what structural considerations should be followed?
21. What are the common types of scapula winging?
22. What are Kocher criteria for a pediatric painful hip?
23. Increasing irradiation doses for ultra-high-molecular-weight polyethylene treatments leads to what changes in mechanical properties of the material?
24. What is the most common complication associated with a tibial spine avulsion fracture?
25. Name 3 natural products associated with platelet inhibition.
26. What is the earliest age at which the femoral epiphysis is ossified enough to clearly assess on plain x-rays?
27. What is the appropriate therapy protocol after reduction of a simple elbow dislocation?
28. What is the best treatment for a 9-month-old with arthrogryposis (amyoplasia) and bilateral hip dislocations?
29. What planar deformity is the strongest predictor of disability in adult patients with scoliosis?
30. During the Henry approach to the radius, what nerve is at risk in the mid to upper third of the radial shaft?
31. What are the 3 common patterns of passage of the recurrent motor branch of the median nerve?
32. What synthetic bone graft has the highest compressive strength?
33. The strength of a tendon repair is most closely related to what property of the repair?
34. What is the most common concern/complication after hip resurfacing?
35. During retrograde nailing for an ankle arthrodesis, what neurovascular structures are often at risk?
36. Locking plates are associated with what percentage of screw-cut when treating 3-part proximal humerus fractures?
37. What is the treatment of choice for cervical myelopathy at multiple levels with concomitant kyphosis?
38. What is the best indicator of a patient's resuscitation level after a major trauma?
39. Chronic bisphosphonate therapy has been associated with what adverse event?
40. What anatomical structures are associated with ulnar nerve compression?
41. What finding is associated with the greatest risk of curve progression with congenital kyphosis?
42. What is the DNA sequence found within genes that is involved in the regulation of patterns of morphogenesis in animals called?
43. Vertical placement of the tibial tunnel in ACL reconstruction is associated with what finding?
44. What is the ring avulsion classification?
45. What is the name of the act that states that patients may not be transferred from one emergency department to another unless the benefits of transfer outweigh risks?
46. What is the pathophysiology and activity that incites lower back pain in adolescents/children with a spondylotic defect, typically L4 level?
47. What is the role of receptor activator of nuclear factor kappa-B in bone metastases?
48. Describe the ASIA (American Spinal Injury Association) classification.
49. What are the classic pathological findings associated with the condition known as tennis elbow, or lateral epicondylitis?
50. What are the zones of the physis?
51. What is the typical translocation associated with Ewing's sarcoma?
52. What are the contraindications for a unicompartmental knee arthroplasty?
53. What is the most common treatment for odontoid fractures in children?
54. Compression of the ulnar nerve in zone 2 of Guyon's canal will produce what type of deficit?
55. What conditions are commonly associated with the formation of postoperative heterotopic ossification?
56. What is pelvic incidence?
57. What are some common cardiac abnormalities found in athletes?
58. What are the tests for continuous variables in a statistical analysis?
59. When doing a lateral retinacular release during a standard TKA, it is important to preserve what vessel?

60. What are the laboratory test values and physiologic markers that lead to poor healing of an amputation wound?
61. What are the differences between vascular and neurogenic claudication?
62. Interference with the hormone-related peptide and transforming growth factor-β1 proteins (both decrease rate of maturation of chondrocytes and endochondral bone formation) occurs with what condition or an open exposure to what?
63. What type of above-knee amputation prosthesis allows you to change the cadence of one's gait?
64. What are some laboratory markers of disease activity in Paget's disease?
65. True or false: The acromioclavicular ligaments primarily function to resist anteroposterior motion of the acromioclavicular joint.
66. What is the best treatment for a lower lumbar burst fracture with minimal canal retropulsion and a normal neurological exam?
67. What is the modified Stoppa approach?
68. During McMurray's test, what maneuver is performed to differentiate between lateral and medial meniscal injuries?
69. What are the typical constituents of bone cement?
70. List tests that analyze categorical data.
71. What is the inheritance pattern of hereditary multiple exostoses?
72. What is the recommended treatment for grade I and II acute posterior collateral ligament injuries in young athletes?
73. What is the most sensitive means to measure polyethylene wear or migration in total joint arthroplasties?
74. What is the best predictor of a patient's ability to ambulate after a closed head injury?
75. What are the radiographic deformities seen on x-rays of patients with a cavus foot deformity?
76. What is the characteristic histological finding of a chondroblastoma?
77. In the case of moderate hallus valgus (intermetatarsal angle of 15 degrees and hallux valgus angle of 33 degrees), what is the best treatment option?
78. List the absolute criteria for limb amputation in the setting of a trauma.
79. What are the common causes for Charcot arthropathy?
80. Define type II error.
81. What autosomal-dominant disorder is the result of a mutation replacing a glycine amino acid to a larger side group, impairing the triple helix formation of type I collagen?
82. What are the characteristics of X-linked hypophosphatemic rickets?
83. What are the indications for arthrodesis takedown of the hip?
84. What is the most appropriate management for a type III AC joint injury in a 10-year-old child?
85. Mineralization of the posteroinferior glenoid often found in overhead throwing athletes is termed what?
86. What are common methods to treat hypercalcemia?
87. Which modality has a higher rate of nonunion: intramedullary nailing or plating of a humeral shaft fracture?
88. What are the 3 most common causes for the inability to reduce a lateral subtalar dislocation?
89. True or false: When performing a quadriceps snip, the range of motion and weight bearing must be restricted postoperatively.
90. During the dial test, increased external rotation at 30 degrees but not 90 degrees indicates an injury to what structure?
91. What is the Blauth classification?
92. Corrosion related to an electrochemical current developed between 2 metals in a conductive/electrolyte solution is called what?
93. The following characteristics are typical of what skeletal dysplasia: extreme short-limb dwarfism, cauliflower ears, scoliosis, hitchhiker thumbs, club feet, normal intelligence, autosomal recessive trait, coxa vara, and delayed epiphyseal ossification.
94. What technical issues should be followed to optimize conditions for patella tracking during a total knee arthroplasty?
95. What are the common characteristics of Apert's syndrome?
96. What type of sacral fracture is associated with the greatest rate of nerve injury?
97. True or false: Alternative bearings, such as ceramic-on-ceramic, metal-on-metal, and cross-linked polyethylene, generate larger wear particles than standard polyethylene bearings.

98. What are the contraindications of Pavlik harness use for managing hip dislocations?
99. What 2 common techniques can be implemented to minimize free radical formation in polyethylene sterilization via the gamma irradiation process?
100. What is the treatment of choice for a noninfected plantar ulcer in a patient with diabetes mellitus with an equinus contracture?
101. What type of bone stimulator functions to raise local tissue pH by reducing the tissue oxygen concentration (increased consumption and hydroxyl radical formation), ultimately leading to decreased osteoclast activity and increased osteoblast activity?
102. What are the hallmark radiographic signs of a SL ligament injury?
103. Define what the power analysis of a study ensures.
104. What are the 4 types of myelodysplasia (spina bifida)?
105. What muscles are innervated by the anterior interosseous nerve?
106. How many types of collagen are there, and where are they found?
107. Name some common complications of tension band fixation of an olecranon fracture.
108. What are common problems associated with below-knee amputation prostheses?
109. What nerve is at risk with anterior placement of a sacroiliac screw?
110. What are the typical provocative maneuvers and the associated pathology of the hand and wrist?
111. What are the most common causes of in-toeing in children?
112. Type II beta errors can be minimized by performing what test?
113. What is the most appropriate diagnostic test to detect a proximal deep vein thrombosis?
114. What is the Salter-Harris classification of physeal injuries?
115. What is the most common benign bone tumor in childhood?
116. What is the energy requirement necessary to ambulate with an above-knee amputation?
117. What are the 2 types of Blount disease?
118. What is the rotator interval with regard to the shoulder?
119. What are the common causes of flap failures in the hand?
120. List the common risk factors that are associated with heterotopic ossification after a total knee arthroplasty.
121. What is the appropriate treatment of an acute Jones fracture?
122. What are the common anatomic abnormalities typically found with hip dysplasia?
123. What length of time after an Achilles tendon rupture is it considered a chronic injury and what are the implications?
124. What is Albers-Schönberg disease?
125. What are the constituents of the 3 layers on the medial and lateral sides of the knee?
126. What is the acceptable amount of deformity in treating fractures of the tibial plateau?
127. What are the 5 lubrication regimes described during motion of a joint?
128. A vertical medial malleolar fracture pattern is commonly seen with what mechanism of ankle fracture?
129. What factors most often lead to clubfoot recurrence?
130. What 2 bone morphogenetic proteins do not have osteogenic activity?
131. A 26-month-old child refuses to walk because of left hip pain with full ROM; he has a normal complete blood count, erythrocyte sedimentation rate, and C-reactive protein. What is the most likely diagnosis, and should you aspirate this hip?
132. What is the gold standard technique for meniscal repair?
133. Define type I error.
134. What factors play a role in receiving the largest dose of radiation from a C-arm procedure?
135. Name a difference often seen in children with a trigger finger compared with adults.
136. What is the most appropriate management of a segmental, closed humeral shaft fracture in a 16-month-old child?
137. Name some common complications of external beam radiation therapy for tumors.
138. What is the second leading cause of death in football players?
139. Hydrofluoric acid and white phosphorous burns can be treated with what chemicals?
140. What are the 3 types of tibial bowing in children?
141. What hematopoietic factors are associated with a hypercoagulable state during surgery?
142. What are the risk factors for a type II odontoid fracture nonunion?

143. When a tibial intramedullary nail for a shaft fracture goes on to nonunion, what is the best treatment option to manage this?
144. Name the different types of liposarcoma.
145. What are the typical contractures associated with clubfoot?
146. What is the anatomical difference in regard to the physis with a distal femur Salter-Harris I fracture compared with other parts of the body?
147. What is the sequential order of sensory nerve functional recovery?
148. Define a 3-point gait.
149. What is the name of the ligament that divides the greater from the lesser sciatic notch?
150. What 2 bone morphogenetic proteins do not have osteoinductive activity?
151. What is the most sensitive and specific modality for determining the presence of spondylolysis that is not seen on plain x-rays?
152. Describe the typical patient and findings for an eosinophilic granuloma.
153. What is the common fracture pattern associated with loss of fracture reduction after sacroiliac screw fixation of a pelvic ring injury?
154. What fragility fracture most consistently predicts a patient's increased risk for a hip fracture?
155. What are the borders of the cubital tunnel?
156. Steppage gait is associated with what physical abnormality?
157. True or false: Pulsatile lavage is better at reducing bacterial counts in wounds than bulb syringe irrigation during an irrigation and debridement.
158. For operative cases of thoracic and double major curves, what is the ideal treatment?
159. What is the mechanism of action of etanercept, infliximab, and adalimumab?
160. Nonoperative management of a tibial shaft fracture is acceptable with what fracture alignment?
161. What are the 3 main types of osteosarcoma?
162. What tests are allogeneic blood screened for during routine laboratory testing?
163. What is the appropriate treatment for 16-year-old boy with a displaced proximal humerus fracture without neurovascular injury?
164. The sciatic nerve typically lies where compared with the piriformis muscle?
165. What are the common portals for elbow arthroscopy and associated structures at risk?
166. What is the role of zona orbicularis?
167. What is the typical treatment for a stage 1 or 2 giant cell tumor of bone?
168. What are the modes of cemented femoral component loosening?
169. What are the general age guidelines for surgical management of the pediatric femoral shaft fracture?
170. What is the definition of Scheuermann's disease?
171. With a brachial plexus birth palsy, what portends a low likelihood of return of function?
172. What type of sternoclavicular injury requires vascular surgery on standby?
173. What test should be ordered in a patient who is 50 years old after sustaining a low-energy fracture?
174. What is the mechanism of action of the bisphosphonate drugs?
175. What structural abnormality of the capsule is commonly found with an overhead throwing athlete?
176. During open reduction and internal fixation of a comminuted tibial plateau fracture, what fragment often necessitates a separate approach for operative fixation?

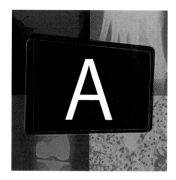

ANSWERS TO
"CRUNCH-TIME" SELF-TEST

1. Limited active ROM and passive ROM of the shoulder are the hallmarks of a frozen shoulder. Treatment consists of stretching because this is a self-limited disease with good to excellent outcomes in 90% of cases.
2. Distal tibia, distal femur, and distal ulna. Distal radius and proximal humerus growth arrest rarely occur.
3. Lateral collateral ligament (LCL), popliteofibular ligament, and biceps femoris. The popliteus does not insert on the LCL.
4. The lumbricals originate on the flexor digitorum profundus and insert on the radial lateral band of the extensor expansion, radial 2 are innervated by the median nerve and ulnar 2 by the ulnar nerve. These muscles also flex the metacarpophalangeal joints and extend the proximal interphalangeal joints.
5. False. The anterolateral portion is tight in flexion and the posteromedial portion is tight in extension. The ligament is approximately 38 mm in length and 13 mm in diameter, and mechanoreceptors provide a proprioceptive function. Meniscofemoral ligaments attach to the PCL anteriorly (Humphrey) and posteriorly (Wrisberg) and extend from the lateral meniscus.
6. Elbow flexion and full forearm supination can enhance stability of the fracture by tightening the interosseous membrane.
7. With aging, we see a decrease in water content, proteoglycans, chondroitin sulfate, and chondrocyte number. Alternatively, there is an increase in keratin sulfate, chondrocyte size, and modulus of elasticity. For osteoarthritic cartilage changes, there is an increase in water, proteoglycan synthesis, proteoglycan degradation (cathepsins B and D and metalloproteinases are increased), and chondroitin sulfate (shorter chains and increased chondroitin-to-keratin sulfate ratio). Concomitantly, there is a decrease in collagen content, proteoglycan content, keratin sulfate concentration, and modulus of elasticity.
8. Humerus, tibia, and femur. Should order skeletal survey when suspicious. Delayed development, multiple fractures, and spiral fractures should raise the level of suspicion for child abuse. Furthermore, fractures in preambulatory children, corner fractures, posterior rib, and a diaphysis greater than the metaphysis are indicators for abuse. Skin involvement is often the number one indicator.

Levine BR. *Acing the Orthopedic Board Exam:*
The Ultimate Crunch-Time Resource (pp 431-442).
© 2016 SLACK Incorporated.

9.   Preoperative intra-arterial embolization to prevent intraoperative hemorrhage because renal cell carcinoma is not radiosensitive.

10.   According to the Bado classification:
    o   Type I: anterior radial head dislocation and proximal one-third ulna fracture (apex anterior); most common (60%); open reduction and internal fixation cast in 110 degrees of flexion.
    o   Type II: posterior radial head dislocation and proximal one-third ulna fracture (apex posterior); 15%; open reduction and internal fixation; cast in 70 degrees of flexion.
    o   Type III: lateral radial head dislocation and ulnar metaphyseal fracture; open reduction and internal fixation with cast in 110 degrees of flexion.
    o   Type IV: anterior radial head dislocation with proximal one-third both-bone fracture; open reduction and internal fixation with cast in 110 degrees of flexion.

11.   Hyperextension of the proximal interphalangeal joint and flexion of the distal interphalangeal joint. Improper balance of forces at proximal interphalangeal joint occurs often secondary to metacarpophalangeal joint volar subluxation, mallet finger, laceration of flexor digitorum superficialis, and intrinsic contracture.

12.   Arcuate ligament (flexor carpi ulnaris aponeurosis), flexor-pronator aponeurosis, cubital tunnel, and arcade of Struthers.

13.   Sacral lateral: Safe zone for screw insertion is between the alar cortex and the sacral neural foramen.

14.   Can be bilateral in Paget's disease, Marfan syndrome, rheumatoid arthritis, ankylosing spondylitis, and osteomalacia.

15.   Less than 10 degrees of change in palmar tilt, less than 2 mm of radial shortening, less than 5 degrees of change in radial angle, less than 1 to 2 mm of articular step-off.

16.   Osteosarcoma occurs in a bimodal pattern in the second or sixth decade. Most commonly found in the metaphysis of the distal femur, proximal tibia, proximal humerus, and pelvis (remember, Codman triangle).

17.   Teres minor, superiorly; teres major, inferiorly; long head of triceps, medially; and humeral shaft, laterally. In the cocking position of throwing, the axillary nerve and posterior humeral circumflex artery may be compressed, causing posterior shoulder pain. The axillary nerve and posterior circumflex artery are found in this space.

18.   Level I: randomized, controlled trial; Level II: prospective cohort study; Level III: retrospective, case-controlled study; Level IV: case series (no control); Level V: expert opinion.

19.   The central slip of the extensor tendon: proximal interphalangeal joint develops a flexion deformity and distal interphalangeal joint and extension deformity.

20.   Iliotibial band: release if tight in extension; popliteus: release if tight in extension; posterior lateral capsule: release if tight in flexion; LCL: corrects flexion and extension and is often the first ligament released in balancing the valgus total knee arthroplasty.

21.   Lateral winging: trapezius palsy, spinal accessory nerve; medial winging: serratus anterior palsy, long thoracic nerve; and a rhomboid palsy, dorsal scapular nerve injury.

22.   Septic arthritis is most common in ages 0 to 2 years. The following are criteria for diagnosis: nonweight bearing on affected side, erythrocyte sedimentation rate greater than 40 mm/hr, fever, and a white blood cell count greater than 12,000 mm^3.
    o   When 4/4 criteria are met, there is a 99% chance that the child has septic arthritis.
    o   When 3/4 criteria are met, there is a 93% chance of septic arthritis.
    o   When 2/4 criteria are met, there is a 40% chance of septic arthritis.
    o   When 1/4 criteria are met, there is a 3% chance of septic arthritis.

23.   Reduced mechanical properties occur with increased irradiation of ultra-high-molecular-weight polyethylene: decrease in ultimate tensile strength, fracture toughness, and resistance to crack propagation. Wear resistance is improved with irradiation, with minimal improvements noted greater than the dose of 10 Mrads. Radiation leads to free radicals that must be quenched (remelting, annealing, or antioxidant doping).

24.   Knee stiffness is the most common complication.

25.   Ginseng, ginko, and garlic can increase the risk of bleeding; garlic and ginseng (irreversible inhibitors) should be stopped 1 week before surgery; and ginko should be stopped within 36 hours before a procedure.

26.   Usually by 6 months, the femoral head is visible on plain x-rays. This may vary with the presence of hip dysplasia, and ultrasound is used prior to this time frame.

27. Early active range of motion (ROM) is indicated through a stable arc. Passive ROM is associated with heterotopic ossification, and more than 3 weeks of immobilization is associated with stiffness.

28. Bilateral open reduction through a medial approach is the preferred response. Typically with arthrogryposis (a nonprogressive disorder with multiple congenitally rigid joints), closed reduction and/or traction will likely be unsuccessful. Open reduction through an anterior approach is reserved for older patients.

29. Sagittal plane imbalance is associated with the inability to maintain neutral upright stance and is correlated with adverse health outcomes and pain; more than curve magnitude, location, or coronal imbalance. Also difficult to control in juveniles.

30. Posterior interosseous nerve.

31. Extraligamentous (50%), subligamentous (30%), transligamentous (20%).

32. Calcium phosphate. Calcium sulfate is quickly resorbed (yet has been associated with increased wound drainage), and fresh allograft has the highest risk of disease transmission for allografts.

33. Tendon repair strength is proportional to the number of sutures bridging the repair. To initiate an active motion therapy protocol, a strong or 4-strand repair technique is needed. Epitendinous sutures help support the repair and add strength.

34. Femoral neck fracture (notching increases the risk for this complication).

35. Lateral plantar artery and nerve.

36. Twenty-three percent, particularly in patients older than 60 years. It is a more common complication than osteonecrosis, nerve injury, infection, and nonunion. An anatomic neck fracture is a relative contraindication for a locked plate.

37. Patients with cervical myelopathy (look for neurologic signs, clumsiness, hyperreflexia, Hoffman's sign, and clonus) at multiple levels and greater than 13 degrees of kyphosis will not see the typical posterior shift of the spinal cord with a direct posterior decompression. Therefore, an anterior decompression and kyphosis correction is needed.

38. Base deficit, lactic acid levels, or both.

39. Alendronate has been associated with low-energy subtrochanteric and diaphyseal femur fractures despite decreasing the risk of femoral neck and vertebral fractures. Look at x-rays carefully for thickened cortices and black line.

40. Intermuscular septum, Osborne's ligament, fascia of the flexor carpi ulnaris, and the deep flexor-pronator aponeurosis.

41. Anterolateral bar with a contralateral quadrant vertebrae.

42. Homeobox genes: Products of these genes play a critical role in axial skeleton development, particularly maintaining a standard sequential activation.

43. Vertical tunnel malposition leads to increased rotational instability and subsequent degenerative changes of the knee, whereas posterior placement of the tibial tunnel is associated with early graft rupture.

44. Class 1: Circulation is intact. Can treat bone and soft tissue in standard manner. Class 2: Poor circulation, needs vessel repair. 2A: No additional bone-tendon-nerve injury. 2B: Bone-tendon-nerve injuries are present. Class 3: Complete degloving or amputation. Types 2B and 3 are better treated with amputation, and cold intolerance occurs in 30% to 70%.

45. EMTALA: The Emergency Medical Treatment and Active Labor Act.

46. Repetitive hyperextension causes impaction of the inferior articular process of cephalad vertebrae into the pars of the caudad vertebrae, and single-limb stance typically exacerbates the lower back pain.

47. RANK is a type I membrane protein that is found on the surface of osteoclasts. Once bound by RANKL (ligand), osteoclasts are activated and proceed with bone destruction associated with metastatic bone disease.

48. A—Complete, no motor or sensory function is preserved; B—Incomplete, sensory but not motor is preserved below neurological level; C—Incomplete, motor function is preserved below the neurological level and more than 50% of the key muscles have less than or equal to 3/5 strength; D—Incomplete, at least 50% of key muscles have a grade of 3/5 or more; E—Normal.

49. Angiofibroblastic hyperplasia: characterized by fibroblast hypertrophy, disorganized collagen, and vascular hyperplasia.

50. Reserve zone:
    - ○ Low oxygen (anaerobic), matrix production, and storage of lipids.
    - ○ Disorders: Gaucher's (beta-glucocerebrosidase deficiency), diastrophic dysplasia (sulfate transport protein defect), Kniest (type II collagen defect), pseudoachondroplasia (cartilage oligomeric matrix protein defect).

    Proliferative zone:
    - ○ Longitudinal growth with stacking of chondrocytes and increased oxygen tension. This zone functions in cellular proliferation (like name!) and matrix production.
    - ○ Disorders: Achondroplasia (fibroblast growth factor receptor 3 defect), gigantism, hypochondroplasia, malnutrition, irradiation injury.

    Hypertrophic zone:
    - ○ Broken down into 3 zones: Chondrocyte growth is controlled by systemic hormones and local factors. For example, chondrocyte maturation is inhibited by parathyroid-related peptide.
    - ○ Maturation: Chondrocytes grow and are prepared for matrix calcification.
    - ○ Degenerative: Chondrocytes are 5 times the size while accumulating calcium.
    - ○ Provisional calcification: Cells die and release calcium, matrix is calcified.
    - ○ Disorders: Slipped capital femoral epiphysis (not associated with renal disease), rickets (provisional calcification zone), spondyloepiphyseal dysplasia (type II collagen defect), multiple epiphyseal dysplasia, Schmid (Type X collagen defect), Kniest, mucopolysaccharidosis (Hurler's and Morquio's syndromes), enchondromas, physeal fractures.

    Metaphysis:
    - ○ Primary spongiosa: Calcified cartilage bars are formed from aligning osteoblasts, which generate woven bone that can be remodeled.
    - ○ Disorders: Metaphyseal chondrodysplasia (Jansen, parathyroid hormone-related protein defect, and Schmid), acute osteomyelitis.
    - ○ Secondary spongiosa: Remodeling of above woven bone in response to stress.
    - ○ Disorders: Osteopetrosis, osteogenesis imperfect, scurvy, metaphyseal dysplasia (Pyle's disease), renal, slipped capital femoral epiphysis.

51. The t11:22 translocation (EWS/FLI1) is associated with the second most common primary bone tumor in children. There is a male:female predominance (3:2), and it is typically found in the pelvis, long bone diaphysis, and scapula. Small, round, blue cells on histology with CD99+ characteristic.

52. Inflammatory arthritis, flexion contracture greater than 15 degrees, greater than 10 degrees varus or 5-degree valgus angular deformity, absence of anterior cruciate ligament, adjacent compartment degenerative changes, and possibly body mass index greater than 32 kg/m^2.

53. Odontoid fractures most often occur at the basilar synchondrosis at the base of the dens. Closed reduction with neck extension and immobilization for 6 to 8 weeks is usually sufficient.

54. Zone 2 affects the deep branch of the nerve and produces a pure motor deficit affecting the intrinsic muscles: motor to the hypothenar, 2 medial lumbricals, interossei, and adductor pollicis. Zone 1 injuries occur prior to the nerve bifurcation and give a mixed sensory and motor deficit. Zone 3 compression leads to compression of the superficial branch of the nerve giving a motor deficit to the palmaris brevis and sensory to the small and ring fingers.

55. Prior formation of heterotopic ossification, diffuse idiopathic skeletal hyperostosis, hypertrophic osteoarthrosis, posttraumatic arthritis, and ankylosing spondylitis; best treated with a single dose (700 cgy) of pre- or postoperative radiation.

56. This is the angle formed by a line perpendicular to the sacral endplate and a line drawn from the midpoint of the sacral endplate to the center of the femoral heads. Increased pelvic incidence correlates with the presence and severity of spondylolisthesis.

57. Hypertrophic cardiomyopathy (young), coronary artery disease (older), and commotion cordis (cardiac contusion from a direct blow to the chest).

58. One-sample t test, paired t test, and analysis of variance test. The first compares the sample mean to a known mean of a standard, the 2-sample compares the mean from 2 independent groups, and a paired t test compares 2 dependent samples. Analysis of variance is used when there are more than 2 independent groups being compared.

59. The superior lateral genicular artery. As with a standard medial parapatellar approach, the 3 medial arteries are cut to the patella (superior and inferior medial genicular arteries and the middle genicular). The inferior lateral genicular artery is taken with the lateral meniscus, leaving the superior lateral artery as the remaining blood supply to the patella. Sacrifice of this artery can lead to osteonecrosis of the patella, anterior knee pain, patella fracture, and premature failure of the patella component.

60. Serum albumin less than 3.5 g/dL, lymphocyte count less than 1500/mm^3, hemoglobin less than 10 g/dL, ischemic index less than 0.5, Doppler pressure less than 70 mm Hg, transcutaneous partial pressure of oxygen less than 20 mm Hg.

61.

Vascular	*Neurogenic*
Walking: Distal-proximal pain, calf pain	Proximal-distal, thigh pain
Uphill walking: Symptoms come sooner	Symptoms come later
Rest: Relief with sitting or bending	No significant relief noted
Bicycling: Symptoms develop	No symptoms
Lying flat: Relief of symptoms	May exacerbate symptoms

62. Blomstrand syndrome and lead poisoning.

63. A polycentric design with hydraulic swing control. These provide the function closest to a normal knee; pneumatic systems are less efficient, and constant-friction devices can only walk at one speed (the same is essentially true for single-axis [hinge] designs). Manual locking knee is ideal for weak or unstable patients but requires excessive energy to power.

64. Alkaline phosphatase, serum bone specific alkaline phosphatase, procollagen I N-terminal peptide, urinary N-telopeptide, and alpha-C-telopeptide are sensitive markers of bone formation and resorption in Paget's disease.

65. True. The coracoclavicular ligaments prevent inferior translation of the coracoid and acromion from the clavicle.

66. Thoracolumbosacral orthosis and early mobilization: nonoperative treatment.

67. The Stoppa approach is an extended Pfannenstiel approach that provides the best exposure to the quadrilateral surface of the acetabulum. Incision is made above the pubic symphysis with a midline split of the rectus abdominis. Provides access to the pubic body, superior pubic ramus, pubic root, ilium, quadrilateral plate, sciatic buttress, and anterior sacroiliac joint.

68. External rotation is used to test the medial meniscus and internal rotation the lateral meniscus. This is done after the knee is forcibly flexed, then rotated, and, lastly, extended slowly. A palpable and audible noise will occur with a positive test.

69. Powder consists of prepolymerized polymethylmethacrylate, radio-opacifier (zirconium dioxide or barium sulphate), and an initiator (di-benzoyl peroxide). The liquid consists of methylmethacrylate monomer, stabilizer (hydroquinone prevents premature polymerization), and an accelerator (N,N-dimethyl-p-toluidine). Typically mixed at a roughly 2:1 ratio, and antibiotics can be added to the powder portion.

70. Chi-square test and Fisher exact test for 2 or more samples with different individuals or McNemar's or Cochran Q-test when samples are related. For ordered categorical or continuous and non-normal tests, include the Mann-Whitney U test and Wilcoxon rank sum test for 2 samples and the Kruskal-Wallis or Friedman statistic for more than 3 samples.

71. Also known as familial osteochondromatosis. This is an autosomal-dominant disorder that stems from a mutation in the chromosomes 8q23-q24 (EXT1), 11p11-p12 (EXT2), and 19p (EXT3).

72. Partial, isolated ruptures, grades I and II, are treated with early rest and limited activity followed by a regimen of quads strengthening (think quad strength to help keep the tibia anterior in PCL injuries and hamstrings to keep tibia posterior in anterior cruciate ligament injuries)

73. Radiostereometric analysis; accuracy has been found to be 0.02 mm.

74. Balance is the key predictor; maximum motor recovery can be expected by 6 months for a stroke and by 12 to 18 months for a traumatic brain injury.

75. Plantarflexed first metatarsal, elevated arch, dorsiflexion of the calcaneus, and posterior positioning of the fibula relative to tibia.

76. Chicken wire appearance = calcification around cells. Most commonly found in distal femur, proximal humerus, or proximal tibia in ages 10 to 25 years. Histology shows sheets of chondroblasts.

77. A Myerson/Ludloff procedure is the common test answer; this is a proximal first metatarsal osteotomy with a lateral metatarsophalangeal joint soft tissue release. Distal osteotomies are reserved for more mild deformities.

78. Warm ischemia time of greater than 6 hours, a defect that cannot be reconstructed, or if further attempts at saving the limb may lead to increased risk of death (remember, life over limb!).

79. Diabetes mellitus (foot/ankle), tabes dorsalis (lower extremity, secondary to syphilis), syringomyelia (most common cause of upper extremity neuropathic arthropathy), Hansen's disease (upper extremities), myelomeningocele (foot/ankle), spinal cord injury, and congenital insensitivity to pain.)

80. Beta error is the failure to reject a false null hypothesis (a false negative).

81. Osteogenesis imperfecta: COL1A1 and COL1A2 genes on chromosome 17.

82. This is an x-linked, dominant form of rickets that is caused by a mutation in the PHEX gene (basically disrupts phosphate excretion). The increased excretion of phosphate leads to impaired bone mineralization. On laboratory tests, there will be low serum phosphate (high urine phosphate levels), normal or near normal calcium (different from normal rickets), and low calcitriol (vitamin D3). X-rays show bowing of long bones and physeal cupping and widening.

83. Painful pseudarthrosis (0% to 10%); mechanical low back pain (most common, often due to increased abduction or excessive limb-length discrepancy with initial fusion); knee pain/instability (ipsilateral knee with adducted position of fusion and contralateral with abduction); and contralateral hip pain. Remember, fusion should be in neutral abduction (or 0 to 5 degrees of adduction, 0 to 15 degrees of external rotation, and 25 to 30 degrees of flexion).

84. Type III is superior displacement of the lateral clavicle with disruption of the periosteal tube; it is treated symptomatically with a sling, as are types I and II. Types IV through VI require an open reduction and repair of the periosteal sleeve.

85. A Bennett lesion: found in 22% of asymptomatic major league pitchers.

86. Fluid resuscitation, loop diuretics, dialysis, weight bearing/activity, and drug therapy: bisphosphonates, mithramycin, calcitonin, and gallium nitrate.

87. The nonunion, iatrogenic radial nerve injury, and infection rates are higher with plating, but nails have a higher rate of reoperation and shoulder impingement. Overall functional scores and pain ratings are equivalent between these treatment options.

88. Inadequate sedation, interposed soft tissues (namely posterior tibial tendon or flexor hallucis longus), and protrusion of the osseous structures (buttonholing).

89. False. This is the advantage of the quad-snip over turndown and VY-plasty for exposure. For tibial tubercle osteotomy, some will not restrict ROM or weight bearing, but this can be controversial.

90. Posterior lateral corner, while laxity at both indicates a posterior cruciate ligament (PCL) and PLC injury.

91. This is used to describe the hypoplastic thumb; remember, the most important factor of a reconstructable thumb is the presence of a stable carpometacarpal joint. Type I, minimal shortening and narrowing (no treatment); type II, thumb-index webspace narrowing, hypoplastic thenar muscles, metacarpophalangeal joint instability (stabilize metacarpophalangeal joint, release webspace, and opponensplasty); type IIIA, type II + extrinsic tendon abnormalities, stable carpometacarpal and hypoplastic metacarpal (same treatment as type II); type IIIB, type II + partial metacarpal aplasia and unstable carpometacarpal; type IV, floating thumb; type V, absent thumb (last 3 treated with thumb amputation and pollicization).

92. Galvanic corrosion.

93. Diastrophic dwarfism.

94. External rotation of the femoral and tibial components, lateralize the femoral implant, avoid excessive valgus alignment of the limb, place the patella in a medial and superior position, avoid too large of a cut on the distal femur (raises the joint line).

95. This is an autosomal-dominant disorder related to a mutation of the FGFr2 gene leading to the following structural disorders: complex syndactyly (rosebud or spoon hand; index, middle, and ring fingers share a common nail), symphalangism, cranial synostosis, acrocephaly, radioulnar synostosis, and hypertelorism.

96. Denis: Zone 3 (medial to the neural foramen). These are the least common fractures but are associated with a nearly 60% rate of nerve injury often resulting in bowel, bladder, and sexual dysfunction.

97. False. Smaller particles of greater volume tend to be generated with newer bearings; some believe these smaller particles are below the osteolysis threshold, which has led to a reduced incidence of osteolysis with these modern bearings.

98. Teratologic hip dislocations should not be managed with a Pavlik harness. The harness has been associated with femoral nerve palsy with excessive flexion as well as osteonecrosis from impingement of the posterosuperior retinacular branch of the medial femoral circumflex artery.

99. Traditionally, annealing and remelting of the polyethylene can reduce free radicals; a more modern option is the process of using vitamin E–infused polyethylene to quench free radicals.

100. The key is the equinus contracture; if you see this, the answer is total contact casting with an Achilles lengthening. The release affords decreased peak plantar pressures on the forefoot and lower ulcer recurrence rates.

101. Implantable direct current bone stimulators vs pulsed ultrasound, which works by simulation nanomotion/mechanical stimulation of the fracture site.

102. Greater than 2 mm SL interval, cortical ring sign (proximal and distal poles of scaphoid overlap), greater than 70-degree SL angle on lateral. Persistent dissociation leads to a dorsal intercalated segment instability deformity.

103. The power of a study is the probability of finding a significant association in a study when one truly exists (essentially, the probability of not committing a type II error).

104. Congenital abnormalities associated with failure of closure of the spinal cord. Related to folate deficiency, increased alpha fetoprotein in utero, and chromosomal abnormalities (trisomy 13 and 18). Sudden changes, such as increased curvature of scoliosis, spasticity, neurologic deficits, or frequent urinary tract infections, are signs in a vignette to look for a tethered cord, hydrocephalus, or hydromyelia. Defined by lowest functioning level: L3 and below can ambulate.
    - ○ Spina bifida occulta: Defect in the vertebral arch, with neural elements confined
    - ○ Meningocele: Sac protrudes out but with no neural elements
    - ○ Myelomeningocele: Sac protrudes out with the neural elements
    - ○ Rachischisis: Neural elements are exposed with no sac covering them

105. The anterior interosseous nerve arises from the median nerve and innervates the flexor pollicis longus, pronator quadratus, and flexor digitorum profundus of the index and long fingers.

106. There are 13 types of collagen. Type I: bone, tendon skin, meniscus, vertebral disk annulus; type II: nucleus pulposus and articular cartilage; type III: skin and blood vessels; type IV: basement membrane; types V and VI: articular cartilage; types VII and VIII: basement membranes; type IX: articular cartilage; type X: hypertrophic cartilage/associated with calcification of cartilage; type XI: articular cartilage; type XII: tendon; and type XIII: endothelial cells.

107. K-wire migration and local skin complications can lead to removal of hardware in up to 81%; common with intramedullary placement of wires. To prevent this, wires can be directed out of the volar ulnar cortex. Beware: this can lead to reduced forearm rotation; it is suggested to start more lateral on the olecranon and direct the wires toward the ulnar midshaft to avoid this complication.

108. Pistoning of the prosthesis while walking (swing phase) is caused by a failure of the suspension system: too soft of a foot affords excessive knee extension, and too hard of a foot leads to knee flexion and lateral rotation of the toes. Malalignment and poor socket fit can lead to irritation and pain, which can limit use of the prosthesis.

109. The L5 nerve root is at risk if the superior/anterior cortex is violated.

110. Watson's test: scapholunate (SL) interval instability; Regan test: lunotriquetral interval instability; Kleinman test: dynamic assessment of lunotriquetral instability; Lichtman test: dynamic assessment of midcarpal instability; triangular fibrocartilage complex (TFCC) grind: assesses for TFCC pathology; extensor carpi ulnaris (ECU) snap: assesses for TFCC pathology; ECU snap: assesses for unstable ECU; and piano key sign—DRUJ instability.

111. Internal tibial torsion (normal 6 to 10 degrees of external rotation), metatarsus adductus (resolves spontaneously in ~90%), and excessive femoral anteversion. Less common pathological conditions include clubfoot, skewfoot, hip disorders, and neuromuscular diseases.

112. Power analysis.

113. Venous ultrasonography is the gold standard, with sensitivities from 95% to 100%.

114. Type I: transverse fracture through physis; type II: fracture through the physis with exit through the metaphysis; type III: fracture through the physis and epiphysis; type IV: fracture through the epiphysis, physis, and metaphysis; type V: crush injury to the physis; type VI: injury to the perichondral ring.

115. Nonossifying fibroma: found in approximately 30% of children; common in the metaphyseal region of long bones, particularly around the knee and distal tibia. Jaffe-Campanacci syndrome consists of multiple nonossifying fibromas. The histology of these lesions includes fibroblastic cells in a whirled or storiform pattern with giant cells and hemosiderin. It's usually treated nonoperatively unless there is an impending fracture.

116. 65% energy above baseline for an above-knee amputation; 10% for a long transtibial; 25% for an average transtibial and bilateral below-knee amputation/short unilateral below-knee amputation require an approximate 40% increase in energy to ambulate.

117. Infantile Blount: More common, often bilateral, overweight, early walking children (younger than 1 year), and associated with tibial torsion. Check for metaphyseal beaking, epiphyseal-metaphyseal angle, metaphyseal-diaphyseal angle (Drennan angle greater than 16 degrees is abnormal). Early Langenskiold stages are braced with later disease, requiring surgery.

Adolescent Blount: Less severe, often on one side; try to treat with lateral epiphysiodesis if growth remains; if not, then osteotomy and possible distraction osteogenesis will be necessary.

118. The interval between the subscapularis and the supraspinatus tendons. The glenohumeral and coracohumeral ligaments are found in this interval. Closing it down results in a decrease in external rotation of the adducted arm but not the abducted arm.

119. Inflow issues include inadequate arterial blood flow, vasospasm, hypotension, hematoma, compression, edema, infection, hypothermia, and use of nicotine. Outflow issues such as venous congestion can lead to a purple discoloration of the flap.

120. The incidence of heterotopic ossification after total knee arthroplasty ranges from 1% to 42%. Common risk factors include trauma, neurologic injury, and burn injuries. Comorbidities that can be associated with heterotopic ossification formation include ankylosing spondylitis, diffuse idiopathic skeletal hyperostosis, infection, hypertrophic osteoarthritis, prior heterotopic ossification, obesity, and male sex.

121. An acute fracture of the base of the proximal fifth metatarsal (Jones fracture) is best treated with a short leg nonweight-bearing cast for 6 weeks; screw fixation can be offered to a high-performance athlete.

122. Common abnormalities of the femur include a small femoral head, short and anteverted femoral neck, small femoral canal, valgus femoral neck, and posterior greater trochanter. Acetabulum findings include shallow depth, lateralized position, anteverted, and deficient in the anterior-superior quadrant. Overall femoral head-acetabulum contact area is decreased, with increased stress over a small area and the potential for future degenerative joint disease.

123. Greater than 3 months = chronic injury; at this time frame, a repair may require a turndown or V-Y advancement (<4 cm defects) or tendon transfer (flexor hallucis longus/flexor digitorum longus/PB) if the defect is greater than 5 cm.

124. This is the autosomal-dominant tarda, or benign, form of osteopetrosis. Generalized osteosclerosis with pathologic fractures through brittle bones are common. This is different from the malignant, infantile form that leads to hepatosplenomegaly and aplastic anemia, which often results in an early death. It is autosomal recessive and requires an early bone marrow transport. The pathophysiology is related to decreased osteoclast and chondroclast function.

125.

Medial	Lateral
Layer I: sartorius and fascia	Layer I: iliotibial tract, biceps, fascia
Layer II: superficial medial collateral ligament, posterior oblique ligament, semimembranosus	Layer II: patellar retinaculum, patellofemoral ligament
Layer III: deep medial collateral ligament, capsule	Layer III: arcuate ligament, fabellofibular ligament, capsule, lateral collateral ligament

126. Up to 5 degrees of mechanical axis deviation, 3 mm of articular incongruency, 5 mm of condylar widening, and 10 degrees of ligamentous laxity.

127. The coefficient of friction for a human joint is 0.002 to 0.04. Cartilage damage (fibrillation) during fluid film formation increases this coefficient; synovial fluid and elastic deformation of articular cartilage lower it.
     - Elastohydrodynamic: Low coefficient of friction with thin fluid film between surfaces. The coefficient of friction is a property of the lubricant, not the surfaces. Articular surfaces typically capable of deforming to allow optimal lubrication.
     - Boundary: The lubrication only partially separates the surfaces because the bearing surfaces do not deform (often seen with modern day total joint arthroplasties).
     - Boosted: Areas of lubrication are trapped between contact points of the articular surfaces. This generates a higher coefficient of friction with this regime.
     - Hydrodynamic: Fluid separates the surfaces under a loading force.
     - Weeping: Fluid shifts to loaded areas.
128. Supination adduction pattern of injury.
129. Compliance with postcorrection bracing (external rotation in boots and bars); of note, 80% require a tendo-Achilles lengthening and 25% require an anterior tibialis transfer to correct residual equinus and forefoot adduction/supination, respectively.
130. BMP3 and BMP12.
131. Toxic synovitis: At this age and with a negative infection workup, this is the likely diagnosis that will resolve in a self-limited manner. Ultrasound may show a joint effusion, but time is the cure. Aspiration is not necessary; although you would not be faulted for doing it in reality, the test answer would be not to.
132. The inside-out technique is the gold standard with vertical mattress sutures. Beware the saphenous nerve with medial repairs and the peroneal nerve with lateral ones.
133. Alpha error is the incorrect rejection of a true null hypothesis (a false positive).
134. The large C-arm gives off more radiation than the smaller (mini) machine; placing a body part closer to the radiation source imparts more radiation, and attempting to expose a larger cross-sectional area requires greater radiation. Remember, larger machine, closer to the machine, and larger the body part examined = more radiation.
135. Children have a higher rate of distal triggering at the sublimis decussation. Adults typically have pain and tenderness at the A1 pulley where the triggering is occurring. In adults, this is often associated with rheumatoid arthritis, amyloidosis, and diabetes mellitus, with the ring finger being affected most commonly.
136. Placement of a coaptation splint/cuff and collar with securing the arm to the thorax. Internal fixation is reserved for multitrauma cases, and external fixation is used to treat fractures associated with a significant soft tissue injury.
137. Postirradiation sarcoma: Typically a spindle cell sarcoma in the area of radiation treatment (Ewing's, lymphoma, myeloma, metastatic disease) with histologic findings consistent with an osteosarcoma, fibrosarcoma, or malignant fibrous histiocytoma. The incidence is approximately 13%.
     Stress fractures: Can occur in weight-bearing bones, often in the subtrochanteric and diaphyseal regions of the femur.
     Others: Skin breakdown, burns, infection, joint stiffness, and fibrosis.
138. Heat stroke: Characterized by collapse, neurological deficits, tachycardia, tachypnea, hypotension and anhidrosis; rapidly cool the patient to treat this condition.
139. Calcium gluconate and 1% copper sulfate solution, respectively.
140. Posteromedial: Typically a physiological bowing related to intrauterine positioning (commonly found in calcaneovalgus feet); will correct spontaneously; often results in shortening of up to 3 to 4 cm (this is typically a symptomatic LLD).
     Anteromedial: Usually found with fibular hemimelia (bowing, ankle instability, equinovarus foot, absent lateral rays, tarsal coalition, shortening of the femur, and proximal focal femoral deficiency/coxa vara). On ball-and-socket ankle on x-rays, a skin dimple is often clinically found. Treatment is based on foot deformity and degree if limb shortening (bracing vs amputation).
     Anterolateral: Congenital pseudarthrosis of the tibia leads to anterolateral bowing and is often found with neurofibromatosis. Treatment involves total contact casting, intramedullary fixation of fractures, vascularized grafting, or amputation (Syme's). Osteotomies to correct the deformity are contraindicated.
141. Deficiencies in protein C, protein S, and antithrombin III; presence of lupus anticoagulant, factor V Leiden, activated protein C resistance, prothrombin G 20210A mutation; excess homocysteine, lipoprotein A, anticardiolipin antibody; factor VIII, IX, or XI; increased platelet with myeloproliferative disorders.

142. This is the most common odontoid fracture through the base of the bone. Nonunion can occur in 30% to 50% of cases. It includes a fracture gap greater than 1 mm, posterior displacement greater than 5 mm (posterior displacement worse than anterior), delayed treatment of greater than 4 days, posterior redisplacement of greater than 2 mm, angulation greater than 10 degrees, older patient age, and comminution at the base of the odontoid.

143. Reamed, locked exchange nailing; a tibial nonunion fracture older than 6 months; or no evidence of healing in 3 consecutive months. When a dynamization procedure (axial stable fractures with minimal callus at 3 months) is the choice, you will need to osteotomize the fibula if healed.

144. Well-differentiated liposarcoma: low grade (< 10% chance of metastasis); 3 types: lipoma-like, sclerosing, and inflammatory.
Myxoid liposarcoma: intermediate grade, 10% to 30% chance of metastasis.
Dedifferentiated liposarcoma: high grade, greater than 50% chance of metastasis.
Round cell liposarcoma: high grade, greater than 50% chance of metastasis.
Pleomorphic liposarcoma: high grade, greater than 50% chance of metastasis.

145. Congenital talipes equinovarus is associated with forefoot adductus (tight tibialis posterior), forefoot supination (tight tibialis anterior), midfoot cavus (tight intrinsics, flexor hallucis longus, flexor digitorum longus), hindfoot varus (tight Achilles and tibialis posterior), and hindfoot equinus (tight Achilles). This is corrected with serial casting to rotate the foot laterally around a fixed talus. The following steps are taken: midfoot cavus, forefoot adductus, hindfoot varus, hindfoot equinus (90% success rate). Last cast corrects the equinus and should be placed in 70 degrees of abduction.

146. The distal femoral physis is undulating, and a fracture through the growth plate typically involves multiple layers of the physis. Typically, Salter-Harris I fractures occur through the zone of provisional calcification of the zone of hypertrophy (in the physis).

147. Anesthesia → proprioception → pain → moving touch → moving 2-point discrimination → static 2-point discrimination → monofilament and vibration testing.

148. This is when a patient walks with both crutches moving forward at the same time with the affected limb; all weight is placed on the crutches and the unaffected limb swings forward (typically used when one lower extremity is to be nonweight bearing).

149. Sacrospinous ligament.

150. Bone morphogenic proteins (BMP) 3 and 12 have no osteoinductive activity, whereas 2, 4, 6, and 7 all have activity within the transforming growth factor–β superfamily.

151. Bone scan with single-photon emission computed tomography is better than magnetic resonance imaging or oblique x-rays. Look for pain with back extension (often in football players) in the vignette description.

152. It is most common in children (younger than 20 years), occurs more often in males than females, can occur in any bone (more commonly in the skull, ribs, clavicle, scapula, vertebrae, long bones, and pelvis), and looks like a punched-out lesion, and histology shows histiocytes with coffee bean nuclei and eosinophilic cytoplasm (lots of small round, blue cells with pink-orange cytoplasm) with scattered giant cells.

153. A vertical shear pattern of fracture with vertical sacral fracture.

154. A proximal humerus fracture (hazard ratio of 5.68) is more predictive than vertebral fractures and distal radius fractures.

155. Floor = medial collateral ligament of elbow and roof = 2 heads of flexor carpi ulnaris (Osborne's ligament).

156. This is a common gait after a peroneal nerve palsy/injury or foot drop. It is characterized by lifting the leg high in the air with the toes pointing down. The foot then almost slaps to the ground. It commonly occurs with direct injury, multiple sclerosis, and spinal cord injuries.

157. Bulb syringe with saline-only irrigation has been shown to be the best at reducing bacterial counts in wounds compared to high-pressure lavage techniques.

158. Posterior spinal fusion with instrumentation has been the gold standard, but combined anterior and posterior fusions are indicated for severe deformities (> 75 degrees), around peak growth velocity, and to prevent a crankshaft phenomenon. Anterior fusion alone can save fusion levels with a good correction but can be associated with kyphosis and pseudoarthrosis.

159. These medications are tumor necrosis factor-α inhibitors and are not to be confused with anakinra, which is an interleukin-1 inhibitor.

160. No more than 5 degrees of varus or valgus angulation, sagittal plane angulation less than 10 degrees, at least 50% cortical apposition, rotational alignment within 10 degrees, and less than 1 cm of shortening.

161. Intramedullary osteosarcoma: Can be high or low grade (most common type). Typically occurs about the knee in children or young adults but can also occur in the shoulder, proximal femur, and pelvis. Ninety percent are high grade and penetrate the bony cortex with an associated soft tissue lesion. Telangiectatic osteosarcoma looks like a bag of blood and can be confused with aneurysmal bone cysts. Treated with chemotherapy, resection, and chemotherapy (in that order).

   Parosteal osteosarcoma: Occurs on the metaphyseal surface of long bones (distal femur, proximal tibia, proximal humerus); females are more commonly affected. Typically have some areas of cartilage in the lesion. With local control of the tumor, there is a greater than 95% long-term survival rate.

   Periosteal osteosarcoma: Rare condition found in the diaphysis of long bones (femur and tibia) with chondroblastic look on histological evaluation. Pulmonary mets occur in 20% to 35%.

162. HIV-1, HIV-2, hepatitis C, syphilis, West Nile virus, and hepatitis B. Some not tested for include Lyme disease, malaria, and Chagas' disease.

163. At this age, the child has limited remodeling potential via the growth plate, so closed reduction and pin fixation is likely the best option; arthroplasty and cast management are not options at this age.

164. Complete nerve typically lies posterior to the piriformis muscle, exiting distally in approximately 79% of cases. Two divisions occur in 14.3% (one passes through muscle, the other beneath it), a complete nerve pierces muscle in approximately 2%, and an early split of the nerve occurs in 4.4%.

165. Anterolateral portal (1 cm distal and anterior to the lateral epicondyle): lateral antebrachial cutaneous and radial nerves; anteromedial portal (2 cm distal and anterior to the medial epicondyle): medial antebrachial cutaneous and median nerves; posterolateral portal (2 cm proximal to olecranon).

166. The zona orbicularis represents the terminal fibers of the iliofemoral ligament. This portion of the capsule is an important structure for hip stability in distraction.

167. Curettage and bone grafting or cementation of the lesion: typically, this is done with a high-speed burr to remove 5 mm of normal surrounding bone.

168. Modes:
    - IA: Pistoning → stem subsides in the cement mantle; may see cement mantle fracture.
    - IB: Pistoning → stem and cement mantle subside within the femur.
    - II: Medial stem pivot → superomedial and inferolateral cement failure/insufficiency; may see varus remodeling of the femur.
    - III: Calcar pivot → windshield wiper motion distally with medial and lateral toggle of the distal stem.
    - IV: Cantilever bending → distal cement holds well, but proximal cement fixation is lost; can see fatigue fracture of the implant.

169. Younger than 6 years: spica casting with or without period of traction; 6 to 13 years old: flexible titanium nails with possible casting, ex-fix (higher refracture rate), plate fixation (have to remove at some point); older than 14 years: intramedullary nail.

170. Thoracic kyphosis greater than 45 degrees with 3 sequential vertebrae experiencing anterior wedging of more than 5 degrees. Radiographic findings include disk space narrowing, spondylolysis, scoliosis, Schmorl's nodes, and endplate abnormalities. Typically treated posteriorly unless curves are greater than 75 degrees or correct to less than 55 degrees on extension x-rays, then anterior release and posterior fusion is necessary.

171. Horner syndrome (disruption of the sympathetic chain) is a sign for a worse prognosis: ptosis, miosis, and anhidrosis. Remember, Erb's palsy (C5-C6) leads to a waiter's tip deformity, and Klumpke's (C8-T1) yields a claw hand. However, a positive twitch biceps activity correlates with a good prognosis.

172. Posterior dislocations can be reduced with a towel clip but need vascular surgery on standby. The anterior dislocation can be reduced with a bump between the shoulders. Typical complications include cosmetic bump, degenerative joint disease, and obtrusive bump with mediastinal impingement when dislocation occurs posteriorly.

173. Dual-energy x-ray absorptiometry (DEXA) scan; it's the gold standard to detect osteoporosis. The T-score is the comparison to the bone density to that of a 30-year-old sex-matched patient, and the Z-score is an age/sex/ethnicity-matched bone density score.

174. The nitrogenous drugs bind to the enzyme farnesyl diphosphate synthase in osteoclasts and prevent their function (in HMG-CoA reductase pathway), the R2 long-chain of the drug affects the strength, and the R1 short-chain the pharmacokinetics.

175. Contracture of the posteroinferior capsule is commonly related to the stress loads associated with the follow-through motion of throwing. This motion places the arm in a forward flexed, adducted, and internally rotated position in which the posterior capsule limits posterior translation of the arm.

176. A posteromedial fragment needs to be visualized and reduced through a separate incision and posteromedial approach to the tibial plateau (often asked about because lateral locked plates do not capture this fragment well).

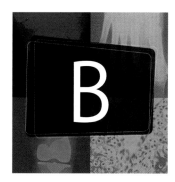

SELF-TEST SCORING GUIDE

Based on percentage of questions you take:

90% to 100%: You likely looked at the answers (aka cheated!).

80% to 89%: It's highly likely you still cheated.

70% to 79%: You are ready to ace your Boards!

50% to 69%: Very respectable score. You are on pace to pass your Boards.

30% to 49%: Not terrible because these are tough questions, but you may want to focus on your weaknesses and hunker down for the test.

15% to 29%: Well below average. You may want to take a review course and certainly must double your efforts in hopes of passing your Boards.

0% to 14%: You may want to delay taking the test and give yourself ample time to get back on track.

Levine BR. *Acing the Orthopedic Board Exam: The Ultimate Crunch-Time Resource* (p 443). © 2016 SLACK Incorporated.

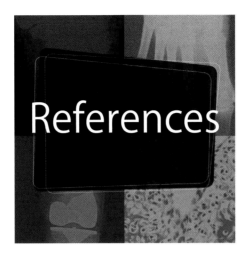

References

1. Zhang Y, Jordan JM. Epidemiology of osteoarthritis. *Rheum Dis Clin North Am*. 2008;34(3):515-529.
2. Roos H, Laurén M, Adalberth T, Roos EM, Jonsson K, Lohmander LS. Knee osteoarthritis after meniscectomy: prevalence of radiographic changes after twenty-one years, compared with matched controls. *Arthritis Rheum*. 1998;41(4):687-693.
3. Papalia R, Del Buono A, Osti L, Denaro V, Maffulli N. Meniscectomy as a risk factor for knee osteoarthritis: a systematic review. *Br Med Bull*. 2011;99:89-106.
4. Sakao K, Takahashi KA, Mazda O, et al. Enhanced expression of interleukin-6, matrix metalloproteinase-13, and receptor activator of NF-kappaB ligand in cells derived from osteoarthritic subchondral bone. *J Orthop Sci*. 2008;13(3):202-210.
5. Richmond J, Hunter D, Irrgang J, et al. Treatment of osteoarthritis of the knee (nonarthroplasty). *J Am Acad Orthop Surg*. 2009;17(9):591-600.
6. Buckwalter JA, Glimcher MJ, Cooper RR, Recker R. Bone biology. II: formation, form, modeling, remodeling, and regulation of cell function. *Instr Course Lect*. 1996;45:387-399.
7. Buckwalter JA, Glimcher MJ, Cooper RR, Recker R. Bone biology. I: structure, blood supply, cells, matrix, and mineralization. *Instr Course Lect*. 1996;45:371-386.
8. Marsell R, Einhorn TA. The biology of fracture healing. *Injury*. 2011;42(6):551-555.
9. Hughes MS, Kazmier P, Burd TA, et al. Enhanced fracture and soft-tissue healing by means of anabolic dietary supplementation. *J Bone Joint Surg Am*. 2006;88(11):2386-2394.
10. Jones KB, Maiers-Yelden KA, Marsh JK, Zimmerman MB, Estin M, Saltzman CL. Ankle fractures in patients with diabetes mellitus. *J Bone Joint Surg Br*. 2005;87(4):489-495.
11. Simon AM, Manigrasso MB, O'Connor JP. Cyclo-oxygenase 2 function is essential for bone fracture healing. *J Bone Miner Res*. 2002;17(6):963-976.
12. van Gaalen FA, Linn-Rasker SP, van Venrooij WJ, et al. Autoantibodies to cyclic citrullinated peptides predict progression to rheumatoid arthritis in patients with undifferentiated arthritis: a prospective cohort study. *Arthritis Rheum*. 2004;50(3):709-715.
13. Savolainen E, Kaipiainen-Seppänen O, Kröger L, Luosujärvi R. Total incidence and distribution of inflammatory joint diseases in a defined population: results from the Kuopio 2000 arthritis survey. *J Rheumatol*. 2003;30(11):2460-2468.
14. Deland JT. Adult-acquired flatfoot deformity. *J Am Acad Orthop Surg*. 2008;16(7):399-406.
15. Bushnell BD, Bynum DK. Malunion of the distal radius. *J Am Acad Orthop Surg*. 2007;15(1):27-40.
16. Park MJ, Cooney WP III, Hahn ME, Looi KP, An KN. The effects of dorsally angulated distal radius fractures on carpal kinematics. *J Hand Surg Am*. 2002;27(2):223-232.
17. Werner FW, Palmer AK, Fortino MD, Short WH. Force transmission through the distal ulna: effect of ulnar variance, lunate fossa angulation, and radial and palmar tilt of the distal radius. *J Hand Surg Am*. 1992;17(3):423-428.
18. Slagel BE, Luenam S, Pichora DR. Management of post-traumatic malunion of fractures of the distal radius. *Orthop Clin North Am*. 2007;38(2):203-216.

19. Marx RG, Axelrod TS. Intraarticular osteotomy of distal radial malunions. *Clin Orthop Relat Res*. 1996;(327):152-157.

20. Zionts LE. Fractures around the knee in children. *J Am Acad Orthop Surg*. 2002;10(5):345-355.

21. Intermountain Joint Replacement Center Writing Committee. A prospective comparison of warfarin to aspirin for thromboprophylaxis in total hip and total knee arthroplasty. *J Arthroplasty*. 2012;27(1):1.e2-9.e2.

22. American College of Chest Physicians. *American College of Chest Physicians (ACCP)'s Guidelines for Diagnosis & Management of DVT/PE*. 9th ed. Glenview, IL: American College of Chest Physicians; 2013.

23. Favorito PJ, Mihalko WM, Krackow KA. Total knee arthroplasty in the valgus knee. *J Am Acad Orthop Surg*. 2002;10(1):16-24.

24. Ranawat AS, Ranawat CS, Elkus M, Rasquinha VJ, Rossi R, Babhulkar S. Total knee arthroplasty for severe valgus deformity. *J Bone Joint Surg Am*. 2005;87 suppl 1(pt 2):271-284.

25. Whiteside LA, Arima J. The anteroposterior axis for femoral rotational alignment in valgus total knee arthroplasty. *Clin Orthop Relat Res*. 1995;(321):168-172.

26. Lee GC, Cushner FD, Scuderi GR, Insall JN. Optimizing patellofemoral tracking during total knee arthroplasty. *J Knee Surg*. 2004;17(3):144-150.

27. Berger RA, Crossett LS, Jacobs JJ, Rubash HE. Malrotation causing patellofemoral complications after total knee arthroplasty. *Clin Orthop Relat Res*. 1998;(356):144-153.

28. Wascher DC. High-velocity knee dislocation with vascular injury. Treatment principles. *Clin Sports Med*. 2000;19(3):457-477.

29. Fanelli GC, Stannard JP, Stuart MJ, et al. Management of complex knee ligament injuries. *J Bone Joint Surg Am*. 2010;92(12):2235-2246.

30. Dejour H, Walch G, Nove-Josserand L, Guier C. Factors of patellar instability: an anatomic radiographic study. *Knee Surg Sports Traumatol Arthrosc*. 1994;2(1):19-26.

31. Micheli LJ, Browne JE, Erggelet C, et al. Autologous chondrocyte implantation of the knee: multicenter experience and minimum 3-year follow-up. *Clin J Sport Med*. 2001;11(4):223-228.

32. Hangody L, Fules P. Autologous osteochondral mosaicplasty for the treatment of full-thickness defects of weight-bearing joints: ten years of experimental and clinical experience. *J Bone Joint Surg Am*. 2003;85 suppl 2:25-32.

33. Gitelis S, Cole BJ. The use of allografts in orthopaedic surgery. *Instr Course Lect*. 2002;51:507-520.

34. Aubin PP, Cheah HK, Davis AM, Gross AE. Long-term followup of fresh femoral osteochondral allografts for post-traumatic knee defects. *Clin Orthop Relat Res*. 2001(391 suppl):S318-S327.

35. Judet R, Judet J, Letournel E. Fractures of the acetabulum: classification and surgical approaches for open reduction: preliminary report. *J Bone Joint Surg Am*. 1964;46:1615-1646.

36. Matta JM. Fractures of the acetabulum: accuracy of reduction and clinical results in patients managed operatively within three weeks after the injury. *J Bone Joint Surg Am*. 1996;78(11):1632-1645.

37. Shadgan B, Menon M, O'Brien PJ, Reid WD. Diagnostic techniques in acute compartment syndrome of the leg. *J Orthop Trauma*. 2008;22(8):581-587.

38. Gustilo RB, Mendoza RM, Williams DN. Problems in the management of type III (severe) open fractures: a new classification of type III open fractures. *J Trauma*. 1984;24(8):742-746.

39. Lonstein JE, Carlson JM. The prediction of curve progression in untreated idiopathic scoliosis during growth. *J Bone Joint Surg Am*. 1984;66(7):1061-1071.

40. Lenke LG, Betz RR, Harms J, et al. Adolescent idiopathic scoliosis: a new classification to determine extent of spinal arthrodesis. *J Bone Joint Surg Am*. 2001;83(8):1169-1181.

41. McCarty EC, Marx RG, DeHaven KE. Meniscus repair: considerations in treatment and update of clinical results. *Clin Orthop Relat Res*. 2002;(402):122-134.

42. Richmond J, Hunter D, Irrgang J, et al. Treatment of osteoarthritis of the knee (nonarthroplasty). *J Am Acad Orthop Surg*. 2009;17(9):591-600.

43. Bartels EM, Lund H, Hagen KB, Dagfinrud H, Christensen R, Danneskiold-Samsøe B. Aquatic exercise for the treatment of knee and hip osteoarthritis. *Cochrane Database Syst Rev*. 2007;(4):CD005523.

44. Moseley B. Arthroscopic surgery did not provide additional benefit to physical and medical therapy for osteoarthritis of the knee. *J Bone Joint Surg Am*. 2009;91(5):1281.

45. Kozinn SC, Scott R. Unicondylar knee arthroplasty. *J Bone Joint Surg Am*. 1989;71(1):145-150.

46. Bellemans J. Multiple needle puncturing: balancing the varus knee. *Orthopedics*. 2011;34(9):e510-e512.

47. Makris CA, Georgoulis AD, Papageorgiou CD, Moebius UG, Soucacos PN. Posterior cruciate ligament architecture: evaluation under microsurgical dissection. *Arthroscopy*. 2000;16(6):627-632.

48. Parsley BS, Conditt MA, Bertolusso R, Noble PC. Posterior cruciate ligament substitution is not essential for excellent postoperative outcomes in total knee arthroplasty. *J Arthroplasty*. 2006;21(6 suppl 2):127-131.

49. Abdel MP, Morrey ME, Jensen MR, Morrey BF. Increased long-term survival of posterior cruciate-retaining versus posterior cruciate-stabilizing total knee replacements. *J Bone Joint Surg Am*. 2011;93(22):2072-2078.

50. Sierra RJ, Berry DJ. Surgical technique differences between posterior-substituting and cruciate-retaining total knee arthroplasty. *J Arthroplasty*. 2008;23(7 suppl):20-23.

51. Schwartz AJ, Della Valle CJ, Rosenberg AG, Jacobs JJ, Berger RA, Galante JO. Cruciate-retaining TKA using a third-generation system with a four-pegged tibial component: a minimum 10-year follow-up note. *Clin Orthop Relat Res.* 2010;468(8):2160-2167.

52. Pagnano MW, Cushner FD, Scott WN. Role of the posterior cruciate ligament in total knee arthroplasty. *J Am Acad Orthop Surg.* 1998;6(3):176-187.

53. Dorr LD, Faugere MC, Mackel AM, Gruen TA, Bognar B, Malluche HH. Structural and cellular assessment of bone quality of proximal femur. *Bone.* 1993;14(3):231-242.

54. Barrack RL, Mulroy RD Jr, Harris WH. Improved cementing techniques and femoral component loosening in young patients with hip arthroplasty: a 12-year radiographic review. *J Bone Joint Surg Br.* 1992;74(3):385-389.

55. Goldner RD, Howson MP, Nunley JA, Fitch RD, Belding NR, Urbaniak JR. One hundred eleven thumb amputations: replantation vs revision. *Microsurgery.* 1990;11(3):243-250.

56. Boulas HJ. Amputations of the fingers and hand: indications for replantation. *J Am Acad Orthop Surg.* 1998;6(2):100-105.

57. Kleinert JM, Graham B. Macroreplantation: an overview. *Microsurgery.* 1990;11(3):229-233.

58. Urbaniak JR, Roth JH, Nunley JA, Goldner RD, Koman LA. The results of replantation after amputation of a single finger. *J Bone Joint Surg Am.* 1985;67(4):611-619.

59. Bayne LG, Klug MS. Long-term review of the surgical treatment of radial deficiencies. *J Hand Surg Am.* 1987;12(2):169-179.

60. Gallant GG, Bora FW Jr. Congenital deformities of the upper extremity. *J Am Acad Orthop Surg.* 1996;4(3):162-171.

61. Manske PR, Goldfarb CA. Congenital failure of formation of the upper limb. *Hand Clin.* 2009;25(2):157-170.

62. Light TR, Gaffey JL. Reconstruction of the hypoplastic thumb. *J Hand Surg Am.* 2010;35(3):474-479.

63. Agins HJ, Alcock NW, Bansal M, et al. Metallic wear in failed titanium-alloy total hip replacements: a histological and quantitative analysis. *J Bone Joint Surg Am.* 1988;70(3):347-356.

64. D'Antonio JA, Sutton K. Ceramic materials as bearing surfaces for total hip arthroplasty. *J Am Acad Orthop Surg.* 2009;17(2):63-68.

65. Klein GR, Parvizi J. Surgical manifestations of Paget's disease. *J Am Acad Orthop Surg.* 2006;14(11):577-586.

66. Kaplan FS, Singer FR. Paget's disease of bone: pathophysiology, diagnosis, and management. *J Am Acad Orthop Surg.* 1995;3(6):336-344.

67. Lees F, Turner JW. Natural history and prognosis of cervical spondylosis. *Br Med J.* 1963;2(5373):1607-1610.

68. Henderson CM, Hennessy RG, Shuey HM Jr, Shackelford EG. Posterior-lateral foraminotomy as an exclusive operative technique for cervical radiculopathy: a review of 846 consecutively operated cases. *Neurosurgery.* 1983;13(5):504-512.

69. Bohlman HH, Emery SE, Goodfellow DB, Jones PK. Robinson anterior cervical discectomy and arthrodesis for cervical radiculopathy: long-term follow-up of one hundred and twenty-two patients. *J Bone Joint Surg Am.* 1993;75(9):1298-1307.

70. Phillips FM, Lee JY, Geisler FH, et al. A prospective, randomized, controlled clinical investigation comparing PCM cervical disc arthroplasty to anterior cervical discectomy and fusion: 2 year results from the US IDE Clinical Trial. *Spine (Phila Pa 1976).* 2013;38(15):E907-E918.

71. Miyasaka KCDD, Stone ML. The incidence of knee ligament injuries in the general population. *Am J Knee Surg.* 1991;4:43-48.

72. Boden BP, Sheehan FT, Torg JS, Hewett TE. Noncontact anterior cruciate ligament injuries: mechanisms and risk factors. *J Am Acad Orthop Surg.* 2010;18(9):520-527.

73. Beynnon BD, Johnson RJ, Abate JA, Fleming BC, Nichols CE. Treatment of anterior cruciate ligament injuries, part 2. *Am J Sports Med.* 2005;33(11):1751-1767.

74. Beynnon BD, Johnson RJ, Abate JA, Fleming BC, Nichols CE. Treatment of anterior cruciate ligament injuries, part I. *Am J Sports Med.* 2005;33(10):1579-1602.

75. Prodromos C HY, Rogowski J, Joyce B, Shi K. *The Anterior Cruciate Ligament: Reconstruction and Basic Science.* Philadelphia, PA: Saunders; 2008.

76. Klenerman L. Fractures of the shaft of the humerus. *J Bone Joint Surg Br.* 1966;48(1):105-111.

77. Papasoulis E, Drosos GI, Ververidis AN, Verettas DA. Functional bracing of humeral shaft fractures: a review of clinical studies. *Injury.* 2010;41(7):e21-e27.

78. Kurup H, Hossain M, Andrew JG. Dynamic compression plating versus locked intramedullary nailing for humeral shaft fractures in adults. *Cochrane Database Syst Rev.* 2011(6):CD005959.

79. Shao YC, Harwood P, Grotz MR, Limb D, Giannoudis PV. Radial nerve palsy associated with fractures of the shaft of the humerus: a systematic review. *J Bone Joint Surg Br.* 2005;87(12):1647-1652.

80. Ekholm R, Tidermark J, Törnkvist H, Adami J, Ponzer S. Outcome after closed functional treatment of humeral shaft fractures. *J Orthop Trauma.* 2006;20(9):591-596.

81. Nielsen AB, Yde J. Epidemiology of acute knee injuries: a prospective hospital investigation. *J Trauma.* 1991;31(12):1644-1648.

82. Greis PE, Bardana DD, Holmstrom MC, Burks RT. Meniscal injury: I. Basic science and evaluation. *J Am Acad Orthop Surg.* 2002;10(3):168-176.

83. Weinstabl R, Muellner T, Vecsei V, Kainberger F, Kramer M. Economic considerations for the diagnosis and therapy of meniscal lesions: can magnetic resonance imaging help reduce the expense? *World J Surg.* 1997;21(4):363-368.

84. Ryzewicz M, Peterson B, Siparsky PN, Bartz RL. The diagnosis of meniscus tears: the role of MRI and clinical examination. *Clin Orthop Relat Res.* 2007;455:123-133.

85. Jeray KJ. Acute midshaft clavicular fracture. *J Am Acad Orthop Surg.* 2007;15(4):239-248.

86. Lazarides S, Zafiropoulos G. Conservative treatment of fractures at the middle third of the clavicle: the relevance of shortening and clinical outcome. *J Shoulder Elbow Surg.* 2006;15(2):191-194.

87. McKee MD, Pedersen EM, Jones C, et al. Deficits following nonoperative treatment of displaced midshaft clavicular fractures. *J Bone Joint Surg Am.* 2006;88(1):35-40.

88. Nordqvist A, Petersson CJ, Redlund-Johnell I. Mid-clavicle fractures in adults: end result study after conservative treatment. *J Orthop Trauma.* 1998;12(8):572-576.

89. Robinson CM, Court-Brown CM, McQueen MM, Wakefield AE. Estimating the risk of nonunion following nonoperative treatment of a clavicular fracture. *J Bone Joint Surg Am.* 2004;86(7):1359-1365.

90. Zlowodzki M, Zelle BA, Cole PA, Jeray K, McKee MD. Treatment of acute midshaft clavicle fractures: systematic review of 2144 fractures: on behalf of the Evidence-Based Orthopaedic Trauma Working Group. *J Orthop Trauma.* 2005;19(7):504-507.

91. Canadian Orthopaedic Trauma Soceity. Nonoperative treatment compared with plate fixation of displaced midshaft clavicular fractures: a multicenter, randomized clinical trial. *J Bone Joint Surg Am.* 2007;89(1):1-10.

92. Ring D, Jupiter JB. *Injuries to the Shoulder Girdle.* Vol 2. Philadelphia, PA: WB Saunders; 2003.

93. Lee DH, Claussen GC, Oh S. Clinical nerve conduction and needle electromyography studies. *J Am Acad Orthop Surg.* 2004;12(4):276-287.

94. Levine MJ, Albert TJ, Smith MD. Cervical radiculopathy: diagnosis and nonoperative management. *J Am Acad Orthop Surg.* 1996;4(6):305-316.

95. Noonan KJ, Price CT. Forearm and distal radius fractures in children. *J Am Acad Orthop Surg.* 998;6(3):146-156.

96. Kim HK. Legg-Calvée-Perthes disease. *J Am Acad Orthop Surg.* 2010;18(11):676-686.

97. Hosalkar HS, Pandya NK, Cho RH, Glaser DA, Moor MA, Herman MJ. Intramedullary nailing of pediatric femoral shaft fracture. *J Am Acad Orthop Surg.* 2011;19(8):472-481.

98. Kocher MS, Sink EL, Blasier RD, et al. Treatment of pediatric diaphyseal femur fractures. *J Am Acad Orthop Surg.* 2009;17(11):718-725.

99. Flynn JM, Schwend RM. Management of pediatric femoral shaft fractures. *J Am Acad Orthop Surg.* 2004;12(5):347-359.

100. Gomez JA, Lee JK, Kim PD, Roye DP, Vitale MG. "Growth friendly" spine surgery: management options for the young child with scoliosis. *J Am Acad Orthop Surg.* 2011;19(12):722-727.

101. Gillingham BL, Fan RA, Akbarnia BA. Early onset idiopathic scoliosis. *J Am Acad Orthop Surg.* 2006;14(2):101-112.

102. DiGiovanni CW, Kang L, Manuel J. Patient compliance in avoiding wrong-site surgery. *J Bone Joint Surg Am.* 2003;85(5):815-819.

103. Paprosky WG, Perona PG, Lawrence JM. Acetabular defect classification and surgical reconstruction in revision arthroplasty: a 6-year follow-up evaluation. *J Arthroplasty.* 1994;9(1):33-44.

104. Cronen G, Ringus V, Sigle G, Ryu J. Sterility of surgical site marking. *J Bone Joint Surg Am.* 2005;87(10):2193-2195.

105. Cowell HR. Wrong-site surgery. *J Bone Joint Surg Am.* 1998;80(4):463.

106. Wong DA, Herndon JH, Canale ST, et al. Medical errors in orthopaedics: results of an AAOS member survey. *J Bone Joint Surg Am.* 2009;91(3):547-557.

107. Dalury DF, Fisher DA, Adams MJ, Gonzales RA. Unicompartmental knee arthroplasty compares favorably to total knee arthroplasty in the same patient. *Orthopedics.* 2009;32(4).

108. Laurencin CT, Zelicof SB, Scott RD, Ewald FC. Unicompartmental versus total knee arthroplasty in the same patient: a comparative study. *Clin Orthop Relat Res.* 1991;(273):151-156.

109. Chassin EP, Mikosz RP, Andriacchi TP, Rosenberg AG. Functional analysis of cemented medial unicompartmental knee arthroplasty. *J Arthroplasty.* 1996;11(5):553-559.

110. Weale AE, Murray DW, Crawford R, et al. Does arthritis progress in the retained compartments after Oxford medial unicompartmental arthroplasty? A clinical and radiological study with a minimum ten-year follow-up. *J Bone Joint Surgery Br.* 1999;81(5):783-789.

111. Hernigou P, Deschamps G. Patellar impingement following unicompartmental arthroplasty. *J Bone Joint Surg Am.* 2002;84(7):1132-1137.

112. Pearse AJ, Hooper GJ, Rothwell A, Frampton C. Survival and functional outcome after revision of a unicompartmental to a total knee replacement: the New Zealand National Joint Registry. *J Bone Joint Surg Br.* 2010;92(4):508-512.

113. Gill T, Schemitsch EH, Brick GW, Thornhill TS. Revision total knee arthroplasty after failed unicompartmental knee arthroplasty or high tibial osteotomy. *Clin Orthop Relat Res.* 1995;(321):10-18.

114. Levine WN, Ozuna RM, Scott RD, Thornhill TS. Conversion of failed modern unicompartmental arthroplasty to total knee arthroplasty. *J Arthroplasty.* 1996;11(7):797-801.

115. Padgett DE, Stern SH, Insall JN. Revision total knee arthroplasty for failed unicompartmental replacement. *J Bone Joint Surg Am.* 1991;73(2):186-190.

116. Skyrme AD, Mencia MM, Skinner PW. Early failure of the porous-coated anatomic cemented unicompartmental knee arthroplasty: a 5- to 9-year follow-up study. *J Arthroplasty.* 2002;17(2):201-205.

117. Berger RA, Meneghini RM, Jacobs JJ, et al. Results of unicompartmental knee arthroplasty at a minimum of ten years of follow-up. *J Bone Joint Surg Am.* 2005;87(5):999-1006.

118. Emerson RH Jr, Hansborough T, Reitman RD, Rosenfeldt W, Higgins LL. Comparison of a mobile with a fixed-bearing unicompartmental knee implant. *Clin Orthop Relat Res*. 2002;(404):62-70.

119. Parratte S, Pauly V, Aubaniac JM, Argenson JN. No long-term difference between fixed and mobile medial unicompartmental arthroplasty. *Clin Orthop Relat Res*. 2012;470(1):61-68.

120. Svärd UC, Price AJ. Oxford medial unicompartmental knee arthroplasty: a survival analysis of an independent series. *J Bone Joint Surg Br*. 2001;83(2):191-194.

121. Harris WH, McCarthy JC Jr, O'Neill DA. Femoral component loosening using contemporary techniques of femoral cement fixation. *J Bone Joint Surg Am*. 1982;64(7):1063-1067.

122. Gruen TA, McNeice GM, Amstutz HC. "Modes of failure" of cemented stem-type femoral components: a radiographic analysis of loosening. *Clin Orthop Relat Res*. 1979;(141):17-27.

123. Engh CA, Massin P, Suthers KE. Roentgenographic assessment of the biologic fixation of porous-surfaced femoral components. *Clin Orthop Relat Res*. 1990;(257):107-128.

124. D'Antonio JA. Periprosthetic bone loss of the acetabulum. Classification and management. *Orthop Clin North Am*. 1992;23(2):279-290.

125. D'Antonio J, McCarthy JC, Bargar WL, et al. Classification of femoral abnormalities in total hip arthroplasty. *Clin Orthop Relat Res*. 1993;(296):133-139.

126. Paprosky WG, Perona PG, Lawrence JM. Acetabular defect classification and surgical reconstruction in revision arthroplasty: a 6-year follow-up evaluation. *J Arthroplasty*. 1994;9(1):33-44.

127. Della Valle CJ, Paprosky WG. The femur in revision total hip arthroplasty evaluation and classification. *Clin Orthop Relat Res*. 2004;(420):55-62.

128. Tausche AK, Jansen TL, Schröder HE, Bornstein SR, Aringer M, Müller-Ladner U. Gout: current diagnosis and treatment. *Dtsch Arztebl Int*. 2009;106(34-35):549-555.

129. Eggebeen AT. Gout: an update. *Amer Fam Physician*. 2007;76(6):801-808.

130. Ekman EF. The role of the orthopaedic surgeon in minimizing mortality and morbidity associated with fragility fractures. *J Am Acad Orthop Surg*. 2010;18(5):278-285.

131. Lane JM, Nydick M. Osteoporosis: current modes of prevention and treatment. *J Am Acad Orthop Surg*. 1999;7(1):19-31.

132. Hamilton H, Jamieson J. Deep infection in total hip arthroplasty. *Can J Surg*. 2008;51(2):111-117.

133. Fulkerson E, Valle CJ, Wise B, Walsh M, Preston C, Di Cesare PE. Antibiotic susceptibility of bacteria infecting total joint arthroplasty sites. *J Bone Joint Surg Am*. 2006;88(6):1231-1237.

134. Chiu FY, Chen CM. Surgical debridement and parenteral antibiotics in infected revision total knee arthroplasty. *Clin Orthop Relat Res*. 2007;461:130-135.

135. Dubost JJ, Soubrier M, Sauvezie B. Pyogenic arthritis in adults. *Joint Bone Spine*. 2000;67(1):11-21.

136. Horowitz DL, Katzap E, Horowitz S, Barilla-LaBarca ML. Approach to septic arthritis. *Am Fam Physician*. 2011;84(6):653-660.

137. Margaretten ME, Kohlwes J, Moore D, Bent S. Does this adult patient have septic arthritis? *JAMA*. 2007;297(13):1478-1488.

138. McGillicuddy DC, Shah KH, Friedberg RP, Nathanson LA, Edlow JA. How sensitive is the synovial fluid white blood cell count in diagnosing septic arthritis? *Am J Emerg Med*. 2007;25(7):749-752.

139. Ateschrang A, Albrecht D, Schröter S, Hirt B, Weise K, Dolderer JH. Septic arthritis of the knee: presentation of a novel irrigation-suction system tested in a cadaver study. *BMC Musculoskelet Disord*. 2011;12:180.

140. Lynch JR, Waitayawinyu T, Hanel DP, Trumble TE. Medial collateral ligament injury in the overhand-throwing athlete. *J Hand Surg Am*. 2008;33(3):430-437.

141. Meyers A, Palmer B, Baratz ME. Ulnar collateral ligament reconstruction. *Hand Clin*. 2008;24(1):53-67.

142. Rohrbough JT, Altchek DW, Hyman J, Williams RJ III, Botts JD. Medial collateral ligament reconstruction of the elbow using the docking technique. *Am J Sports Med*. 2002;30(4):541-548.

143. Lachiewicz PF, Kauk JR. Anterior iliopsoas impingement and tendinitis after total hip arthroplasty. *J Am Acad Orthop Surg*. 2009;17(6):337-344.

144. Bricteux S, Beguin L, Fessy MH. Iliopsoas impingement in 12 patients with a total hip arthroplasty [in French]. *Rev Chir Orthop Reparatrice Appar Mot*. 2001;87(8):820-825.

145. Trousdale RT, Cabanela ME, Berry DJ. Anterior iliopsoas impingement after total hip arthroplasty. *J Arthroplasty*. 1995;10(4):546-549.

146. Sankar WN, Weiss J, Skaggs DL. Orthopaedic conditions in the newborn. *J Am Acad Orthop Surg*. 2009;17(2):112-122.

147. Vitale MG, Skaggs DL. Developmental dysplasia of the hip from six months to four years of age. *J Am Acad Orthop Surg*. 2001;9(6):401-411.

148. Lane JM, Nydick M. Osteoporosis: current modes of prevention and treatment. *J Am Acad Orthop Surg*. 1999;7(1):19-31.

149. Kwon YW, Hurd JL. Arthritis and arthroplasty of the shoulder. In Lieberman JR, ed. *AAOS Comprehensive Orthopaedic Review*. Rosemont, IL: American Academy of Orthopaedic Surgeons; 2009:827-833.

150. Walch G, Badet R, Boulahia A, Khoury A. Morphologic study of the glenoid in primary glenohumeral osteoarthritis. *J Arthroplasty*. 1999;14(6):756-760.

151. Chen AL, Joseph TN, Zuckerman JD. Rheumatoid arthritis of the shoulder. *J Am Acad Orthop Surg*. 2003;11(1):12-24.

152. Bryant D, Litchfield R, Sandow M, Gartsman GM, Guyatt G, Kirkley A. A comparison of pain, strength, range of motion, and functional outcomes after hemiarthroplasty and total shoulder arthroplasty in patients with osteoarthritis of the shoulder. A systematic review and meta-analysis. *J Bone Joint Surg Am*. 2005;87(9):1947-1956.

153. Murthi AM. Rotator cuff tears and cuff tear arthropathy. In Lieberman JR, ed. *AAOS Comprehensive Orthopaedic Review*. Rosemont, IL: American Academy of Orthopaedic Surgeons; 2009:817-820.

154. Ditunno JF, Little JW, Tessler A, Burns AS. Spinal shock revisited: a four-phase model. *Spinal Cord*. 2004;42(7):383-395.

155. Chesnut RM, Marshall LF, Klauber MR, et al. The role of secondary brain injury in determining outcome from severe head injury. *J Trauma*. 1993;34(2):216-222.

156. Dietrich WD III. Therapeutic hypothermia for spinal cord injury. *Crit Care Med*. 2009;37(7 suppl):S238-S242.

157. Kwon BK, Mann C, Sohn HM, et al. Hypothermia for spinal cord injury. *Spine J*. 2008;8(6):859-874.

158. Miller M, Sekiya J. Acromioclavicular, sternoclavicular and clavicle injuries. In: Miller M, Sekiya J, eds. *Core Knowledge in Orthopaedics: Sports Medicine*. Philadelphia, PA: Mosby, Inc; 2006.

159. Simovitch R, Sanders B, Ozbaydar M, Lavery K, Warner JJ. Acromioclavicular joint injuries: diagnosis and management. *J Am Acad Orthop Surg*. 2009;17(4):207-219.

160. Green A. Traumatic conditions of the shoulder. In: Lieberman JR, ed. *AAOS Comprehensive Orthopaedic Review*. Rosemont, IL: American Academy of Orthopaedic Surgeons; 2009:843-858.

161. Parvizi J, Leunig M, Ganz R. Femoroacetabular impingement. *J Am Acad Orthop Surg*. 2007;15(9):561-570.

162. Audenaert EA, Mahieu P, Pattyn C. Three-dimensional assessment of cam engagement in femoroacetabular impingement. *Arthroscopy*. 2011;27(2):167-171.

163. Notzli HP, Siebenrock KA, Hempfing A, Ramseier LE, Ganz R. Perfusion of the femoral head during surgical dislocation of the hip. Monitoring by laser Doppler flowmetry. *J Bone Joint Surg Br*. 2002;84(2):300-304.

164. Meyer DC, Beck M, Ellis T, Ganz R, Leunig M. Comparison of six radiographic projections to assess femoral head/neck asphericity. *Clin Orthop Relat Res*. 2006;445:181-185.

165. Pape HC, Giannoudis PV, Krettek C, Trentz O. Timing of fixation of major fractures in blunt polytrauma: role of conventional indicators in clinical decision making. *J Orthop Trauma*. 2005;19(8):551-562.

166. McGee S, Abernethy WB III, Simel DL. The rational clinical examination: is this patient hypovolemic? *JAMA*. 1999;281(11):1022-1029.

167. Roberts CS, Pape HC, Jones AL, Malkani AL, Rodriguez JL, Giannoudis PV. Damage control orthopaedics: evolving concepts in the treatment of patients who have sustained orthopaedic trauma. *Instr Course Lect*. 2005;54:447-462.

168. Pape HC, Giannoudis P, Krettek C. The timing of fracture treatment in polytrauma patients: relevance of damage control orthopedic surgery. *Am J Surg*. 2002;183(6):622-629.

169. Harwood PJ, Giannoudis PV, van Griensven M, Krettek C, Pape HC. Alterations in the systemic inflammatory response after early total care and damage control procedures for femoral shaft fracture in severely injured patients. *J Trauma*. 2005;58(3):446-452.

170. Stein BES. *Shoulder Conditions in the Athlete*. Rosemont, IL: American Academy of Orthopaedic Surgeons; 2009.

171. Keener JD, Brophy RH. Superior labral tears of the shoulder: pathogenesis, evaluation, and treatment. *J Am Acad Orthop Surg*. 2009;17(10):627-637.

172. Buddoff JE. Glenohumeral instability, adhesive capsulitis and superior labral anteroposterior lesions. In: Miller M, Sekiya J, eds. *Core Knowledge in Orthopaedics: Sports Medicine*. Philadelphia, PA: Mosby, Inc; 2006.

173. Mileski RA, Snyder SJ. Superior labral lesions in the shoulder: pathoanatomy and surgical management. *J Am Acad Orthop Surg*. 1998;6(2):121-131.

174. Miller M, Sekiya J. SLAP tears and internal impingement. In: Miller M, Sekiya J, eds. *Core Knowledge in Orthopaedics: Sports Medicine*. Philadelphia, PA: Mosby, Inc; 2006.

175. Matava MJ. Patellar tendon ruptures. *J Am Acad Orthop Surg*. 1996;4(6):287-296.

176. Zernicke RF, Garhammer J, Jobe FW. Human patellar-tendon rupture. *J Bone Joint Surg Am*. 1977;59(2):179-183.

177. Siwek CW, Rao JP. Ruptures of the extensor mechanism of the knee joint. *J Bone Joint Surg Am*. 1981;63(6):932-937.

178. Matava MJ. Patellar Tendon Ruptures. *J Am Acad Orthop Surg*. 1996;4(6):287-296.

179. Allen BL Jr, Ferguson RL, Lehmann TR, O'Brien RP. A mechanistic classification of closed, indirect fractures and dislocations of the lower cervical spine. *Spine (Phila Pa 1976)*. 1982;7(1):1-27.

180. Initial closed reduction of cervical spine fracture-dislocation injuries. *Neurosurgery*. 2002;50(3 suppl):S44-S50.

181. Warner JJ. Frozen shoulder: diagnosis and management. *J Am Acad Orthop Surg*. 1997;5(3):130-140.

182. Rill BK, Fleckenstein CM, Levy MS, Nagesh V, Hasan SS. Predictors of outcome after nonoperative and operative treatment of adhesive capsulitis. *Am J Sports Med*. 2011;39(3):567-574.

183. Alanay Y, Lachman RS. A review of the principles of radiological assessment of skeletal dysplasias. *J Clin Res Pediatr Endocrinol*. 2011;3(4):163-178.

184. Brook CG, de Vries BB. Skeletal dysplasias. *Arch Dis Child*. 1998;79(3):285-289.

185. Phornphutkul C, Gruppuso PA. Disorders of the growth plate. *Curr Opin Endocrinol Diabetes Obes*. 2009;16(6):430-434.

186. Ritter MA, Faris PM, Keating EM. Anterior femoral notching and ipsilateral supracondylar femur fracture in total knee arthroplasty. *J Arthroplasty*. 1988;3(2):185-187.

187. Platzer P, Schuster R, Luxl M, et al. Management and outcome of interprosthetic femoral fractures. *Injury.* 2011;42(11):1219-1225.

188. Lombardi AV Jr, Mallory TH, Vaughn BK, et al. Dislocation following primary posterior-stabilized total knee arthroplasty. *J Arthroplasty.* 1993;8(6):633-639.

189. Leopold SS, McStay C, Klafeta K, Jacobs JJ, Berger RA, Rosenberg AG. Primary repair of intraoperative disruption of the medical collateral ligament during total knee arthroplasty. *J Bone Joint Surg Am.* 2001;83(1):86-91.

190. Kurtz SM. A primer on UHMWPE. In: Kurtz SM, ed. *The UHMWPE Handbook.* San Diego, CA: Elsevier; 2004:1-9.

191. Charnley J, Halley DK. Rate of wear in total hip replacement. *Clin Orthop Relat Res.* 1975;(112):170-179.

192. Gordon AC, D'Lima DD, Colwell CW Jr. Highly cross-linked polyethylene in total hip arthroplasty. *J Am Acad Orthop Surg.* 2006;14(9):511-523.

193. D'Antonio JA, Sutton K. Ceramic materials as bearing surfaces for total hip arthroplasty. *J Am Acad Orthop Surg.* 2009;17(2):63-68.

194. Heier KA, Infante AF, Walling AK, Sanders RW. Open fractures of the calcaneus: soft-tissue injury determines outcome. *J Bone Joint Surg Am.* 2003;85(12):2276-2282.

195. Buckley RE, Tough S. Displaced intra-articular calcaneal fractures. *J Am Acad Orthop Surg.* 2004;12(3):172-178.

196. Carr JB. Mechanism and pathoanatomy of the intraarticular calcaneal fracture. *Clin Orthop Relat Res.* 1993;(290):36-40.

197. Paley D, Hall H. Intra-articular fractures of the calcaneus: a critical analysis of results and prognostic factors. *J Bone Joint Surg Am.* 1993;75(3):342-354.

198. Potter MQ, Nunley JA. Long-term functional outcomes after operative treatment for intra-articular fractures of the calcaneus. *J Bone Joint Surg Am.* 2009;91(8):1854-1860.

199. Pilliar RM, Lee JM, Maniatopoulos C. Observations on the effect of movement on bone ingrowth into porous-surfaced implants. *Clin Orthop Relat Res.* 1986;(208):108-113.

200. Kienapfel H, Sprey C, Wilke A, Griss P. Implant fixation by bone ingrowth. *J Arthroplasty.* 1999;14(3):355-368.

201. Illgen R II, Rubash HE. The optimal fixation of the cementless acetabular component in primary total hip arthroplasty. *J Am Acad Orthop Surg.* 2002;10(1):43-56.

202. Strickland JW. Flexor tendon injuries: I. Foundations of treatment. *J Am Acad Orthop Surg.* 1995;3(1):44-54.

203. Leddy JP. Avulsions of the flexor digitorum profundus. *Hand Clin.* 1985;1(1):77-83.

204. Boyer MI, Ditsios K, Gelberman RH, Leversedge F, Silva M. Repair of flexor digitorum profundus tendon avulsions from bone: an ex vivo biomechanical analysis. *J Hand Surg Am.* 2002;27(4):594-598.

205. Brustein M, Pellegrini J, Choueka J, Heminger H, Mass D. Bone suture anchors versus the pullout button for repair of distal profundus tendon injuries: a comparison of strength in human cadaveric hands. *J Hand Surg Am.* 2001;26(3):489-496.

206. Amadio PC, Wood MB, Cooney WP III, Bogard SD. Staged flexor tendon reconstruction in the fingers and hand. *J Hand Surg Am.* 1988;13(4):559-562.

207. LaSalle WB, Strickland JW. An evaluation of the two-stage flexor tendon reconstruction technique. *J Hand Surg Am.* 1983;8(3):263-267.

208. Pulido L, Ghanem E, Joshi A, Purtill JJ, Parvizi J. Periprosthetic joint infection: the incidence, timing, and predisposing factors. *Clin Orthop Relat Res.* 2008;466(7):1710-1715.

209. Bedair H, Ting N, Jacovides C, et al. The Mark Coventry Award: diagnosis of early postoperative TKA infection using synovial fluid analysis. *Clin Orthop Relat Res.* 2011;469(1):34-40.

210. Cheung EV, Adams R, Morrey BF. Primary osteoarthritis of the elbow: current treatment options. *J Am Acad Orthop Surg.* 2008;16(2):77-87.

211. Kokkalis ZT, Schmidt CC, Sotereanos DG. Elbow arthritis: current concepts. *J Hand Surg Am.* 2009;34(4):761-768.

212. Cohen AP, Redden JF, Stanley D. Treatment of osteoarthritis of the elbow: a comparison of open and arthroscopic debridement. *Arthroscopy.* 2000;16(7):701-706.

213. Tang PC, Ravji K, Key JJ, Mahler DB, Blume PA, Sumpio B. Let them walk! Current prosthesis options for leg and foot amputees. *J Am Coll Surg.* 2008;206(3):548-560.

214. Laferrier JZ, Gailey R. Advances in lower-limb prosthetic technology. *Phys Med Rehabil Clin N Am.* 2010;21(1):87-110.

215. Meyerding HW. Spondylolisthesis. *Surg Gynecol Obstet.* 1932;54:371-377.

216. Agabegi SS, Fischgrund JS. Contemporary management of isthmic spondylolisthesis: pediatric and adult. *Spine J.* 2010;10(6):530-543.

217. Petraco DM, Spivak JM, Cappadona JG, Kummer FJ, Neuwirth MG. An anatomic evaluation of L5 nerve stretch in spondylolisthesis reduction. *Spine (Phila Pa 1976).* 1996;21(10):1133-1138.

218. Schlenzka D, Remes V, Helenius I, et al. Direct repair for treatment of symptomatic spondylolysis and low-grade isthmic spondylolisthesis in young patients: no benefit in comparison to segmental fusion after a mean follow-up of 14.8 years. *Eur Spine J.* 2006;15(10):1437-1447.

219. Drakos MC, Rudzki JR, Allen AA, Potter HG, Altchek DW. Internal impingement of the shoulder in the overhead athlete. *J Bone Joint Surg Am.* 2009;91(11):2719-2728.

220. Kazár B, Relovszky E. Prognosis of primary dislocation of the shoulder. *Acta Orthop Scand.* 1969;40(2):216-224.

221. Thomas SC, Matsen FA III. An approach to the repair of avulsion of the glenohumeral ligaments in the management of traumatic anterior glenohumeral instability. *J Bone Joint Surg Am.* 1989;71(4):506-513.

222. Turkel SJ, Panio MW, Marshall JL, Girgis FG. Stabilizing mechanisms preventing anterior dislocation of the glenohumeral joint. *J Bone Joint Surg Am*. 1981;63(8):1208-1217.

223. Taylor DC, Arciero RA. Pathologic changes associated with shoulder dislocations: arthroscopic and physical examination findings in first-time, traumatic anterior dislocations. *Am J Sports Med*. 1997;25(3):306-311.

224. Hovelius L, Olofsson A, Sandstrom B, et al. Nonoperative treatment of primary anterior shoulder dislocation in patients forty years of age and younger: a prospective twenty-five-year follow-up. *J Bone Joint Surg Am*. 2008;90(5):945-952.

225. Sayegh FE, Kenanidis EI, Papavasiliou KA, Potoupnis ME, Kirkos JM, Kapetanos GA. Reduction of acute anterior dislocations: a prospective randomized study comparing a new technique with the Hippocratic and Kocher methods. *J Bone Joint Surg Am*. 2009;91(12):2775-2782.

226. Bottoni CR, Wilckens JH, DeBerardino TM, et al. A prospective, randomized evaluation of arthroscopic stabilization versus nonoperative treatment in patients with acute, traumatic, first-time shoulder dislocations. *Am J Sports Med*. 2002;30(4):576-580.

227. Sulaiman AR, Nawaz H, Munajat I, Sallehudin AY. Proximal femoral focal deficiency as a manifestation of Antley-Bixler syndrome: a case report. *J Orthop Surg (Hong Kong)*. 2007;15(1):84-86.

228. Parakh A, Nagar G. Proximal femoral focal deficiency. *Indian Pediatr*. 2006;43(4):349-350.

229. Zywiel MG, McGrath MS, Seyler TM, Marker DR, Bonutti PM, Mont MA. Osteonecrosis of the knee: a review of three disorders. *Orthop Clin North Am*. 2009;40(2):193-211.

230. Duany NG, Zywiel MG, McGrath MS, et al. Joint-preserving surgical treatment of spontaneous osteonecrosis of the knee. *Arch Orthop Trauma Surg*. 2010;130(1):11-16.

231. Cohen MS, Hastings H II. Acute elbow dislocation: evaluation and management. *J Am Acad Orthop Surg*. 1998;6(1):15-23.

232. Ebrahimzadeh MH, Amadzadeh-Chabock H, Ring D. Traumatic elbow instability. *J Hand Surg Am*. 2010;35(7):1220-1225.

233. Troyer J, Levine BR. Proximal tibia reconstruction with a porous tantalum cone in a patient with Charcot arthropathy. *Orthopedics*. 2009;32(5):358.

234. Fullerton BD, Browngoehl LA. Total knee arthroplasty in a patient with bilateral Charcot knees. *Arch Phys Med Rehabil*. 1997;78(7):780-782.

235. Klenerman L. The Charcot joint in diabetes. *Diabet Med*. 1996;13 suppl 1:S52-S54.

236. Newman AP. Articular cartilage repair. *Am J Sports Med*. 1998;26(2):309-324.

237. Sophia Fox AJ, Bedi A, Rodeo SA. The basic science of articular cartilage: structure, composition, and function. *Sports Health*. 2009;1(6):461-468.

238. Ulrich-Vinther M, Maloney MD, Schwarz EM, Rosier R, O'Keefe RJ. Articular cartilage biology. *J Am Acad Orthop Surg*. 2003;11(6):421-430.

239. Greis PE, Bardana DD, Holstrom MC, Burks RT. Meniscal injury: I. Basic science and evaluation. *J Am Acad Orthop Surg*. 2002;10(3):168-176.

240. Hutchinson ID, Moran CJ, Potter HG, Warren RF, Rodeo SA. Restoration of the meniscus: form and function. *Am J Sports Med*. 2014;42(4):987-998.

241. Charnley J, Halley DK. Rate of wear in total hip replacement. *Clin Orthop Relat Res*. 1975;(112):170-179.

242. McGovern TF, Ammeen DJ, Collier JP, Currier BH, Engh GA. Rapid polyethylene failure of unicondylar tibial components sterilized with gamma irradiation in air and implanted after a long shelf life. *J Bone Joint Surg Am*. 2002;84(6):901-906.

243. Hood RW, Wright TM, Burstein AH. Retrieval analysis of total knee prostheses: a method and its application to 48 total condylar prostheses. *J Biomed Mater Res*. 1983;17(5):829-842.

244. Jacobs JJ, Campbell PA, T Konttinen Y; Implant Wear Symposium 2007 Biologic Work Group. How has the biologic reaction to wear particles changed with newer bearing surfaces? *J Am Acad Orthop Surg*. 2008;16 suppl 1:S49-S55.

245. Thompson ML, Martin C. Management of necrotizing fasciitis infections. *Orthopedics*. 2011;34(2):111-115.

246. Stoneback JW, Hak DJ. Diagnosis and management of necrotizing fasciitis. *Orthopedics*. 2011;34(3):196.

247. Kaushik AP, Das A, Cui Q. Osteonecrosis of the femoral head: an update in year 2012. *World J Orthop*. 2012;3(5):49-57.

248. Lavernia CJ, Sierra RJ, Grieco FR. Osteonecrosis of the femoral head. *J Am Acad Orthop Surg*. 1999;7(4):250-261.

249. Beaulée PE, Amstutz HC. Management of Ficat stage III and IV osteonecrosis of the hip. *J Am Acad Orthop Surg*. 2004;12(2):96-105.

250. Berry DJ, von Knoch M, Schleck CD, Harmsen WS. The cumulative long-term risk of dislocation after primary Charnley total hip arthroplasty. *J Bone Joint Surg Am*. 2004;86(1):9-14.

251. Bozic KJ, Kurtz SM, Lau E, Ong K, Vail TP, Berry DJ. The epidemiology of revision total hip arthroplasty in the United States. *J Bone Joint Surg Am*. 2009;91(1):128-133.

252. Parvizi J, Picinic E, Sharkey PF. Revision total hip arthroplasty for instability: surgical techniques and principles. *J Bone Joint Surg Am*. 2008;90(5):1134-1142.

253. Frisbie DD, Cross MW, McIlwraith CW. A comparative study of articular cartilage thickness in the stifle of animal species used in human pre-clinical studies compared to articular cartilage thickness in the human knee. *Vet Comp Orthop Traumatol*. 2006;19(3):142-146.

254. Temple-Wong MM, Bae WC, Chen MQ, et al. Biomechanical, structural, and biochemical indices of degenerative and osteoarthritic deterioration of adult human articular cartilage of the femoral condyle. *Osteoarthritis Cartilage*. 2009;17(11):1469-1476.

255. Abzug JM, Herman MJ. Management of supracondylar humerus fractures in children: current concepts. *J Am Acad Orthop Surg*. 2012;20(2):69-77.

256. Gaston RG, Cates TB, Devito D, et al. Medial and lateral pin versus lateral-entry pin fixation for Type 3 supracondylar fractures in children: a prospective, surgeon-randomized study. *J Pediatr Orthop*. 2010;30(8):799-806.

257. Skaggs DL, Cluck MW, Mostofi A, Flynn JM, Kay RM. Lateral-entry pin fixation in the management of supracondylar fractures in children. *J Bone Joint Surg Am*. 2004;86(4):702-707.

258. Moosmayer S, Lund G, Seljom U, et al. Comparison between surgery and physiotherapy in the treatment of small and medium-sized tears of the rotator cuff: a randomised controlled study of 103 patients with one-year follow-up. *J Bone Joint Surg Br*. 2010;92(1):83-91.

259. Nho SJ, Shindle MK, Sherman SL, Freedman KB, Lyman S, MacGillivray JD. Systematic review of arthroscopic rotator cuff repair and mini-open rotator cuff repair. *J Bone Joint Surg Am*. 2007;89 suppl 3:127-136.

260. Chambers HG, Sutherland DH. A practical guide to gait analysis. *J Am Acad Orthop Surg*. 2002;10(3):222-231.

261. Weinstein JN, Lurie JD, Tosteson TD, et al. Surgical versus nonoperative treatment for lumbar disc herniation: four-year results for the Spine Patient Outcomes Research Trial (SPORT). *Spine (Phila Pa 1976)*. 2008;33(25):2789-2800.

262. Barth M, Weiss C, Thomé C. Two-year outcome after lumbar microdiscectomy versus microscopic sequestrectomy: part 1: evaluation of clinical outcome. *Spine (Phila Pa 1976)*. 2008;33(3):265-272.

263. Carragee EJ, Spinnickie AO, Alamin TF, Paragioudakis S. A prospective controlled study of limited versus subtotal posterior discectomy: short-term outcomes in patients with herniated lumbar intervertebral discs and large posterior anular defect. *Spine (Phila Pa 1976)*. 2006;31(6):653-657.

264. Jonsson T, Althoff B, Peterson L, Renstrom P. Clinical diagnosis of ruptures of the anterior cruciate ligament: a comparative study of the Lachman test and the anterior drawer sign. *Am J Sports Med*. 1982;10(2):100-102.

265. Lane CG, Warren R, Pearle AD. The pivot shift. *J Am Acad Orthop Surg*. 2008;16(12):679-688.

266. Serover ST, Bach BR. *Graft Choice in ACL Reconstruction*. Thorofare, NJ: SLACK Incorporated; 2010.

267. Zelle BA, Brucker PU, Feng MT, Fu FH. Anatomical double-bundle anterior cruciate ligament reconstruction. *Sports Med*. 2006;36(2):99-108.

268. Blauth M, Bastian L, Krettek C, Knop C, Evans S. Surgical options for the treatment of severe tibial pilon fractures: a study of three techniques. *J Orthop Trauma*. 2001;15(3):153-160.

269. Patterson MJ, Cole JD. Two-staged delayed open reduction and internal fixation of severe pilon fractures. *J Orthop Trauma*. 1999;13(2):85-91.

270. Abdul-Karim FW, el-Naggar AK, Joyce MJ, Makley JT, Carter JR. Diffuse and localized tenosynovial giant cell tumor and pigmented villonodular synovitis: a clinicopathologic and flow cytometric DNA analysis. *Hum Pathol*. 1992;23(7):729-735.

271. Simon M. *Surgical Margins*. Philadelphia, PA: Lippincott-Raven; 1998.

272. Frassica F. *Orthopaedic Pathology*. Philadelphia, PA: WB Saunders; 1996.

273. Rosemont, IL: American Academy of Orthopaedic Surgeons; 2007.

274. *Diseases of Synovial Membrane*. Philadelphia, PA: WB Saunders; 1998.

275. Rindfleisch JA, Muller D. Diagnosis and management of rheumatoid arthritis. *Am Fam Physician*. 2005;72(6):1037-1047.

276. Gardner GC, Kadel NJ. Ordering and interpreting rheumatologic laboratory tests. *J Am Acad Orthop Surg*. 2003;11(1):60-67.

277. Howe CR, Gardner GC, Kadel NJ. Perioperative medication management for the patient with rheumatoid arthritis. *J Am Acad Orthop Surg*. 2006;14(9):544-551.

278. Chalmers PN, Sherman SL, Raphael BS, Su EP. Rheumatoid synovectomy: does the surgical approach matter? *Clin Orthop Relat Res*. 2011;469(7):2062-2071.

279. Anglen J. Distal humerus fractures. *J Am Acad Orthop Surg*. 2005;13(5):291-297.

280. Galano GJ, Ahmad CS, Levine WN. Current treatment strategies for bicolumnar distal humerus fractures. *J Am Acad Orthop Surg*. 2010;18(1):20-30.

281. Cobb TK, Morrey BF. Total elbow arthroplasty as primary treatment for distal humeral fractures in elderly patients. *J Bone Joint Surg Am*. 1997;79(6):826-832.

282. McKee MD, Veillette CJ, Hall JA, et al. A multicenter, prospective, randomized, controlled trial of open reduction-internal fixation versus total elbow arthroplasty for displaced intra-articular distal humeral fractures in elderly patients. *J Shoulder Elbow Surg*. 2009;18(1):3-12.

283. Blomfeldt R, Tornkvist H, Eriksson K, Soderqvist A, Ponzer S, Tidermark J. A randomised trial comparing bipolar hemiarthroplasty with total hip replacement for displaced intracapsular fractures of the femoral neck in elderly patients. *J Bone Joint Surg Br*. 2007;89(2):160-165.

284. Lee BP, Berry DJ, Harmsen WS, Sim FH. Total hip arthroplasty for the treatment of an acute fracture of the femoral neck: long-term results. *J Bone Joint Surg Am*. 1998;80(1):70-75.

285. Moran CG, Wenn RT, Sikand M, Taylor AM. Early mortality after hip fracture: is delay before surgery important? *J Bone Joint Surg Am*. 2005;87(3):483-489.

286. Ring D, Jupiter JB, Waters PM. Monteggia fractures in children and adults. *J Am Acad Orthop Surg*. 1998;6(4):215-224.

287. Dreyer SJ, Boden SD. Natural history of rheumatoid arthritis of the cervical spine. *Clin Orthop Relat Res*. 1999;(366):98-106.

288. Boden SD, Dodge LD, Bohlman HH, Rechtine GR. Rheumatoid arthritis of the cervical spine: a long-term analysis with predictors of paralysis and recovery. *J Bone Joint Surg Am*. 1993;75(9):1282-1297.

289. Fithian DC, Paxton EW, Stone ML, et al. Epidemiology and natural history of acute patellar dislocation. *Am J Sports Med.* 2004;32(5):1114-1121.

290. Colvin AC, West RV. Patellar instability. *J Bone Joint Surg Am.* 2008;90(12):2751-2762.

291. Maenpaa H, Lehto MU. Patellar dislocation. The long-term results of nonoperative management in 100 patients. *Am J Sports Med.* 1997;25(2):213-217.

292. O'Driscoll SW, Bell DF, Morrey BF. Posterolateral rotatory instability of the elbow. *J Bone Joint Surg Am.* 1991;73(3):440-446.

293. Cohen MS. Lateral collateral ligament instability of the elbow. *Hand Clin.* 2008;24(1):69-77.

294. Bertrand J, Cromme C, Umlauf D, Frank S, Pap T. Molecular mechanisms of cartilage remodelling in osteoarthritis. *Int J Biochem Cell Biol.* 2010;42(10):1594-1601.

295. Lories RJ. Joint homeostasis, restoration, and remodeling in osteoarthritis. *Best Pract Res Clin Rheumatol.* 2008;22(2):209-220.

296. Lories RJ, Luyten FP. The bone-cartilage unit in osteoarthritis. *Nat Rev Rheumatol.* 2011;7(1):43-49.

297. Loeser RF, Goldring SR, Scanzello CR, Goldring MB. Osteoarthritis: a disease of the joint as an organ. *Arthritis Rheum.* 2012;64(6):1697-1707.

298. Sun HB. Mechanical loading, cartilage degradation, and arthritis. *Ann N Y Acad Sci.* 2010;1211:37-50.

299. Loeser RF, Olex AL, McNulty MA, et al. Microarray analysis reveals age-related differences in gene expression during the development of osteoarthritis in mice. *Arthritis Rheum.* 2012;64(3):705-717.

300. American Academy of Orthopaedic Surgeons. AAOS clinical practice guideline: treatment of osteoarthritis of the knee. AAOS website. http://www.aaos.org/research/guidelines/TreatmentofOsteoarthritisoftheKneeGuideline.pdf. Accessed August 8, 2013.

301. Kubiak EN, Moskovich R, Errico TJ, Di Cesare PE. Orthopaedic management of ankylosing spondylitis. *J Am Acad Orthop Surg.* 2005;13(4):267-278.

302. Alebiosu CO, Raimi TH, Badru AI, Amore OO, Ogunkoya JO, Odusan O. Reiters syndrome: a case report and review of literature. *Afr Health Sci.* 2004;4(2):136-138.

303. Vaughan-Jackson OJ. Rupture of extensor tendons by attrition at the inferior radio-ulnar joint; report of two cases. *J Bone Joint Surg Br.* 1948;30(3):528-530.

304. Schindele SF, Herren DB, Simmen BR. Tendon reconstruction for the rheumatoid hand. *Hand Clin.* 2011;27(1):105-113.

305. Rizzo M, Cooney WP III. Current concepts and treatment for the rheumatoid wrist. *Hand Clin.* 2011;27(1):57-72.

306. Millender LH, Nalebuff EA, Albin R, Ream JR, Gordon M. Dorsal tenosynovectomy and tendon transfer in the rheumatoid hand. *J Bone Joint Surg Am.* 1974;56(3):601-610.

307. Braga-Silva J. Anatomic basis of dorsal finger skin cover. *Tech Hand Up Extrem Surg.* 2005;9(3):134-141.

308. Friedrich JB, Katolik LI, Vedder NB. Soft tissue reconstruction of the hand. *J Hand Surg Am.* 2009;34(6):1148-1155.

309. Abdel MP, Lewallen DG, Berry DJ. Periprosthetic femur fractures treated with modular fluted, tapered stems. *Clin Orthop Relat Res.* 2014;472(2):599-603.

310. Berry DJ. Treatment of Vancouver B3 periprosthetic femur fractures with a fluted tapered stem. *Clin Orthop Relat Res.* 2003;(417):224-231.

311. Lindahl H, Malchau H, Odéen A, Garellick G. Risk factors for failure after treatment of a periprosthetic fracture of the femur. *J Bone Joint Surg Br.* 2006;88(1):26-30.

312. Haidukewych GJ, Langford J, Liporace FA. Revision for periprosthetic fractures of the hip and knee. *J Bone Joint Surg Am.* 2013;95(4):368-376.

313. Kolstad K. Revision THR after periprosthetic femoral fractures. An analysis of 23 cases. *Acta Orthop Scand.* 1994;65(5):505-508.

314. Bozic KJ, Ong K, Lau E, et al. Estimating risk in Medicare patients with THA: an electronic risk calculator for periprosthetic joint infection and mortality. *Clin Orthop Relat Res.* 2013;471(2):574-583.

315. Parvizi J, Adeli B, Zmistowski B, Restrepo C, Greenwald AS. Management of periprosthetic joint infection: the current knowledge: AAOS exhibit selection. *J Bone Joint Surg Am.* 2012;94(14):e104.

316. Della Valle CJ, Paprosky WG. The femur in revision total hip arthroplasty evaluation and classification. *Clin Orthop Relat Res.* 2004;(420):55-62.

317. Bedair H, Ting N, Jacovides C, et al. The Mark Coventry Award: diagnosis of early postoperative TKA infection using synovial fluid analysis. *Clin Orthop Relat Res.* 2011;469(1):34-40.

318. Yi PH, Cross MB, Moric M, Sporer SM, Berger RA, Della Valle CJ. The 2013 Frank Stinchfield Award: diagnosis of infection in the early postoperative period after total hip arthroplasty. *Clin Orthop Relat Res.* 2014;472(2):424-429.

319. Parvizi J, Zmistowski B, Berbari EF, et al. New definition for periprosthetic joint infection: from the Workgroup of the Musculoskeletal Infection Society. *Clin Orthop Relat Res.* 2011;469(11):2992-2994.

320. Sherrell JC, Fehring TK, Odum S, et al. The Chitranjan Ranawat Award: fate of two-stage reimplantation after failed irrigation and débridement for periprosthetic knee infection. *Clin Orthop Rrelat Res.* 2011;469(1):18-25.

321. Skues MA, Welchew EA. Anaesthesia and rheumatoid arthritis. *Anaesthesia.* 1993;48(11):989-997.

322. Clarke HD, Fuchs R, Scuderi GR, Scott WN, Insall JN. Clinical results in valgus total knee arthroplasty with the "pie crust" technique of lateral soft tissue releases. *J Arthroplasty.* 2005;20(8):1010-1014.

323. Easley ME, Insall JN, Scuderi GR, Bullek DD. Primary constrained condylar knee arthroplasty for the arthritic valgus knee. *Clin Orthop Relat Res.* 2000;(380):58-64.

324. Griffin FM, Insall JN, Scuderi GR. The posterior condylar angle in osteoarthritic knees. *J Arthroplasty*. 1998;13(7):812-815.

325. Gill GS, Mills D, Joshi AB. Mortality following primary total knee arthroplasty. *J Bone Joint Surg Am*. 2003;85(3):432-435.

326. Kirksey M, Chiu YL, Ma Y, et al. Trends in in-hospital major morbidity and mortality after total joint arthroplasty: United States 1998-2008. *Anesth Analgesia*. 2012;115(2):321-327.

327. Nho SJ, Strauss EJ, Lenart BA, et al. Long head of the biceps tendinopathy: diagnosis and management. *J Am Acad Orthop Surg*. 2010;18(11):645-656.

328. Rudzki JR, Shaffer BS. *Arthroscopic Treatment of Biceps Tendonopathy*. Vol 1. Philadelphia, PA: Wolters Kluwer/Lippincott Williams & Wilkins; 2011.

329. Waters RL, Hu SS. Penetrating injuries of the spinal cord: stab and gunshot injuries. In: Frymoyer JW, ed. *The Adult Spine: Principles and Practice*. Vol 1. New York, NY: Raven Press; 1991:815-826.

330. DeMuth WE Jr. Bullet velocity and design as determinants of wounding capability: an experimental study. *J Trauma*. 1966;6(2):222-232.

331. Waters RL, Sie IH. Spinal cord injuries from gunshot wounds to the spine. *Clin Orthop Relat Res*. 2003;(408):120-125.

332. Lin SS, Vaccaro AR, Reisch S, Devine M, Cotler JM. Low-velocity gunshot wounds to the spine with an associated transperitoneal injury. *J Spinal Disord*. 1995;8(2):136-144.

333. Quigley KJ, Place HM. The role of debridement and antibiotics in gunshot wounds to the spine. *J Trauma*. 2006;60(4):814-819.

334. Isiklar ZU, Lindsey RW. Low-velocity civilian gunshot wounds of the spine. *Orthopedics*. 1997;20(10):967-972.

335. Browne JE, Branch TP. Surgical alternatives for treatment of articular cartilage lesions. *J Am Acad Orthop Surg*. 2000;8(3):180-189.

336. Curl WW, Krome J, Gordon ES, Rushing J, Smith BP, Poehling GG. Cartilage injuries: a review of 31,516 knee arthroscopies. *Arthroscopy*. 1997;13(4):456-460.

337. Levy AS, Lohnes J, Sculley S, LeCroy M, Garrett W. Chondral delamination of the knee in soccer players. *Am J Sports Med*. 1996;24(5):634-639.

338. Kocher MS, Tucker R, Ganley TJ, Flynn JM. Management of osteochondritis dissecans of the knee: current concepts review. *Am J Sports Med*. 2006;34(7):1181-1191.

339. Berry GE, Adams S, Harris MB, et al. Are plain radiographs of the spine necessary during evaluation after blunt trauma? Accuracy of screening torso computed tomography in thoracic/lumbar spine fracture diagnosis. *J Trauma*. 2005;59(6):1410-1413.

340. Gale SC, Gracias VH, Reilly PM, Schwab CW. The inefficiency of plain radiography to evaluate the cervical spine after blunt trauma. *J Trauma*. 2005;59(5):1121-1125.

341. Griffen MM, Frykberg ER, Kerwin AJ, et al. Radiographic clearance of blunt cervical spine injury: plain radiograph or computed tomography scan? *J Trauma*. 2003;55(2):222-226.

342. Holmes JF, Akkinepalli R. Computed tomography versus plain radiography to screen for cervical spine injury: a meta-analysis. *J Trauma*. 2005;58(5):902-905.

343. Khan SN, Erickson G, Sena MJ, Gupta MC. Use of flexion and extension radiographs of the cervical spine to rule out acute instability in patients with negative computed tomography scans. *J Orthop Trauma*. 2011;25(1):51-56.

344. Maak TG, Grauer JN. The contemporary treatment of odontoid injuries. *Spine (Phila Pa 1976)*. 2006;31(11 suppl):S53-S60.

345. Koivikko MP, Kiuru MJ, Koskinen SK, Myllynen P, Santavirta S, Kivisaari L. Factors associated with nonunion in conservatively-treated type-II fractures of the odontoid process. *J Bone Joint Surg Br*. 2004;86(8):1146-1151.

346. Smith TO, Sexton D, Mitchell P, Hing CB. Opening- or closing-wedged high tibial osteotomy: a meta-analysis of clinical and radiological outcomes. *Knee*. 2011;18(6):361-368.

347. Warden SJ, Morris HG, Crossley KM, Brukner PD, Bennell KL. Delayed- and non-union following opening wedge high tibial osteotomy: surgeons' results from 182 completed cases. *Knee Surg Sports Traumatol Arthrosc*. 2005;13(1):34-37.

348. Billings A, Scott DF, Camargo MP, Hofmann AA. High tibial osteotomy with a calibrated osteotomy guide, rigid internal fixation, and early motion: long-term follow-up. *J Bone Joint Surg Am*. 2000;82(1):70-79.

349. Hernigou P, Ma W. Open wedge tibial osteotomy with acrylic bone cement as bone substitute. *Knee*. 2001;8(2):103-110.

350. Hui C, Salmon LJ, Kok A, et al. Long-term survival of high tibial osteotomy for medial compartment osteoarthritis of the knee. *Am J Sports Med*. 2011;39(1):64-70.

351. Erak S, Naudie D, MacDonald SJ, McCalden RW, Rorabeck CH, Bourne RB. Total knee arthroplasty following medial opening wedge tibial osteotomy: technical issues early clinical radiological results. *Knee*. 2011;18(6):499-504.

352. Parvizi J, Hanssen AD, Spangehl MJ. Total knee arthroplasty following proximal tibial osteotomy: risk factors for failure. *J Bone Joint Surg Am*. 2004;86(3):474-479.

353. Shao YC, Harwood P, Grotz MR, Limb D, Giannoudis PV. Radial nerve palsy associated with fractures of the shaft of the humerus: a systematic review. *J Bone Joint Surg Br*. 2005;87(12):1647-1652.

354. Sammer DM, Chung KC. Tendon transfers: part I. Principles of transfer and transfers for radial nerve palsy. *Plast Reconstr Surg*. 2009;123(5):169e-177e.

355. Ratner JA, Peljovich A, Kozin SH. Update on tendon transfers for peripheral nerve injuries. *J Hand Surg Am*. 2010;35(8):1371-1381.

356. Baumgaertner MR, Curtin SL, Lindskog DM, Keggi JM. The value of the tip-apex distance in predicting failure of fixation of peritrochanteric fractures of the hip. *J Bone Joint Surg Am*. 1995;77(7):1058-1064.

357. Haidukewych GJ. Intertrochanteric fractures: ten tips to improve results. *J Bone Joint Surg Am.* 2009;91(3):712-719.

358. Sadowski C, Lüubbeke A, Saudan M, Riand N, Stern R, Hoffmeyer P. Treatment of reverse oblique and transverse inter-trochanteric fractures with use of an intramedullary nail or a 95 degrees screw-plate: a prospective, randomized study. *J Bone Joint Surg Am.* 2002;84(3):372-381.

359. Vaccaro AR, Lehman RA Jr, Hurlbert RJ, et al. A new classification of thoracolumbar injuries: the importance of in-jury morphology, the integrity of the posterior ligamentous complex, and neurologic status. *Spine (Phila Pa 1976).* 2005;30(20):2325-2333.

360. McCormack T, Karaikovic E, Gaines RW. The load sharing classification of spine fractures. *Spine (Phila Pa 1976).* 1994;19(15):1741-1744.

361. Wood K, Buttermann G, Mehbod A, Garvey T, Jhanjee R, Sechriest V. Operative compared with nonoperative treatment of a thoracolumbar burst fracture without neurological deficit: a prospective, randomized study. *J Bone Joint Surg Am.* 2003;85(5):773-781.

362. Esses SI, McGuire R, Jenkins J, et al. The treatment of symptomatic osteoporotic spinal compression fractures. *J Am Acad Orthop Surg.* 2011;19(3):176-182.

363. Agabegi SS, Asghar FA, Herkowitz HN. Spinal orthoses. *J Am Acad Orthop Surg.* 2010;18(11):657-667.

364. Gillette BP, Maradit Kremers H, Duncan CM, et al. Economic impact of tranexamic acid in healthy patients undergoing primary total hip and knee arthroplasty. *J Arthroplasty.* 2013;28(8 suppl):137-139.

365. Temple-Wong MM, Bae WC, Chen MQ, et al. Biomechanical, structural, and biochemical indices of degenerative and osteoarthritic deterioration of adult human articular cartilage of the femoral condyle. *Osteoarthritis Cartilage.* 2009;17(11):1469-1476.

366. Whitehouse MR, Stefanovich-Lawbuary NS, Brunton LR, Blom AW. The impact of leg length discrepancy on patient satisfaction and functional outcome following total hip arthroplasty. *J Arthroplasty.* 2013;28(8):1408-1414.

367. DeHart MM, Riley LH Jr. Nerve injuries in total hip arthroplasty. *J Am Acad Orthop Surg.* 1999;7(2):101-111.

368. Hoover NW. Injuries of the popliteal artery associated with fractures and dislocations. *Surg Clin North Am.* 1961;41:1099-1112.

369. Kennedy JC. Complete dislocation of the knee joint. *J Bone Joint Surg Am.* 1963;45:889-904.

370. Bone LB, Johnson KD, Weigelt J, Scheinberg R. Early versus delayed stabilization of femoral fractures: a prospective randomized study. *J Bone Joint Surg Am.* 1989;71(3):336-340.

371. Ricci WM, Gallagher B, Haidukewych GJ. Intramedullary nailing of femoral shaft fractures: current concepts. *J Am Acad Orthop Surg.* 2009;17(5):296-305.

372. Boden SD, Kaplan FS. Calcium homeostasis. *Orthop Clin North Am.* 1990;21(1):31-42.

373. Tejwani NC, Schachter AK, Immerman I, Achan P. Renal osteodystrophy. *J Am Acad Orthop Surg.* 2006;14(5):303-311.

374. Jolles BM, Bogoch ER. Posterior versus lateral surgical approach for total hip arthroplasty in adults with osteoarthritis. *Cochrane Database Syst Rev.* 2006;(3):CD003828.

375. Geerdink CH, Grimm B, Rahmy AI, Vencken W, Heyligers IC, Tonino AJ. Correlation of Technetium-99m scintigraphy, progressive acetabular osteolysis and acetabular component loosening in total hip arthroplasty. *Hip Int.* 2010;20(4):460-465.

376. Palestro CJ, Love C, Tronco GG, Tomas MB, Rini JN. Combined labeled leukocyte and technetium 99m sulfur colloid bone marrow imaging for diagnosing musculoskeletal infection. *Radiographics.* 2006;26(3):859-870.

377. Joseph TN, Mutjaba M, Chen AL, et al. Efficacy of combined technetium-99m sulfur colloid/indium-111 leukocyte scans to detect infected total hip and knee arthroplasties. *J Arthroplasty.* 2001;16(6):753-758.

378. Chen CA, Chen W, Goodman SB, et al. New MR imaging methods for metallic implants in the knee: artifact correction and clinical impact. *J Magn Reson Imaging.* 2011;33(5):1121-1127.

379. Berger RA, Crossett LS, Jacobs JJ, Rubash HE. Malrotation causing patellofemoral complications after total knee arthro-plasty. *Clin Orthop Relat Res.* 1998;(356):144-153.

380. Wyrick JD. Proximal row carpectomy and intercarpal arthrodesis for the management of wrist arthritis. *J Am Acad Orthop Surg.* 2003;11(4):277-281.

381. Cohen MS, Kozin SH. Degenerative arthritis of the wrist: proximal row carpectomy versus scaphoid excision and four-corner arthrodesis. *J Hand Surg Am.* 2001;26(1):94-104.

382. Enna M, Hoepfner P, Weiss AP. Scaphoid excision with four-corner fusion. *Hand Clin.* 2005;21(4):531-538.

383. Stover MD, Beaulé PE, Matta JM, Mast JW. Hip arthrodesis: a procedure for the new millennium? *Clin Orthop Relat Res.* 2004;(418):126-133.

384. Matta JM, Siebenrock KA, Gautier E, Mehne D, Ganz R. Hip fusion through an anterior approach with the use of a ventral plate. *Clin Orthop Relat Res.* 1997;(337):129-139.

385. Callaghan JJ, Brand RA, Pedersen DR. Hip arthrodesis: a long-term follow-up. *J Bone Joint Surg Am.* 1985;67(9):1328-1335.

386. Sponseller PD, McBeath AA, Perpich M. Hip arthrodesis in young patients: a long-term follow-up study. *J Bone Joint Surg Am.* 1984;66(6):853-859.

387. Jain S, Giannoudis PV. Arthrodesis of the hip and conversion to total hip arthroplasty: a systematic review. *J Arthro-plasty.* 2013;28(9):1596-1602.

388. Hardy RH, Clapham JC. Observations on hallux valgus; based on a controlled series. *J Bone Joint Surg Br.* 1951;33(3):376-391.

389. Mann RA. Bunion surgery: decision making. *Orthopedics.* 1990;13(9):951-957.

390. Richardson EG, Graves SC, McClure JT, Boone RT. First metatarsal head-shaft angle: a method of determination. *Foot Ankle*. 1993;14(4):181-185.

391. Coughlin MJ, Freund E. Roger A. Mann Award. The reliability of angular measurements in hallux valgus deformities. *Foot Ankle Int*. 2001;22(5):369-379.

392. Faber FW, Kleinrensink GJ, Verhoog MW, et al. Mobility of the first tarsometatarsal joint in relation to hallux valgus deformity: anatomical and biomechanical aspects. *Foot Ankle Int*. 1999;20(10):651-656.

393. Torkki M, Malmivaara A, Seitsalo S, Hoikka V, Laippala P, Paavolainen P. Surgery vs orthosis vs watchful waiting for hallux valgus: a randomized controlled trial. *JAMA*. 2001;285(19):2474-2480.

394. Easley ME, Trnka HJ. Current concepts review: hallux valgus part II: operative treatment. *Foot Ankle Int*. 2007;28(6):748-758.

395. Gerber C, Schneeberger AG, Vinh TS. The arterial vascularization of the humeral head: an anatomical study. *J Bone Joint Surg Am*. 1990;72(10):1486-1494.

396. Wijgman AJ, Roolker W, Patt TW, Raaymakers EL, Marti RK. Open reduction and internal fixation of three and four-part fractures of the proximal part of the humerus. *J Bone Joint Surg Am*. 2002;84(11):1919-1925.

397. Robinson CM, Page RS. Severely impacted valgus proximal humeral fractures: results of operative treatment. *J Bone Joint Surg Am*. 2003;85(9):1647-1655.

398. Frankle MA, Mighell MA. Techniques and principles of tuberosity fixation for proximal humeral fractures treated with hemiarthroplasty. *J Shoulder Elbow Surg*. 2004;13(2):239-247.

399. *Orthopaedic Knowledge Update: Shoulder and Elbow 2*. Rosemont, IL: American Academy of Orthopaedic Surgeons; 2002.

400. Frankle MA, Ondrovic LE, Markee BA, Harris ML, Lee WE III. Stability of tuberosity reattachment in proximal humeral hemiarthroplasty. *J Shoulder Elbow Surg*. 2002;11(5):413-420.

401. Lane JM, Nydick M. Osteoporosis: current modes of prevention and treatment. *J Am Acad Orthop Surg*. 1999;7(1):19-31.

402. Favus MJ. Bisphosphonates for osteoporosis. *N Engl J Med*. 2010;363(21):2027-2035.

403. Lu L, Kaufman KR, Yaszemski MJ. Biomechanics. In: Einhorn TA, O'Keefe RJ, Buckwalter JA, eds. *Orthopaedic Basic Science: Foundations of Clinical Practice*. 3rd ed. Rosemont, IL: American Academy of Orthopaedic Surgeons; 2007:49-64.

404. Levangie PK, Norkin CC. *Joint Structure and Function: A Comprehensive Analysis*. 3rd ed. Philadelphia, PA: F.A. Davis Company; 2001.

405. Vincent KA. Tarsal coalition and painful flatfoot. *J Am Acad Orthop Surg*. 1998;6(5):274-281.

406. Cowell HR, Elener V. Rigid painful flatfoot secondary to tarsal coalition. *Clin Orthop Relat Res*. 1983;(177):54-60.

407. Swiontkowski MF, Scranton PE, Hansen S. Tarsal coalitions: long-term results of surgical treatment. *J Pediatr Orthop*. 1983;3(3):287-292.

408. Cooperman DR, Janke BE, Gilmore A, Latimer BM, Brinker MR, Thompson GH. A three-dimensional study of calcaneonavicular tarsal coalitions. *J Pediatr Orthop*. 2001;21(5):648-651.

409. Maquirriain J. Posterior ankle impingement syndrome. *J Am Acad Orthop Surg*. 2005;13(6):365-371.

410. Healy WL, Siliski JM, Incavo SJ. Operative treatment of distal femoral fractures proximal to total knee replacements. *J Bone Joint Surg Am*. 1993;75(1):27-34.

411. Korompilias AV, Karantanas AH, Lykissas MG, Beris AE. Transient osteoporosis. *J Am Acad Orthop Surg*. 2008;16(8):480-489.

412. Horlocker TT, Wedel DJ, Rowlingson JC, et al. Regional anesthesia in the patient receiving antithrombotic or thrombolytic therapy: American Society of Regional Anesthesia and Pain Medicine Evidence-Based Guidelines (Third Edition). *Reg Anesth Pain Med*. 2010;35(1):64-101.

413. Weinstein JN, Tosteson TD, Lurie JD, et al. Surgical versus nonsurgical therapy for lumbar spinal stenosis. *N Engl J Med*. 2008;358(8):794-810.

414. Atlas SJ, Keller RB, Wu YA, Deyo RA, Singer DE. Long-term outcomes of surgical and nonsurgical management of lumbar spinal stenosis: 8 to 10 year results from the Maine lumbar spine study. *Spine (Phila Pa 1976)*. 2005;30(8):936-943.

415. Atlas SJ, Deyo RA, Keller RB, et al. The Maine Lumbar Spine Study, Part III: 1-year outcomes of surgical and nonsurgical management of lumbar spinal stenosis. *Spine (Phila Pa 1976)*. 1996;21(15):1787-1794.

416. Weinstein JN, Lurie JD, Tosteson TD, et al. Surgical versus nonsurgical treatment for lumbar degenerative spondylolisthesis. *N Engl J Med*. 2007;356(22):2257-2270.

417. Glassman SD, Berven S, Bridwell K, Horton W, Dimar JR. Correlation of radiographic parameters and clinical symptoms in adult scoliosis. *Spine (Phila Pa 1976)*. 2005;30(6):682-688.

418. Antoniou J, Duckworth DT, Harryman DT II. Capsulolabral augmentation for the the management of posteroinferior instability of the shoulder. *J Bone Joint Surg Am*. 2000;82(9):1220-1230.

419. Kim SH, Park JS, Jeong WK, Shin SK. The Kim test: a novel test for posteroinferior labral lesion of the shoulder—a comparison to the jerk test. *Am J Sports Med*. 2005;33(8):1188-1192.

420. Burkhead WZ Jr, Rockwood CA Jr. Treatment of instability of the shoulder with an exercise program. *J Bone Joint Surg Am*. 1992;74(6):890-896.

421. Boykin RE, Anz AW, Bushnell BD, Kocher MS, Stubbs AJ, Philippon MJ. Hip instability. *J Am Acad Orthop Surg*. 2011;19(6):340-349.

422. Schoenecker PL, Clohisy JC, Millis MB, Wenger DR. Surgical management of the problematic hip in adolescent and young adult patients. *J Am Acad Orthop Surg*. 2011;19(5):275-286.

423. Garvin KL, Konigsberg BS. Infection following total knee arthroplasty: prevention and management. *J Bone Joint Surg Am.* 2011;93(12):1167-1175.

424. Parvizi J, Della Valle CJ. AAOS Clinical Practice Guideline: diagnosis and treatment of periprosthetic joint infections of the hip and knee. *J Am Acad Orthop Surg.* 2010;18(12):771-772.

425. Della Valle C, Parvizi J, Bauer TW, et al. Diagnosis of periprosthetic joint infections of the hip and knee. *J Am Acad Orthop Surg.* 2010;18(12):760-770.

426. Zywiel MG, Daley JA, Delanois RE, Naziri Q, Johnson AJ, Mont MA. Advance pre-operative chlorhexidine reduces the incidence of surgical site infections in knee arthroplasty. *Int Orthop.* 2011;35(7):1001-1006.

427. Hacek DM, Robb WJ, Paule SM, Kudrna JC, Stamos VP, Peterson LR. *Staphylococcus aureus* nasal decolonization in joint replacement surgery reduces infection. *Clin Orthop Relat Res.* 2008;466(6):1349-1355.

428. Freeman MG, Fehring TK, Odum SM, Fehring K, Griffin WL, Mason JB. Functional advantage of articulating versus static spacers in 2-stage revision for total knee arthroplasty infection. *J Arthroplasty.* 2007;22(8):1116-1121.

429. Van Thiel GS, Berend KR, Klein GR, Gordon AC, Lombardi AV, Della Valle CJ. Intraoperative molds to create an articulating spacer for the infected knee arthroplasty. *Clin Orthop Relat Res.* 2011;469(4):994-1001.

430. Chiu FY, Chen CM. Surgical débridement and parenteral antibiotics in infected revision total knee arthroplasty. *Clin Orthop Relat Res.* 2007;461:130-135.

431. von Foerster G, Klüuber D, Käabler U. Mid- to long-term results after treatment of 118 cases of periprosthetic infections after knee joint replacement using one-stage exchange surgery [in German]. *Orthopade.* 1991;20(3):244-252.

432. Zervos M. Treatment options for uncomplicated community-acquired skin and soft tissue infections caused by methicillin-resistant Staphylococcus aureus: oral antimicrobial agents. *Surg Infect (Larchmt).* 2008;9 suppl 1:s29-s34.

433. Gustilo RB, Anderson JT. Prevention of infection in the treatment of one thousand and twenty-five open fractures of long bones: retrospective and prospective analyses. *J Bone Joint Surg Am.* 1976;58(4):453-458.

434. Holtom PD. Antibiotic prophylaxis: current recommendations. *J Am Acad Orthop Surg.* 2006;14(10 spec no.):S98-S100.

435. Bates SM, Greer IA, Pabinger I, Sofaer S, Hirsh J; American College of Chest Physicians. Venous thromboembolism, thrombophilia, antithrombotic therapy, and pregnancy: American College of Chest Physicians Evidence-Based Clinical Practice Guidelines (8th Edition). *Chest.* 2008;133(6 suppl):844S-886S.

436. Shimoyama Y, Sawai T, Tatsumi S, et al. Perioperative risk factors for deep vein thrombosis after total hip arthroplasty or total knee arthroplasty. *J Clin Anesth.* 2012;24(7):531-536.

Bibliography

Anderson RB, Hunt KJ, McCormick JJ. Management of common sports-related injuries about the foot and ankle. *J Am Acad Orthop Surg.* 2010;18(9):546-556.

Arvind CH, Hargreaves DG. Table top relocation test--new clinical test for posterolateral rotatory instability of the elbow. *J Shoulder Elbow Surg.* 2006;15(4):500-501.

Cohen MS, Hastings H II. Rotatory instability of the elbow: the anatomy and role of the lateral stabilizers. *J Bone Joint Surg Am.* 1997;79(2):225-233.

Completo A, Simões JA, Fonseca F. Revision total knee arthroplasty: the influence of femoral stems in load sharing and stability. *Knee.* 2009;16(4):275-279.

Deben SE, Pomeroy GC. Subtle cavus foot: diagnosis and management. *J Am Acad Orthop Surg.* 2014;22(8):512-520.

DeFranco MJ, Nho S, Romeo AA. Scapulothoracic fusion. *J Am Acad Orthop Surg.* 2010;18(4):236-242.

DiCaprio MR, Enneking WF. Fibrous dysplasia: pathophysiology, evaluation, and treatment. *J Bone Joint Surg Am.* 2005;87(8):1848-1864.

Egol KA, Sheikhazadeh A, Mogatederi S, Barnett A, Koval KJ. Lower-extremity function for driving an automobile after operative treatment of ankle fracture. *J Bone Joint Surg Am.* 2003;85(7):1185-1189.

Forsberg JA, Potter BK, Cierny G III, Webb L. Diagnosis and management of chronic infection. *J Am Acad Orthop Surg.* 2011;19 suppl 1:S8-S19.

Gilbert NF, Cannon CP, Lin PP, Lewis VO. Soft tissue sarcoma. *J Am Acad Orthop Surg.* 2009;17(1):40-47.

Gill LH. Plantar fasciitis: diagnosis and conservative management. *J Am Acad Orthop Surg.* 1997;5(2):109-117.

Henderson JJ, Bamford DJ, Noble J, Brown JD. The value of skeletal scintigraphy in predicting the need for revision surgery in total knee replacement. *Orthopedics.* 1996;19(4):295-299.

Herring A. *Tachdjian's Pediatric Orthopaedics: from the Texas Scottish Rite Hospital for Children.* 4th ed. Philadelphia, PA: Saunders Elsevier; 2008.

Hosalkar HS, Torbert JT, Fox EJ, Delaney TF, Aboulafia AJ, Lackman RD. Musculoskeletal desmoid tumors. *J Am Acad Orthop Surg.* 2008;16(4):188-198.

Howard A, Mulpuri K, Abel MF, et al. The treatment of pediatric supracondylar humerus fractures. *J Am Acad Orthop Surg.* 2012;20(5):320-327.

Howard JL, Kudera J, Lewallen DG, Hanssen AD. Early results of the use of tantalum femoral cones for revision total knee arthroplasty. *J Bone Joint Surg Am.* 2011;93(5):478-484.

Janisse DJ, Janisse E. Shoe modification and the use of orthoses in the treatment of foot and ankle pathology. *J Am Acad Orthop Surg*. 2008;16(3):152-158.

Johnson DL, Urban WP Jr, Caborn DN, Vanarthos WJ, Carlson CS. Articular cartilage changes seen with magnetic resonance imaging detected bone bruises associated with acute anterior cruciate ligament rupture. *Am J Sports Med*. 1998;26:409-414.

Krishnan SG, Hawkins RJ, Michelotti JD, Litchfield R, Willis RB, Kim YK. Scapulothoracic arthrodesis: indications, technique, and results. *Clin Orthop Relat Res*. 2005;(435):126-133.

Lafferty PM, Min W, Tejwani NC. Stress radiographs in orthopaedic surgery. *J Am Acad Orthop Surg*. 2009;17(8):528-539.

Lareau CR, Sawyer GA, Wang JH, DiGiovanni CW. Plantar and medial heel pain: diagnosis and management. *J Am Acad Orthop Surg*. 2014;22(6):372-380.

Levine B, Sporer S, Della Valle CJ, Jacobs JJ, Paprosky W. Porous tantalum in reconstructive surgery of the knee: a review. *J Knee Surg*. 2007;20(3):185-194.

Mabry TM, Hanssen AD. The role of stems and augments for bone loss in revision knee arthroplasty. *J Arthroplasty*. 2007;22(4 suppl 1):56-60.

Maheshwari AV, Cheng EY. Ewing sarcoma family of tumors. *J Am Acad Orthop Surg*. 2010;18(2):94-107.

Mann RA. Disorders of the first metatarsophalangeal joint. *J Am Acad Orthop Surg*. 1995;3(1):34-43.

Marco RA, Gitelis S, Brebach GT, Healey JH. Cartilage tumors: evaluation and treatment. *J Am Acad Orthop Surg*. 2000;8(5):292-304.

Mendenhall WM, Zlotecki RA, Gibbs CP, Reith JD, Scarborough MT, Mendenhall NP. Aneurysmal bone cyst. *Am J Clin Oncol*. 2006;29(3):311-315.

Messerschmitt PJ, Garcia RM, Abdul-Karim FW, Greenfield EM, Getty PJ. Osteosarcoma. *J Am Acad Orthop Surg*. 2009;17(8):515-527.

Michelson JD. Ankle fractures resulting from rotational injuries. *J Am Acad Orthop Surg*. 2003;11(6):403-412.

Neufeld SK, Cerrato R. Plantar fasciitis: evaluation and treatment. *J Am Acad Orthop Surg*. 2008;16(6):338-346.

Patil N, Lee K, Huddleston JI, Harris AH, Goodman SB. Patellar management in revision total knee arthroplasty: is patellar resurfacing a better option? *J Arthroplasty*. 2010;25(4):589-593.

Sah AP, Shukla S, Della Valle CJ, Rosenberg AG, Paprosky WG. Modified hybrid stem fixation in revision TKA is durable at 2 to 10 years. *Clin Orthop Relat Res*. 2011;469(3):839-846.

Schwend RM, Drennan JC. Cavus foot deformity in children. *J Am Acad Orthop Surg*. 2003;11(3):201-211.

Shirzad K, Kiesau CD, DeOrio JK, Parekh SG. Lesser toe deformities. *J Am Acad Orthop Surg*. 2011;19(8):505-514.

Sullivan JA. Pediatric flatfoot: evaluation and management. *J Am Acad Orthop Surg*. 1999;7(1):44-53.

Thomas DM, Skubitz KM. Giant cell tumour of bone. *Curr Opin Oncol*. 2009;21(4):338-344.

Tyler WK, Vidal AF, Williams RJ, Healey JH. Pigmented villonodular synovitis. *J Am Acad Orthop Surg*. 2006;14(6):376-385.

van der Ven A, Chapman CB, Bowker JH. Charcot neuroarthropathy of the foot and ankle. *J Am Acad Orthop Surg*. 2009;17(9):562-571.

Watson TS, Shurnas PS, Denker J. Treatment of Lisfranc joint injury: current concepts. *J Am Acad Orthop Surg*. 2010;18(12):718-728.

Weber KL. Evaluation of the adult patient (aged >40 years) with a destructive bone lesion. *J Am Acad Orthop Surg*. 2010;18(3):169-179.

Weinstein SL, Zavala DC, Ponseti IV. Idiopathic scoliosis: long-term follow-up and prognosis in untreated patients. *J Bone Joint Surg Am*. 1981;63(5):702-712.

White RH, McKittrick T, Hutchinson R, Twitchell J. Temporary discontinuation of warfarin therapy: changes in the international normalized ratio. *Ann Intern Med*. 1995;122(1):40-42.

Whittaker JP, Dharmarajan R, Toms AD. The management of bone loss in revision total knee replacement. *J Bone Joint Surg Br*. 2008;90(8):981-987.

Younger AS, Hansen ST Jr. Adult cavovarus foot. *J Am Acad Orthop Surg*. 2005;13(5):302-315.

Zalavras C, Thordarson D. Ankle syndesmotic injury. *J Am Acad Orthop Surg*. 2007;15(6):330-339.

Zionts LE, McKellop HA, Hathaway R. Torsional strength of pin configurations used to fix supracondylar fractures of the humerus in children. *J Bone Joint Surg Am*. 1994;76(2):253-256.

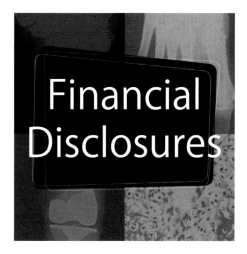

Financial Disclosures

Dr. Amir M. Abtahi has no financial or proprietary interest in the materials presented herein.

Dr. Frank R. Avilucea has not disclosed any financial or proprietary interest in the materials presented herein.

Dr. James T. Beckmann has no financial or proprietary interest in the materials presented herein.

Dr. Michael J. Beebe has no financial or proprietary interest in the materials presented herein.

Dr. Sanjeev Bhatia is a reviewer for the *American Journal of Sports Medicine*.

Dr. Andrew A. Brief has no financial or proprietary interest in the materials presented herein.

Dr. Nicholas M. Brown has no financial or proprietary interest in the materials presented herein.

Dr. Peter N. Chalmers has no financial or proprietary interest in the materials presented herein.

Dr. Dan J. Del Gaizo receives paid research support from Stryker and Zimmer, is a consultant for SPR Therapeutics and Biom'up, and is on the editorial board of the *Journal of Arthroplasty*.

Dr. Michael B. Ellman has no financial or proprietary interest in the materials presented herein.

Dr. Brandon J. Erickson has no financial or proprietary interest in the materials presented herein.

Dr. Jonathan M. Frank has no financial or proprietary interest in the materials presented herein.

Dr. Rachel Frank has no financial or proprietary interest in the materials presented herein.

Dr. James M. Gregory has no financial or proprietary interest in the materials presented herein.

Dr. Christopher E. Gross has no financial or proprietary interest in the materials presented herein.

Dr. Wyatt Lee Hadley has no financial or proprietary interest in the materials presented herein.

Dr. Justin M. Haller has no financial or proprietary interest in the materials presented herein.

Dr. Marc Haro has not disclosed any financial or proprietary interest in the materials presented herein.

Dr. Bryan D. Haughom has no financial or proprietary interest in the materials presented herein.

Dr. Andrew R. Hsu has no financial or proprietary interest in the materials presented herein.

Dr. Benjamin R. Koch has no financial or proprietary interest in the materials presented herein.

Dr. Monica Kogan has no financial or proprietary interest in the materials presented herein.

Dr. Erik N. Kubiak has financial relationships with Zimmer, DePuy, Connections, Orthogrid, and FOT BOD.

Dr. Simon Lee is a Board or committee member at the American Orthopaedic Foot and Ankle Society and is on the Editorial or governing board of Foot and Ankle International.

Dr. Brett Lenart has no financial or proprietary interest in the materials presented herein.

Dr. Brett R. Levine is a consultant for Zimmer, Link, McGraw-Hill, and Janssen; receives research funds from Zimmer, Biomet, and Artelon; and receives royalties from Human Kinetics.

Dr. David Levy has no financial or proprietary interest in the materials presented herein.

Dr. Randy Mascarenhas has no financial or proprietary interest in the materials presented herein.

Dr. Benjamin J. Miller has no financial or proprietary interest in the materials presented herein.

Dr. Shane J. Nho is a consultant for Stryker and Ossur; receives research support from Stryker, Allosource, and the Arthroscopy Association of North America; and receives royalties from Springer.

Dr. Dan K. Park is a consultant for Stryker and K2M.

Dr. David L. Rothberg has no financial or proprietary interest in the materials presented herein.

Dr. Zachary M. Working has no financial or proprietary interest in the materials presented herein.

Dr. Thomas Wuerz is a consultant for Conmed.

Dr. Robert Wysocki has no financial or proprietary interest in the materials presented herein.

Dr. Adam B. Yanke has no financial or proprietary interest in the materials presented herein.

Dr. Joseph D. Zuckerman has no financial or proprietary interest in the materials presented herein.

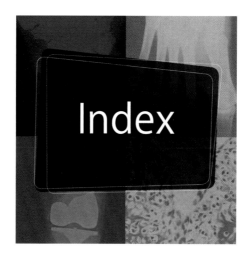

Index